STUTTERING
Theory and Treatment

The Irvington Speech and Hearing Series

GENERAL EDITOR, Hayes A. Newby

CHAIRMAN, DEPARTMENT OF HEARING AND SPEECH SCIENCES

UNIVERSITY OF MARYLAND

Marcel E. Wingate

STUTTERING

Theory and Treatement

IRVINGTON PUBLISHERS, INC., New York

HALSTED PRESS DIVISION
JOHN WILEY & SONS, INC.

New York London Sydney Toronto

To the memory of my father

For information, write to Irvington Publishers, Inc.,
551 Fifth Avenue, New York, New York 10017

Distributed by HALSTED PRESS
A division of JOHN WILEY & SONS, Inc., New York

Library of Congress Cataloging in Publication Data
Wingate, Marcel Edward, 1923-
Stuttering.

(Speech and hearing series)
1. Stuttering. I. Title. [DNLM: 1. Stuttering. WM475 W769s]
RC424.W56 616.8'554 76-18766
ISBN 0-470-15171-4

Printed in The United States of America

Overview Contents

Analytical Contents

Part II: Mitigation of Stuttering

Part III: Therapy: The Objective and The Approach

Part IV: Management

List of Illustrations

List of Tables

PREFACE

This book is concerned primarily with the identification of principles fundamental to a coherent and realistic approach to the management of stuttering. These principles are educed through a careful analysis of a broad range of empirical findings, research data, and casual reports. The management rationale developed and the treatment procedures advocated are based on integration of evidence from many sources.

It might help the reader appreciate the intent of the book to know something of the circumstances of its preparation. My formal professional training was primarily as a clinical psychologist and secondarily as a speech pathologist. For several years after my initial exposure to stuttering I remained quite assured, following the bent of my training as a psychologist, that the disorder was essentially of psychodynamic origin and that the characteristics of stuttering were "symptoms" of underlying emotional conflicts having the classic features of cause, significance, and economy. Working psychotherapeutically with stutterers was both rewarding and disappointing. It was rewarding in the sense that some changes in adjustment were frequently realized, but disappointing in that such changes were not regularly associated with a commensurate change in the stuttering. There was particular reward from those rare instances in which the stuttering could be plausibly linked to some intrapersonal "dynamics," but even here the expected changes in the stuttering were not impressive. Overall, there was more disappointment than reward, simply because in most cases the findings were not consistent with theoretical expectations—except through recourse to devious and presumptive interpretations which generated a feeling of intellectual subterfuge.

This experience increased my interest in theories of stuttering. Through ensuing study it became clear that most of the theories of stuttering were essentially of a prescientific era and did not deserve the acceptance they had received. It was equally evident that an adequate theory of stuttering would not develop until the effort was made to formulate it on the basis of all the facts, to identify and resolve inconsistencies, to eliminate paradox and contradiction, and to search for unifying principles.

The pursuit of such goals constitutes a considerable undertaking, and their attainment lies somewhere in the future. In the meantime, attempts must be made to manage stuttering in the best way possible. Therapy cannot await a comprehensive, consistent theory. Treatment method can develop relatively independently of theory. At the same time the development of stuttering therapy method should follow prerequisites similar to those set forth above for theory. It should have a broad base, be realistic, consistent with sound knowledge, and guided by a search for focal principles.

This book represents an effort to develop an approach to the management of stuttering with a rationale that adheres to these requirements. The rationale is based on a critical analysis of a great deal of empirical research and literature in the field. The result is a position which calls for a considerable reorientation to the whole topic of the management of stuttering.

I

BASIC CONSIDERATIONS

1

INTRODUCTION

Stuttering has attracted considerable interest for centuries. Over a span of more than 2,000 years many different ideas have been offered to explain its nature, cause, and treatment. In spite of this, the disorder is still not very well understood.

Speculation has always figured prominently in what has been said and written about stuttering, and this practice continues. Undoubtedly speculation is encouraged by the fact that the vast literature on stuttering contains many partial truths, equivocal findings, puzzling observations, dramatic testimonies, and appraent contradictions. But after more than 50 years of presumably scientific investigation of stuttering, there is no justifiable basis for so much continued conjecture. Speculation has value when it stimulates investigation, but when it restricts the range of inquiry, determines what facts are to be considered, becomes circular and self-reinforcing, it has congealed into dogma. Dogma currently is concealed in the euphemism of "theory."

Many criticisms can be leveled at the existent "theories" of stuttering, but they can be incorporated into two general statements.

First, present theories of stuttering do not deserve that label in a serious sense of the term; for they are little more than favored speculative notions supported by partial observations, preferred facts, and contrived explanations. Many widely accepted viewpoints embody concepts and principles which are internally inconsistent, contrary to many facts, lacking in support from either research findings or therapeutic results, and most regrettable of all, seemingly impervious to reasoned analysis. For example, the psychoanalytic interpretation of stuttering brings an already established dogma to the subject, where it is applied primarily through the fact that speech involves oral activity. Although the psychoanalytic view of stuttering commands a devoted following, it can claim no persuasive support from research findings, historical data, nor therapeutic results.[1]

A similar criticism can be directed at the "evaluation theory" of Wendell Johnson, and its derivations, which represent the interpretation of stuttering most widely accepted in America today. This viewpoint has had considerable appeal for a number of reasons[2] but probably mostly because of its simplicity and the fact that it has generated a considerable amount of research effort. Advocates of this viewpoint seem to have routinely assumed that the results of the research confirm, or at least support, the "theory," since some of the data may be interpreted in that way. However, careful analysis[3] of the purportedly supportive findings reveals that they are either equivocal in their significance for evaluation theory or actually contradict it.

Second, existent theories of stuttering have unwarranted eminence and influence. We are concerned here mainly with the matter of influence, for theory eventually affects the development and conduct of therapy, regardless of its validity.

Surgical treatment of stuttering, which flourished briefly in the middle of the 19th century, is a dramatic example of how theoretical speculation can lead to unwarranted treatment. That method was abandoned soon after it was recognized to be unsuccessful. Unfortunately, therapeutic failure has not discouraged other approaches that have little better rationale than did surgical intervention.

There is a tendency among both the leaders and followers of any particular viewpoint to assume, or at least imply, that the therapy approach is derived from the theory. Of course, some treatment principles have been developed from a theoretical position. For example: change of handedness to augment the presumed natural gradient of dominance; surgery of the tongue to minimize excessive muscular antagonism; and also certain esoteric procedures encountered in psychodynamic approaches to treatment. However, for the most part, methods in stuttering therapy are tied in only a loose way to any particular theory. This fact is reflected in the observation that many therapy practices are common to the activities of therapists representing different theoretical viewpoints. As Van Riper (1954, p. 410) noted a number of years ago:

> From our consideration of all these points of view, the student would be likely to expect that an equally wide variety of therapeutic methods would be available. Oddly enough, this is not the case. When the actual therapies in use are scrutinized, one is impressed not by the differences but by the similarities of the methods used. Terminologies, emphases and theoretical justifications differ, but the activity remains the same.

In some cases a therapy approach is explained in terms of certain hypotheses which are presented as the core of the therapy, but such explanations are little more than constructions appliqued to therapy procedures which have been developed previously or separately. A good example is Sheehan's (1958) "conflict theory" of stuttering. In this interpretation Sheehan has introduced a new set of words and concepts bearing the apparent sophistication of learning theory and psychodynamics, but the only innovations are the interpretations; the therapy prescriptions remain essentially unchanged. Bloodstein (1958) provides a tacit admission of such maneuvering in his discussion of therapy from the point of view that stuttering is anticipatory struggle reaction.[4] He states that the remedial procedures he is about to describe are based on a method of treatment which has been developed over the preceding twenty years by several individuals, then adds that this method " . . . *may be adapted with little change to accord with* . . . "[5] the theoretical viewpoint he maintains.

A further point to be made here is that most therapy methods have been developed on essentially empirical or pragmatic grounds. Many therapy methods exist independent of any particular theory. One might say that most of the widely used and evidently worthwhile methods owe little of their substance to contributions from theory.

In contrast, theory can be shown to have a confounding effect on the development and implementation of treatment. The ubiquitous notion of "punishment" provides a good illustration of a source of confusion. How is the therapist to deal with punishment in implementing a treatment program? Is stuttering the result of punishment? Or is it reflexive, that is, self-punishing? If so, is it punishing as an effect or as an atonement? Or is it expressive, a means of punishing others: parents, the auditor, people in general? For that matter, to what extent is punishment involved at all in stuttering? In a different vein: should stuttering be punished as a means of modifying it? If so, by whom, how, and when? Moreover, what constitutes "punishment" in this context? There are no cogent answers to these questions, only dubious interpretations and convictions.[6]

A similar situation is created by the notion of "avoidance" which has attained unwarranted prominence in the field of stuttering. Avoidance is dealt with as though it were a reality, but theorists have yet to provide a consistent, coherent, or convincing identification of it. Still, therapists are encouraged to deal with "the stutterer's avoidances," without any reasonably consistent assurance regarding what, if indeed anything, is being "avoided"—or if any aspects of stuttering are reasonably conceivable as "avoidances."

There are many examples in which the management of stuttering is affected by theoretical biases which have no demonstrable value or which may even create problems. For instance, there is simply no substantial justification or evident virtue in the widespread injunction against calling attention to stuttering. Yet because of it many clinicians, particularly in the public schools, avoid working with young stutterers, or implement management in a devious and tentative manner, if at all. Similarly, the proscription against using the word "stuttering" has no justification in reality. Yet large numbers of clinicians have been taught to shun the use of this word as though it has some insidious generative power.

The most influential theories of stuttering impugn parents in some way. But what are the reasonable grounds for presuming to counsel parents regarding "their part" in a child's stuttering, with the implication that their child-rearing practices have caused or contributed to the stuttering, either haplessly or through some deviation in child management policies? One could search in vain for compelling evidence.

Lastly, many potentially useful management techniques are overtly or implicitly repudiated through theoretically derived restrictions. For example, most therapists "know" that advising a stutterer to "slow down" is either useless or harmful, essentially because this supposedly heightens his negative reaction to his speech.[7] The use of rhythm is widely disparaged; since theoretical positions can give little sensible account of the effect of rhythm, it is therefore dismissed as a "distraction" or a "crutch." Probably another reason for repudiating rhythm is that it has been advocated and used by "untrained practitioners" and "charlatans."

In sum, theory has contributed to stuttering therapy in only a devious and patchwork manner, frequently emphasizing principles which are of contestable or dubious value. At the same time it has precluded the development and refinement of certain practical techniques simply because they do not accord with theoretical preconceptions. Yet at least some of such techniques show promise of making a worthwhile contribution to a therapy program. Later on we will identify techniques of this kind and consider how they might justifiably be incorporated into the therapeutic repertoire.

The essential message of this chapter is that, at least for the time being, the only reasonable basis for an approach to stuttering therapy is a rationale that is consistent with the available facts, rather than one determined by some preferred interpretation of these facts. This means that the approach to stuttering therapy should be guided by empirical consideration and pragmatic procedure.

There is no need to make any apology for emphasizing an empirical approach. As indicated earlier, the majority of useful therapy methods have developed in this manner. One can find many examples of a similar history of treatment in other areas. For instance, shock therapy, widely employed in certain kinds of psychiatric disorder, was discovered adventitiously and is used successfully despite the fact that the reason for its effect is still not known; the management of diabetes is reported to have been practiced in primitive cultures where essentially nothing was known about human physiology. Further, commonsense methods should not be dismissed lightly: the modern treatment for certain kinds of burns is to apply cold water or ice to the affected areas; in substance this is the "natural" or "practical" thing to do.

Of course, no particular method should be used indiscriminately, but this too is a commonsense consideration consistent with the rationale mentioned above. More importantly, flexibility in use of methods that "work" should be matched with an equal flexibility in attempting to understand them. In the course of following an empirical approach we should constantly endeavor to reason carefully how certain methods overlap or coordinate with others, and how such relationships articulate with the data available to us. Such endeavor represents a search for common principles and coherent explanation which should lead to a unified system of therapy and eventually assist in the development of a cogent theory.

Notes

1. The reader may be aware of the joke about the stutterer who, after completing his psychoanalysis, admits that he still stutters but adds, "But nnnnow I know wh . . .y!" The credibility of this joke is attested to by reports from several eminent psychoanalysts that their work with stutterers was disappointing. [Brill (1932), Blanton (1931), and Reed and Scripture (cf. Hollingworth, 1930); further, see Froeschels (1943) and Sheehan (1958) regarding Freud's own views on stuttering.]

2. Both evaluation theory and psychoanalysis, as well as other "psychological" interpretations derive implicit appeal and support through their currency with the intellectual climate of the times. This matter is discussed in Chapter 2.

3. See Wingate, 1962a, 1962b, 1962c.

4. Essentially an expression of evaluation theory.

5. O. Bloodstein, "Stuttering as an Anticipatory Struggle Reaction," in J. Eisenson (ed.), *Stuttering: A Symposium*, Harper Bros., New York, 1958, p. 39. (Italics added.)

6. Siegel's (1970) review of the matter of punishment offers an excellent commentary on the confusion surrounding this issue. Attention is drawn in particular to the suggestion (p. 678) that punishment *be defined* as a decrease in per-

formance occasioned by the response-contingent presentation of some stimulus. Siegel is willing to substitute this *ad hoc* definition of punishment for the experiential or commonsense definition of punishment. Thus, instead of considering an event as punishing in terms of our ordinary knowledge of it, we are to identify it as punishing because of the effect it produces. Here the meaning of a word is altered to suit the explanation desired and almost obscures the neat circularity involved, viz: the response decreased because it was punished; it was punished because it decreased. The advocacy of this definition of punishment was evidently motivated by the fact that some research has shown a decrease in stuttering through contingent events which defy identification as "punishing" in the ordinary sense of the term. Altering the definition permits the salvage of a concept—and the theoretical model to which it is central. The relevance to stuttering therapy remains a peripheral concern.

7. We will see later the extent to which this prescription has been misguided.

References

Blanton, S. Stuttering. *Mental Hygiene*, **15,** 271–282, 1931.

Bloodstein, O. Stuttering as an anticipatory struggle reaction. In Eisenson, J. (Ed.), *Stuttering: A Symposium*, Harper Bros., New York, 1958.

Brill, A. A. Speech disturbances in neurosis and mental diseases. *Quart. J. Speech Educ.*, **9** 129–135, 1932.

Froeschels, E. Pathology and therapy of stuttering. *Nervous Child*, **2**, 148–161, 1943.

Hollingworth, H. L. *Abnormal Psychology*, Ronald Press, New York, 1930.

Sheehan, J. G. Conflict theory of stuttering. In Eisenson, J. (Ed.), *Stuttering: A Symposium*, Harper Bros, New York, 1958.

Siegel, G. M. Punishment, stuttering and disfluency. *J. Speech Hearing Research*, **13**, 677–714, 1970.

Van Riper, C. *Speech Correction* (3rd ed.), Prentice-Hall, Englewood Cliffs, 1954.

Wingate, M. E. Evaluation and stuttering: I. Speech characteristics of young children. *J. Speech Hearing Dis.*, **27**, 106–115, 1962a.

———Evaluation and stuttering: II. Environmental stress and critical appraisal of speech. *J. Speech Hearing Dis.*, **27**, 244–257, 1962b.

———Evaluation and stuttering: III. Identification of stuttering and the use of a label. *J. Speech Hearing Dis.*, **27**, 368–377, 1962c.

2

STUTTERING AS A PSYCHOLOGICAL PROBLEM

The most popular accounts of stuttering explain it as some kind of psychological problem. The fact that the source of stuttering remains obscure and that the outlines of the problem are often ill-defined and apparently shifting contributes indirectly, but substantially, to the belief that stuttering is "psychological." As with other beliefs, this conviction gathers strength from the very obscurity and mystery that surround it—as well as from its continued restatement.

Certain observations about stuttering, to be reviewed later, suggest an association between stuttering and apparent changes in the psychological state of the stutterer. Additionally, the findings of a good deal of research have been interpreted as evidence that stuttering is basically a "functional disorder."

The readiness with which stuttering has been accepted as a functional disorder, particularly in the United States, may reflect a pervasive influence which is not often recognized: the heritage of our cultural ideology. Viewpoints of stuttering which present it as a psychological problem are consistent with the strong appeal of the premise that environment holds the keys to human behavior. The American political ideal, and presumed moral tenet, that all men are created equal, seems to have evolved into a tacit belief in a basic equivalence of individual capacities and tendencies. Genetic or constitutional contributions to behavior characteristics are given a sort of peripheral recognition. The prevailing attitude shows a decided preference for environmentally based explanations of individual differences. While due exception is made for certain extreme or structurally obvious deviations from normality, the common tendency is to consider the human organism implicitly as a kind of "quantum" when delivered, with his ultimate nature to be shaped and molded by the effects to which he is exposed during life.

Cogent testimony to the influence of this heritage is reflected in two significant phenomena in 20th century America. It is no historical accident that behavioristic psychology developed and flourished in this nation. Similarly, it is no happenstance that dynamic psychology was received here so hospitably in the early part of this century[1] and has subsequently acquired such a wide and enthusiastic support and following.

In America today, and in the past several decades, almost everyone with a standard education—and the assistance of the mass communications media, particularly motion pictures and television—is reasonably conversant with at least the rationale of dynamic psychology, namely that everyone's behavior patterns are the result of the internalized experiences of his past. The populace is thus a prepared audience, receptive to the behavior explanations of both formally trained experts, many of whom have simply ingested dogma during their years of training, and do-it-yourself "experts" whose only credentials are a vivid imagination and the audacity to display it. A lengthy essay titled "Pop Psych" which appeared in the October 7, 1966, issue of *Time* magazine aptly described the 20th century American preoccupation with the psyche and the facility with which laymen indulge in psychological hypothesizing.

People are prepared to believe that almost any kind of behavior deviation or human problem is "psychological." Almost in contradiction to the fact that we are faced continuously with the inadequately explained differences among vast numbers of "normal" people,[2] there is a powerful undercurrent in our thinking which directs us to accept such differences as the result of environmental influences and events in the individual's development. There is a pronounced tendency to discount, one might even say a wish to ignore, considerations of behavior determinants contributed by the constitutional uniqueness of the individual.

It is reasonable to contend that psychological factors may be involved in stuttering, and certainly anyone seriously interested in the disorder should be prepared to give due consideration to the possible psychological elements operative in any particular case. But this is a position far different from one which operates on the assumption that all cases of stuttering reflect a common psychopathology, or even that the same kind of psychological variables are at work in all cases.

Before going further we should call attention to the denominator common to all psychological interpretations of stuttering, namely, that emotion—of a "negative" character—plays a central role. It is easy to appreciate how emotion has attained prominence in explanations of stuttering. First, many stutterers report that their stuttering varies according to circumstances and is related to how they feel, that is, whether they feel threatened or confident, tense or relaxed, apprehensive or secure.[3] Second, statements of this kind are corroborated by an association between the occurrence of stuttering and an apparent emotional state of the individual. Third, normal speakers can recognize that they too tend to be disfluent under conditions similar to those in which some stuttering is observed and reported.

It cannot be denied that much evidence indicates that stuttering is often associated with "negative" emotions. But, however relevant such evidence may be, it must be tempered by certain considerations which are typically overlooked. First, the personal testimony of self-observation is regularly obtained from older stutterers, and their reports are by no means necessarily applicable to the young child who stutters. Second, while emphasis is placed on the concurrence of stuttering and "negative" emotions (fear, embarrassment, hostility), stuttering is also associated with "positive" emotion (excitement), particularly in youngsters. Third, some stuttering occurs in the absence of any observable indication of emotional arousal—in older as well as young stutterers. Fourth, when the fluency of normal speakers is affected by emotional stress it is evidenced as *normal* disfluencies—a point of particular importance. Fifth, emotional stress can disrupt other skilled motor acts too, and we can accept this without being led to interpret the disturbed performance as "an emotional problem." Sixth, while various kinds of normal function may be disrupted by emotion, abnormal function is also exacerbated by stress. One need only consider, for example, the effect of stress on the performance of the aphasic or the cerebral palsied. Again, we do not therefore conclude that the disturbance in function is "an emotional problem."

In the final analysis, it seems evident that emotion and stuttering are related in some way. But to acknowledge an evident connection is not tantamount to offering an explanation. Unfortunately, the recognition that stuttering is associated with emotion has been probably the most misleading of our observations about stuttering. The deception has derived from a failure to distinguish correlation from causation and to understand stuttering in its proper relation to emotion. The net result has been a wide range of speculation and inference of doubtful credibility.

PSYCHOLOGICAL INTERPRETATIONS OF STUTTERING

There are many approaches to the explanation of stuttering as a psychological problem. However, it is not feasible to attempt a review of these various points of view. Instead, we can develop a brief discussion in terms of two major types of explanation which have developed in this area and single out certain basic limitations which cast doubt on the validity and usefulness of these interpretations.

Psychological explanations of stuttering may be categorized as (1) personality, or (2) learning conceptions. These two categories are not mutually exclusive; there are certain facets of interpretation which are common to differing viewpoints representative of both categories. However, a distinction may be drawn in terms of the major focus of their conception. "Personality" accounts of stuttering are concerned primarily with some presumed underlying disturbance in the personality; the acts of stuttering are viewed as symptoms of the underlying disturbance, to which they are related in a specific manner. In learning interpretations the acts of stuttering are viewed as learned behaviors acquired in the developmental history of the individual, essentially through a common motivational source, namely, fear (or some equivalent of fear such as "anxiety" or "apprehension.")[4]

Stuttering as a Personality Disturbance

In the most widely accepted personality accounts of stuttering the basic problem is believed to be some hidden emotional conflict; the actual stuttering is viewed as an overt manifestation of a covert conflict, either in representational or symbolic form. For example, the stutterer is said to harbor unfulfilled dependency needs which are symbolized in the oral act of stuttering. Or, stuttering is the substitutive expression of deep-seated hostile feelings which the stutterer is unable to express appropriately. Or, stuttering is self-punitive behavior reflecting the need to atone for unconsciously felt guilt.

The intractable persistence of viewpoints which interpret stuttering as a personality problem is augmented by their remarkable flexibility. No matter what the circumstances, the interpretation can be adjusted to fit the observations. For instance, if a stutterer admits to, or is assessed as having, personal problems, it is quickly assumed that his stuttering is a manifestation of these problems. On the other hand, if a stutterer gives all appearance of otherwise being normal and well-adjusted, his "symptoms" (the stuttering) can be interpreted as representing his "solution" to his inner conflicts.

Such interpretative possibilities are manifold—many possible combinations of personality and behavioral variables can be invoked to generate explanations of this type. Interested readers can find a substantial array of such contentions in Murphy and Fitzsimmons (1960). We will consider briefly the evidence which bears on the credibility of all such interpretations.

A great deal of research has been addressed to the investigation of stuttering as a personality disturbance. Goodstein (1958) surveyed the relevant research of the preceding twenty years. He undertook separate reviews of the data bearing on the personality and adjustment of child and adult stutterers. He found little evidence to support the contention that the stuttering child or adult has a particular pattern of personality, or is neurotic or severely maladjusted. Within the substantial accumulated data there was some indication that adult stutterers have more personal problems than adult nonstutterers; however, it was not possible to identify whether such problems were related to the stuttering. In general, personality assessment of stutterers regularly found them to be more like psychologically normal individuals than like psychiatric patients.

In a similar analysis Sheehan (1958) reviewed studies of stutterers which had employed several well-established projective tests (Rorschach, Thematic Apperception Test, Rosenzweig Picture-Frustration, two Level-of-Aspiration tests, and two Self-Concept techniques). These tests have been used successfully to distinguish between various groups of individuals with significant personality problems. In their use with stutterers, however, Sheehan found the findings of various studies to be contradictory and equivocal. Except for a suggestion that stutterers may tend to have a somewhat lower level of aspiration than nonstutterers, the results of these studies failed to show any reliable differences between stutterers and the nonstutterers used as controls. Further, no consistent personality pattern emerged which could be considered to be typical of stutterers. Sheehan concluded that the findings from these "best tools modern clinical psychology has developed" provide no support for theories which claim consistent personality differences between stutterers and nonstutterers, nor for viewpoints which describe stutterers in terms of some unique personality pattern.

Murphy and Fitzsimmons (1960), in a similarly comprehensive review, noted that the assessed needs and motives of stutterers differ so much from one to another that it is not possible to identify a pattern of personality dynamics descriptive of stutterers as a group.

More recently Sheehan (1970) extended his original analysis to include relevant research published in the twelve years subsequent to his initial review. Again the accumulated evidence failed to show reliable differences in personality between stutterers and nonstutterers. Van Riper (1970), surveying personality studies dating from 1928, arrived at the same conclusion.

The failure to uncover a type of personality unique to stutterers, or a recurring pattern of personality dynamics among stutterers, carries profound implications, not only for personality interpretations of stuttering, but also in respect to the conditions that supposedly give rise to stuttering. That is, one should expect to find some evidence of uniqueness if, in fact, children who become stutterers do so because of certain kinds of significant life experiences. One should also expect to find some common theme in the psychological make-up of stutterers if, in fact, being a stutterer and being reactive to it have any kind of consistent effect on the individual. To find that considerable research has failed to yield evidence of such uniqueness thus makes it seem very doubtful that stuttering originates and develops from some "typical" set of experiential circumstances, or that stuttering itself has some regularly occurring effect on the developing person.

Stuttering as Learned Behavior

The belief that stuttering is a habit has a long history. Explanations of this kind have been offered repeatedly in the lengthy recorded history of stuttering (see Klingbeil, 1939). Such views have understandably become more popular in the present century; and, especially in this country, the interpretation of stuttering as learned behavior has developed a particular prominence since the middle 1930's. The popularity of this viewpoint within the profession has been due largely to influences from academic psychology, where a vigorous interest in the learning process has developed steadily since the 1920's. Proponents of the view that stuttering is learned have found what appear to be appropriate analogies in models developed through work in the psychological laboratories. Subsequently, research in stuttering, undertaken in the presumption of conformity to such models, has yielded findings which have been interpreted routinely as support for the view that stuttering is learned.

Readers interested in a detailed criticism involving an extensive review of the research bearing on learning theory interpretations of stuttering are referred to a two-article series (Wingate, 1966a, 1966b) which presents a critical analysis of the relevant concepts and research. For present purposes it is sufficient to state briefly, in summary of that analysis, that contrary to the claims frequently made, the concepts involved in this research and the results obtained are sufficiently inconsistent and contradictory that they cannot be seriously entertained as providing support for the contention that stuttering is learned.

The articles did not deal specifically with two learning theory models which have achieved some prominence in intervening years, namely, the two-factor model (Brutten and Shoemaker, 1967) and the operant model (Shames and Sherrick, 1963; Goldiamond, 1965). In most particulars the criticisms developed in the articles are relevant to these models as well. However, a brief review and criticism of these models seem appropriate here.

The two-factor theory.—Brutten and Shoemaker's adaptation of two-factor theory to an explanation of stuttering follows in the stimulus-response tradition found in Wischner's (1950, 1952a, 1952b) formulations. However, whereas Wischner endeavored to account for the complete act of stuttering (the speech features and possible associated actions) as an instrumental response acquired and maintained through reinforcement, Brutten and Shoemaker attempt to account separately for the speech and the nonspeech aspects of stuttering. The speech aspects of stuttering ("fluency failure") are explained in terms of Classical conditioning (associative learning)[5]; the nonspeech aspects of stuttering (eye blink, breath holding, articulatory posturing) are explained in terms of Instrumental conditioning (reinforcement of certain acts performed by the organism)[6].

According to the two-factor model, the acquisition of the speech aspects of stuttering proceeds in three stages. It is important to bear in mind that throughout this three-stage progression the speech aspects of stuttering, the "fluency failures," retain their original character—namely, the overt manifestations, or result, of negative emotional arousal.

In Stage I the speech features of stuttering are "a form of fluency failure" which is believed to be occasioned by a disruptive emotional state. Thus, "Stuttering is . . .a fluency failure caused by the cognitive and motor disorganization associated with negative emotion." (Brutten and Shoemaker, p. 29.)

In Stage II the negative emotion and resulting fluency failure become linked to certain external stimuli through associative learning. Thus, "This relationship between specific situational stimuli,[7] and negative emotion in essence defines the onset of stuttering, since the fluency failure now depends on learning." (*Ibid.*, p. 33.)

In Stage III there is an extension of the range of stimuli to which the negative emotional response becomes associated. In particular, the stimuli which now become sufficient to evoke the negative emotional response include various aspects of the speech process:

Stage III in the growth of stuttering is defined by the development of conditioned negative emotional reactions to the act of speaking, the words employed, or the speech produced. Generally this speech specific conditioning arises because stuttering is a noxious stimulus to the listener, and consequently, listeners often respond punitively to the stutterer. These punitive responses may take the form of derision, impatience, or a simple decrease in time spent interacting with a stutterer. In addition, the stutterer himself may perceive his speech as inadequate or unacceptable, and may experience negative emotion even though he receives little actual negative reaction from the environment. (*Ibid.*, p. 31.)

Primarily, stuttering is conceived as " . . . that class of fluency failure that results from conditioned negative emotion." (*Ibid.*, p. 38.) In simpler terms, "conditioned negative emotion" means "fear" or "anxiety."

The nonspeech aspects of stuttering are conceived as additions to or embellishments of the fluency failure, acquired as a result of this fluency failure and its associated negative emotion. In the authors' words: " . . . it is posited that these responses are the adjustive or 'problem solving' behaviors that are engendered as a means of coping with the noxious state that was the consequence of fluency failure." (*Ibid.*, p. 38.)

There are a number of serious limitations in this model. The most fundamental is that the model hinges on a confounded definition of stuttering. To contend that stuttering is " . . . that form of fluency failure that results from conditioned negative emotion" is to mix an imprecise objective description of stuttering with a presumed etiologic factor.[8]

To say that stuttering results from conditioned negative emotion assumes the fact. Moreover, it is contradictory to observation: stuttering has been reported to occur in the absence of evident negative emotion and not to occur in circumstances in which negative emotion is evident—a point which the authors themselves acknowledge. (*Ibid.*, p. 43.)

Here we are concerned less with the imprecise identification of stuttering than with the central role assigned to negative emotion. Why should negative emotion be given such a prominent and powerful role in stuttering? In one sense probably because we have heard for so long and from so many sources that some variant of negative emotion is a cause of stuttering. However, we should point out a more immediate motivation. Any learning theory model which incorporates principles derived from the Law of Effect requires a motive source to make the model credible. In the case of stimulus-response learning models of stuttering the "negative emotion" so frequently claimed to be associated with stuttering provides the leverage for a plausible explanation in these terms.

We will soon consider whether negative emotion deserves such a prominent role in conceptions of stuttering. The evidence will have bearing on conceptions of stuttering other than those which invoke learning theory principles. At the moment it is pertinent to point out one other serious problem which is not handled adequately by S–R learning theory models. It is this: the stimuli sufficient to evoke stuttering, or "negative emotion," are only crudely and vaguely specified. Actually they are inferred,[9] essentially on the grounds that if stuttering is a response to stimuli (which it is assumed to be) then there must be adequate and sufficient stimuli.

The operant model.—Recently the operant model of learning has been applied to stuttering with considerable enthusiasm. An apparent advantage of the operant model is that it avoids the necessity of identifying the stimulus, or stimuli, sufficient to elicit stuttering. Instead, stuttering, like any "operant," can be conceived as *emitted* behavior, which occurs for reasons that need not be specified, and which is then stabilized (learned) through the effect of some kind of reinforcement associated with its occurrence. Operant analysis does not ignore the fact that stuttering may be more likely to occur in the context of certain stimuli, but such correspondences can be accounted for *post hoc* by referring to such stimuli as "discriminative cues" to which the response, already established by reinforcement, has become attached.

According to the operant model explanation, stuttering begins as normal disfluencies[10] which are a "natural" and understandable occurrence in children's speech under certain circumstances. (See Shames and Sherrick, 1963; Goldiamond, 1965.) During the initial periods of their occurrence, these disfluencies are encouraged through some schedule of positive reinforcement. These conditions recur, and in time certain aspects of them become discriminative cues which then gradually acquire the power to "control the emission" of the disfluencies. However, negative emotion in the form of punishment soon enters the picture, initially through the agency of social (essentially parental) disapproval of the disfluencies and then, somewhat later, in the form of negative self-reaction when the child's speech has acquired "aversive properties," principally through social disapproval. The effect of the negative emotion is to generate struggle with the nonfluencies, which then degenerates into ("what is called") stuttering. This degeneration is accompanied by the appearance of nonspeech acts. The finally developed pattern of behavior identified as stuttering is thus supposedly learned through complex and intricate schedules of reinforcement.

The operant model represents a form of instrumental learning and, as such, embodies principles based on the Law of Effect. Thus, like S–R models, it requires the conception of some form of motive source. In the application of this model to stuttering both positive and negative aspects of motivation are invoked. Their manner of operation, however, remains conjectural. As Shames and Sherrick admit: "A very important, but as yet undefined, variable in these pardigms is the schedules of punishment and negative and positive reinforcements which are necessary to stabilize a stuttering response." It should be added that we still have no substantial reason to believe that stuttering *is* a response, let alone that it becomes stabilized through certain effects.

As noted earlier, the two-factor and the operant conceptions share inconsistencies and contradictions common to learning theory interpretations of stuttering. In particular, these conceptions lack supporting evidence that stuttering originates as "fluency failure" or "normal nonfluency" which then gets worse.[11] Also they are confounded by the evidence regarding penalty and punishment in stuttering.[12] Further, as we shall see in the next chapter, the evidence relevant to the presumed significance of negative emotion in stuttering is not very persuasive. In fact, there is good reason not only to question its import but to doubt its common existence.

Notes

1. In his visits to this country, Freud was received much more openly and favorably than he was in Europe. Freudian oriented thinking has continued to flourish in this nation as compared to other countries. For a fairly recent statement regarding this situation see W. Sargent, "Psychiatric Treatment Here and in England," *Atlantic Monthly*, Vol. 214, July, 1964, 88–95.
2. An exemplary case in point is provided by the obvious differences in coordinative skill underlying excellence or mediocrity in athletic achievement.
3. This is not true of all stutterers, nor perhaps even most of them, but it is the kind of report much favored in the literature.
4. Bloodstein's (1958, 1961) use of "anticipation" (of difficulty) seems designed to evade the problems posed by the notion of "fear." However, use of this seemingly neutral term does not evade the problem so neatly. It is difficult to understand how one can anticipate a presumed negative experience with other than a negative attitude. In this context, then, "anticipation" reduces to "apprehension" or "fear."
5. The type of learning exemplified by Pavlov's dogs.
6. The kind of learning exemplified when a rat learns to press a lever to receive food, avoid a threatened shock, or escape from an electrified grid.
7. These specific situational stimuli are not explicitly identified by the authors. Presumably they include any stimulus or stimulus complex in the presence of which the fluency failure occurs.
8. Even with the authors' suggestion at one point (p. 61) that " . . . involuntary repetitions and prolongations are uniquely descriptive of stuttering behavior . . .", their definition consists of one criterion ("fluency failure," or "in-

voluntary repetitions and prolongations") that is not sufficiently precise, and another (negative emotion) that is not criterial. This is rather like saying that bananas are (a) yellow things that are (b) found in grocery stores.

9. Even in research showing some variation of stuttering in relation to changes in stimulus conditions, the "responses" do not occur with the regularity or predictability that is expected of stimulus–response connections.

10. Evidently these disfluencies are the equivalent of what Brutten and Shoemaker identify as "fluency failures." A possible distinction might be that Brutten and Shoemaker admit the possibility that some children may have a predisposition to fluency failure; proponents of the operant model adhere to the contention of the essential actuarial and organismic normality of these "early" disfluencies.

11. See McDearmon, 1968; Wingate, 1962.

12. See Siegel, 1970.

References

Bloodstein, O. Stuttering as an anticipatory struggle reaction. In Eisenson J. (Ed.), *Stuttering: A Symposium*, Harper Bros., New York, 1958.

———The development of stuttering: III Theoretical and clinical implications. *J. Speech Hearing Dis.*, **26**, 67–82, 1961.

Brutten, E. J. and D. J. Shoemaker. *The Modification of Stuttering*, Prentice-Hall, Englewood Cliffs, 1967.

Goldiamond, I. Stuttering and fluency as manipulatable operant response classes. In Krasner, L. and L. P. Ullman (Eds.), *Research in Behavior Modification: New Development and Implications*, Holt, Rinehart and Winston, New York, 1965, Chapter 6.

Goodstein, L. D. Functional speech disorders & personality: A survey of the research. *J. Speech Hearing Res.*, **1**, 358–377, 1958.

Klingbeil, G. M. The historical background of the modern speech clinic. *J. Speech Hearing Dis.*, **4**, 115–132, 1939.

McDearmon, J. R. Primary stuttering at the onset of stuttering: A reexamination of data. *J. Speech Hearing Res.*, **11**, 631–637, 1968.

Murphy, A. T. and Ruth M. Fitzsimmons. *Stuttering and Personality Dynamics*, Ronald Press, New York, 1960.

Shames, G. H. and C. H. Sherrick, Jr. A discussion of non-fluency and stuttering as operant behavior. *J. Speech Hearing Dis.*, **28**, 3–18, 1963.

Sheehan, J. G. Projective studies of stuttering. *J. Speech Hearing Dis.*, **23**, 18–25, 1958.

———Personality approaches. In Sheehan, J. G. (Ed.), *Stuttering: Research and Therapy*, Harper & Row, New York, 1970, Chapter 3.

Siegel, G. M. Punishment, stuttering and disfluency. *J. Speech Hearing Res.*, **13**, 677–714, 1970.

Van Riper, C. *The Nature of Stuttering*, Prentice-Hall, Englewood Cliffs, 1970.

Wingate, M. E. Evaluation and Stuttering, Part I: Speech characteristics of young children. *J. Speech Hearing Dis.*, **27**, 106–115, 1962.

———Stuttering adaptation and learning: I. The relevance of adaptation studies to stuttering as "learned behavior." *J. Speech Hearing Dis.*, **31**, 148–156, 1966a.

———Stuttering adaptation and learning: II. The adequacy of learning principles in the interpretation of stuttering. *J. Speech Hearing Dis.*, **31**, 211–218, 1966a.

Wischner, G. J. An experimental approach to expectancy and anxiety in stuttering behavior. *J. Speech Hearing Dis.*, **17**, 139–154, 1952a.

———Anxiety reduction as reinforcement in maladaptive behavior: Evidence in stutterers' representations of the moment of difficulty. *J. Abn. Soc. Psychol.*, **47**, 566–571, 1952b.

———Stuttering behavior and learning: A preliminary theoretical formulation. *J. Speech Hearing Dis.*, **15**, 324–335, 1950.

3

FEAR AND STUTTERING

The motivation concepts invoked as a central feature in stuttering reduce to a common denominator, namely, fear. "Negative emotion," "punishment," "penalty," "noxious consequences," "anticipation," "apprehension," "dread," "anxiety"—all represent alternate ways of referring to fear and its presumed influence in stuttering. Fear has been elevated to a position of prominence and influence that it does not deserve. How has this situation developed?

A powerful source of the status of fear has been the continual restatement of its significance. Throughout the recorded history of stuttering, fear has been mentioned frequently as a major force in the development and maintenance of the disorder. Since the development of speech pathology as a profession, we find constant reference to fear in the literature: in reports of cases, in transcribed testimonials, and particularly in the various theoretical formulations of the nature of stuttering by some of our most influential figures. Impressive reminders of its claimed significance are woven into most therapy approaches, and the practitioner is "programmed" to infer the presence of fear even when it is hardly warranted. In contrast, reporst which minimize the role of fear are ignored. For instance, one hardly ever finds reference to the kind of statement made by Bryngelson (1935):

> Indeed, there are many stutterers who possess neither anxiety nor fear in relation to their broken rhythms in speech. This situation I have found to be quite prevalent in children, as well as in adults who have stuttered since the onset of speech. It is an interesting observation that these folks showed no

marked abnormal reactions to anything about themselves or to their environments in general.

NONSTUTTERERS' ATTITUDES ABOUT SPEAKING

The continued emphasis on the stutterer's fear of speaking and of speech situations has encouraged the tendency to overlook the fact that normal speakers have similar reactions. All of us are familiar with the experience of "stage fright," which occurs in many situations much less formal than being on a stage, and before "audiences" that may be quite small. Clevenger (1959) has reviewed some of the fairly extensive experimental literature on this phenomenon in adult-level age groups. Shaw (1967) studied "speech fright" and speaking ability in 420 children from kindergarten through sixth grade and reported that at least 20 percent of the children were considerably concerned about speech fright. It is of interest that he found no apparent relationship between speech fright and speaking ability.

Normal speakers are known to be fearful of speaking under a wide variety of circumstances. Knower (1938) developed a Speech Attitude Scale consisting of 96 items in its final (shortened) version, many of which referred to quite commonplace and casual speaking experiences. Knower used this scale in investigations involving over 3,000 high school- and college-age normal speakers. He reported that individuals had negative attitudes toward a wide variety of speech activities and, interestingly, that speakers of varying levels of capability had negative attitudes toward the same kinds of speaking experiences.

The existence of intense and pervasive negative reactions to speaking situations among normal speakers has led Phillips (1968) to the identification of "Reticents"—individuals with normal speech who show a pattern of fear of speaking in a wide range of situations. Phillips studied 198 such college-age individuals, most of whom had been referred by advisors or counselors because of their speech problems. These individuals reported physical symptoms during attempts to speak, for example, "butterflies in the stomach," loud or rapid heartbeat, headache, excessive perspiration. Sometimes they found it necessary to break off communication abruptly because of their fears and apprehensions. They tended to relive their failures, suffering again in retrospective contemplation. They expressed an inability to communicate with "important" people, and had a fear of being asked questions. Parents and teachers had called attention to their communicative inadequacies. Most of them had an image of themselves as excessively quiet and typically on the fringe of social gatherings.

Phillips reporter that later additional surveys of fairly sizable college and high school populations suggested that approximately 5 percent of these groups evidenced the major features of this syndrome. Clearly, fear of speaking is not unique to stutterers.

STUTTERERS' ATTITUDES ABOUT SPEAKING

If fluency, normal nonfluency, and stuttering all occur in the presence of fear of speaking, there is no special connection between fear of speaking and stuttering. The role of fear of speaking is not specific. It might well be that stuttering is more likely to occur, or increase, under conditions of fear, but the fear is at best a precipitant and the stuttering must be due to something else.

Some sources might object that a comparison of stutterers to nonstutterers is not justified, because stutterers fear more speech situations than do nonstutterers, or fear them more. This objection begs the question. Fearing more situations still does not mean that there is some unique or special relationship between fear and stuttering. Besides, the relevant experimental evidence is contradictory.

Situation Fears

Knott (1935) had 28 college stutterers identify their most pleasant and most unpleasant speaking experiences and rate them on an eleven-point scale. Results indicated that the speaking experiences of these stutterers were no more pleasant or unpleasant than their nonspeaking experiences. Further, the same could be said in comparison of their stuttering and nonstuttering experiences. Knott concluded that "The average attitude of these stutterers toward speaking situations was apparently entirely normal."

Several studies have compared the attitudes of stutterers and nonstutterers to different kinds of speaking experiences. Brown and Hull (1942) used the Speech Attitude Scale developed by Knower with 59 older stutterers and compared their scores to those reported for the standardization (normative) group. The authors reported that *as a group* the stutterers' scores were significantly lower, which was interpreted to suggest that stutterers were less confident and enthusiastic about speaking, less poised in doing so, and enjoyed it less. Although the methodology of the study (comparing a selected sample with population norms) is questionable, our immediate concern is more with the omission of data on individual variation in the stutterers' scores and reactions. Studies which report this individual variation yield a rather different picture.

Trotter and Bergman (1952) compared the reactions of 100 nonstuttering and 50 stuttering young adults to 40 different speaking situations through a rating scale technique. Comparisons were made from rating scales designed to measure (a) the tendency to avoid a situation, (b) the degree of enjoyment from speaking in a situation, (c) the frequency with which the situation was met, and (d) the amount of nonfluency in a situation. In terms of group comparison, the stutterers' ratings indicated a tendency to avoid situations more and to enjoy speaking in them less than the nonstutterers. At the same time the groups did not differ in the frequency with which they met the situations, indicating that the "tendency to avoid" was not actualized, and suggesting that such discomfort as might be experienced did not affect their acceptance of the situation. Beyond this, the most impressive finding was that " . . . a considerable number of non-stutterers were more avoidant of speaking situations and enjoyed speaking in them less than many stutterers." Also, those nonstutterers most inclined to avoid speaking situations and to enjoy speaking in them less tended to be the less fluent in those situations. Such findings indicate that "fear" of speaking situations is not unique to stutterers or to stuttering.

Erickson (1969) has described the development of a scale designed specifically to assess communication attitudes among stutterers. The final "S-scale" consisted of 39 items retained from an initial Communication Inventory of 466 items. The 39 items were retained on the basis that they discriminated significantly between criterion groups of 50 young adult stutterers and 100 nonstutterers. As might be expected, comparison of the responses of the two groups to the selected items of the final scale yielded a bimodal distribution with a highly significant difference between the mean scores. However, even with this careful and intentional effort to create a measure which would yield a distinction between stutterers and nonstutterers, there was still a considerable amount of overlap in the response distributions of the two groups. The author's own words make the point quite clearly:

> The composition of the S-scale, nevertheless, does not appear to suggest that the basis for differentiation of stutterers and non-stutterers involved grossly disparate attitudes toward communication in general. The great number of Communication Inventory items which do not appear in the S-scale because stutterers and non-stutterers responded to them in an essentially similar fashion provide

additional evidence consistent with this view. In addition, the overlap observed between their S-scale score distributions suggests that communication attitudes of stutterers and non-stutterers may differ, when they differ, primarily in degree. Differences among stutterers in turn may not be qualitatively distinct from those which appear between stutterers and non-stutterers or among non-stutterers.

A number of studies have attempted a direct assessment of the effect of speaking situations on stuttering. The majority of these studies have investigated variation in stuttering frequency or severity with changes in audience size or personnel (Hahn, 1940; Porter, 1939; Sheehan, Hadley, and Gould, 1967; Siegel and Haugen, 1964; Van Riper and Hull, 1955; Young, 1965). Some studies have included other features, such as speaking on the telephone (Dixon, 1955) or speaking in interview about situations of presumably varying difficulty (Lerman and Shames, 1965). Although it is frequently reported in such studies that the situational variables had some relationship to frequency of stuttering when the subjects were considered *as a group*, in those studies which make note of individual reactions (Hahn, 1940; Porter, 1939; Sheehan *et al.* 1967; Van Riper and Hull, 1955) one regularly finds evidence of considerable individual variation. Moreover, in some studies the influence of the situation effect is irregular or equivocal (Porter, 1939; Siegel and Haugen, 1964) or not evidenced (Lerman and Shames, 1965; Young, 1965).

It is frequently said that stutterers do not stutter when they speak alone. This claim is invariably presented as indirect evidence of the import of situation fears—to wit, that when the stutterer is isolated from sources which generate fear, he does not stutter. However, Bryngelson (1955) reported that six of the 13 stutterers he studied reported having difficulty when speaking alone. Hahn (1940), observing 52 stutterers reading aloud when they believed themselves to be alone, noted that all but three of them stuttered in this situation. Hahn had asked the subjects to record their own stuttering while speaking alone. Later comparison of the experimenter's record of stutterings with those of a randomly selected group of 20 cases showed that the stutterers usually underestimated the number of their stutterings (over half of them stuttered from two to eight times as much as they reported). Porter (1939) also observed her subjects when reading alone and noted that only two of the 13 subjects did not stutter in this situation. Razdol'skii (1965) reported a study of the solitary and social-situation speech of 125 stutterers who ranged in age from 2 years to adulthood. The speech of most of the preschool-age children contained about as much stuttering when alone as when they spoke in the presence of other people. Most of the school-age children were observed to stutter less when alone and most of the teenagers and adults stuttered much less when alone. However, only 11 of the 125 subjects evidenced no stuttering in their isolated speaking. In subsequent interrogation subjects of all ages who were sufficiently knowledgeable about their speech defect to comment on it were asked if they stuttered when talking alone. Initially most of them stated that they did not have difficulty when speaking by themselves, but after more careful questioning many reported "occasional brief lapses" under such circumstances.

Word and Sound Fears

Stutterers supposedly fear certain words or certain sounds, and purportedly it is the fear of these words and sounds which causes them to be stuttered. This belief has attained wide acceptance; in fact, certain theoretical formulations have elevated it to the status of a principle, namely "specific word anxiety." Most of what is known about word and sound fears is supplied from anecdotes and "example" case histories (some of which are repeated from one literature source to another). In contrast, there is little in the way of research findings which provides any support for the purported effects of word and sound fears.

The so-called "consistency effect" is often cited as experimental evidence of the influence of word or sound fears. However, a careful look at the consistency effect and the data on which it is based prompts a number of serious reservations about its significance. First, data on the consistency effect have been obtained from repeated readings of prepared material rather than from protocols of spontaneous speech. Second, the average value of "consistency" is about 60 percent, which is not a very impressive figure for its purported function and significance. Third, as Tate and Cullinan (1962) report, the values obtained by the usual methods of computing consistency can be obtained on a purely chance basis. Fourth, there is a great deal of individual variation in the extent of consistency. There are other serious limitations, but it is sufficient to emphasize that consistency is a friable concept based on a phenomenon that is poorly understood and as yet inadequately investigated.

The "expectancy" phenomenon has also been invoked as evidence that stuttering results from word and sound fears. However, like the consistency effect, expectancy is a very ephemeral phenomenon that is little understood. At best, the concurrence of expectancy and stuttering is limited, intermittent, and variable, and any interpretation of the connection between the two events remains conjectural.

Very little is known about the relationship of expectancy to stuttering in spontaneous connected speech. The available research findings have been obtained under quite artificial conditions which are likely to exaggerate the manifestations of expectancy. This is particularly true of certain studies (e.g., Johnson *et al.*, 1937; Johnson and Sinn, 1937), which also happen to have shown the most dramatic occurrence of expectancy. Studies which are somewhat less vulnerable to this criticism have yielded much less impressive results. For instance, Johnson and Solomon (1937) found stuttering to occur on only about 53 percent of the words expected; Johnson and Ainsworth (1938) reported a similar figure; Peins (1961) indicated that her subjects were "not very accurate" in their predictions of stuttering; and Martin and Haroldson (1967) found a concurrence of expectancy and stuttering to be less than 50 percent.

Moreover, studies of expectancy regularly reveal that the subjects also stutter on many words on which they evidently did not expect to stutter. A recent study (Wingate, 1975) which took this into account yielded evidence that true expectancy ratios must be very low for most stutterers. It is pertinent to recall here the evidence from other research (cf. p. 25) that stutterers are often unaware of their stutterings, thus precluding an expectancy effect. Further, there are considerable individual differences: some stutterers, under certain conditions, seem able to predict stutterings reasonably well; others evidently are not.

It bears emphasizing that consistency and expectancy are abstruse phenomena that still require a great deal of investigation. Their relationship to stuttering is by no means clear and their interpreted connection to fear is highly conjectural and tenuous (cf. Lingwall, 1967; Wingate, 1975).

Some research seems to bear more directly on the matter of stuttering and word fears. Several studies have attempted to investigate the concurrence of stuttering and certain physiological measures assumed to reflect "anxiety," such as galvanic skin response and pulse rate. The results of this research have been equivocal: some studies have reported a positive relationship between stuttering and "anxiety" (Brutten, 1963; Kline, 1959; Maxwell, 1965); others have found no correlation (Gray and Brutten, 1965; Karmen, 1964); some have yielded equivocal or contradictory results (Lingwall, 1967; Knott *et al.*, 1959; Shrum, 1967). Moreover, regardless of the findings in such research, there remains the fundamental issue of whether the physiological measures employed can be reasonably assumed to reflect anxiety or fear rather than some more basic organismic arousal. A case in point is provided by the findings of a study by Valyo (1964). He obtained GSR recordings from stutterers and nonstutterers while they alternated speech and silence in one-minute intervals. The GSR recordings of both groups were comparable during the silent periods, but during the speech intervals the amplitude of the GSR of the stutterers doubled while it remained the same among the nonstutterers. Although it seems clear that the stutterers' GSR fluctuated directly in relation to speech or silence, it seems incredible that fear or anxiety should turn on and off sequentially in such brief temporal segments.

There is one further, compelling, reason to doubt the validity of the purported relationship of word and sound fears to stuttering, at least in the sense of some cause-and-effect relationship. This is the lack of any real evidence of generalization of stuttering in relation to words or sounds.

The matter of generalization of stuttering is chronically neglected by learning theory interpretations. This is a curious omission. It is well known, from various areas of psychological investigation, that responses established in association with a certain cue tend to generalize to other perceptually similar cues, particularly if a strong motivational element is involved. Certainly, if stuttering is in any substantial measure due to fear, and if stuttering is "learned behavior," we should expect to find considerable evidence of generalization.

At the most elementary level one could well expect generalization based on speech sounds themselves. Among the various phonemes the features of type, placement, and manner of execution contain overlapping commonalities that should support generalization in several directions.

Generalization should also find a ready avenue for expression in terms of the patterns of sounds common to different words. Homophones (bear, bare; red, read; vein, vane, vain) constitute the extreme instance, but also consider: but, bud; bug, buck; bum, bun; butter, buddy; buggy, buckle. Research in other areas has shown that responses such as salivation and GSR, originally associated with some particular word, will generalize to homophones of that word (Razran, 1939; Reiss, 1940, 1946).

Generalization of stuttering could be expected to occur along semantic lines as well, that is, in terms of word reference or meaning. Again, research in other areas has shown generalization of GSR and salivation to synonyms of words with which these responses were originally associated (Diven, 1937; Razran, 1939; Reiss, 1940).

There is a profound lack of evidence that stuttering generalizes on any of these potential dimensions. It seems clear that generalization of stuttering simply does not occur. Actually, one can project that if generalization of stuttering were to occur in a manner and at a rate consistent with the purported effect of fear, one could reasonably expect that once a child begins to stutter he should become essentially mute within a few years. Obviously this does not happen. In fact we find quite the contrary, as we shall see in a subsequent chapter.

Fear of Speaking

If speaking is so laden with fear for stutterers, they should be much less inclined to talk than nonstutterers. There is considerable evidence to indicate that this is not the case. Moore *et al.* (1952) recorded the answers of 16 young adult male stutterers to questions focusing on six different personal topics. While the amount of stuttering varied somewhat among the different topics, the amount of speaking was equivalent from one topic to another. The authors reported that the " . . . severity of stuttering does not inhibit verbal output." Lerman and Shames (1965) interviewed 20 young adult stutterers concerning their feelings and anticipations about entering into four speaking situations of varying degrees of difficulty. From each interview they obtained measures of frequency of stuttering, the number of words spoken in the interview, and a Discomfort-Relief Quotient. They found no relationship between the amount of stuttering, the number of words spoken, or the degree of "anxiety" in the interview. Knabe *et al.* (1966) investigated several dimensions of the linguistic performance of 16 stuttering and 16 nonstuttering college students matched for age, sex, academic level, and verbal ability on the College Qualification Test. The subjects were asked five personal and five impersonal questions with the instruction to answer each with unlimited response. The groups differed only in the amount of disfluency; there was no difference in the amount of verbalization.

Similar results were obtained by Wingate (1970) in a study of 20 male stutterers and 20 nonstutterers in the adolescent and young adult range matched for age, educational level, and recognition vocabulary. Subjects recorded a story in response to a card selected from the Thematic Apperception Test and later wrote a story about a card selected from Stanford-Binet materials. The two groups did not differ appreciably in the amount of verbalization in either task—actually, stutterers used somewhat more words than nonstutterers in telling a story but fewer words in writing a story. Grubman (1970) had matched groups of nine college-level stutterers and nonstutterers make up 40 sentences constructed around given words. The two groups did not differ in amount of verbalization.

Comparable findings have been reported for similar work done with young children. Meltzer (1935) studied the talkativeness of 50 stuttering and 50 nonstuttering children between the ages of 8 and 17, matched for sex, age, intelligence, grade level, and school. The stuttering youngsters were found to talk significantly more than the nonstutterers. Meltzer noted that similar results had been obtained in a contemporary study by Hawthorne which compared the responses of 68 stuttering children and a control group of 250 nonstuttering youngsters in reply to a set of three questions. Muma and Frick (1967) obtained speech samples from 17 fluent and 17 "dysfluent" four-year-olds matched for age, sex, race, intelligence, sibling status, socioeconomic level, and school experience. While the two groups were considerably different in respect to "dysfluency," they did not differ in terms of the amount of speaking.

Fear of Stuttering

There is no intention here to discredit or deny the claim of many stutterers that, in certain situations at least, they are apprehensive lest they stutter and feel bad when they do. At the same time it is necessary to present evidence which contradicts the belief that fear of stuttering is an integral and determining feature of the problem.

Testimony regarding fear of stuttering is supplied by older stutterers, and it is hardly legitimate to presume that whatever feelings they report are also to be found in stuttering youngsters. But even if we limit our consideration to evidence regarding older stutterers it is quite impressive to discover that the relevant research provides very little support for belief in the ubiquity or consequence of a fear of stuttering.

Johnson and Ammons (1944) developed a Test of Attitude toward Stuttering, a measure in which a respondent indicates his agreement, on a five-point scale ranging from "strongly agree" to "strongly disagree," with various statements about stuttering, stutterers, and their behavior. This scale, consisting of 160 items in its original form, was administered to 40 college freshmen, 40 townspeople, 72 stutterers, and 67 speech clinicians. The results indicated that the most unfavorable reaction was registered by the townspeople and the least unfavorable reaction by the clinicians. The responses of the stutterers and of the college freshmen were comparable and occupied the middle range, showing them to have "a moderate reaction" in comparison to the other groups. Moreover, there was no evident relationship for the stutterers between attitude toward stuttering and self-ratings of stuttering severity or the number of years of remedial speech work.

The original Test of Attitude toward Stuttering was reduced to a scale of 45 items by eliminating those items which did not discriminate well between the extremes. This refined and highly specialized scale, which appears in Johnson, Darley, and Spriestersbach (1952), was administered by Friedman (1955) to 326 stutterers, mostly adolescent and young adults, and 100 nonstuttering speech pathology students. There was no difference between the scores of these two large groups of stutterers and nonstutterers; they "showed about the same degree of non-acceptance of stuttering."

People who have a negative or unfavorable (nonobjective) attitude about a personal handicap can be expected to harbor an undue sensitivity about the problem, particularly if there is an implication of social ridicule. Such was the rationale of two studies which investigated stutterers' reaction to jokes about handicaps. Staats (1955) selected ten "personal" cartoons (ones in which the comedy related primarily to a personal impairment) and ten impersonal cartoons. The two sets were equated for degree of humor through a rating method. The cartoons were presented to a group of 26 male college stutterers, a nonstuttering experimental group of 63 college males and a nonstuttering control group of 57 college males. The subjects were asked to rate each cartoon on a seven-point scale of funniness. The three groups did not differ from each other in their median or mean ratings for each of the 20 cartoons (except for a difference on one cartoon between the two nonstuttering groups). Further, none of the groups differed in their mean ratings of the personal as compared to the nonpersonal cartoons. These findings thus yielded no evidence to suggest that stutterers are inclined to be sensitive about humor involving a personal handicap.

Adler (1956) extended this line of investigation to assess stutterers' reactions to comedy about stuttering. He compiled a group of 21 jokes dealing with various kinds of personal handicaps: 15 involved stuttering, 3 dealt with the deaf, 1 with the deaf and dumb, 1 with a hunchback, and 1 with a blind person. He presented these jokes to 23 adolescent and young adult stutterers and a comparable group of nonstutterers who were asked to rate each joke on a five-point scale which ranged from "not funny" to "very funny." He found no differences in the way the stutterers and the control group rated the 21 jokes. Further, neither group reacted any differently to the stuttering jokes than they did to those involving the other handicaps.

Comparable results have been obtained from studies designed to assess stutterers' sensitivities about stuttering through the use of projective methods. Bloodstein and Bloodstein (1955) prepared a movie consisting of segments showing the facial expressions of ten persons who had been filmed, without their knowledge, while listening to a severe stutterer in a face-to-face contact. Immediately after this experience the listeners were asked to indicate, from a list of eleven reactions, what their reaction had been while listening to the stutterer. The film was shown to 25 stutterers and 25 nonstutterers of adolescent and young adult age, who were advised that the pictures were obtained while the listeners were being spoken to by a severe stutterer. These subjects were asked to indicate, on the same eleven-item checklist, the reaction they perceived in each listeners's expressions. The results revealed no differences between the interpretations of the stutterers and the nonstutterers. The stutterers actually reported perceiving "no unfavorable reaction" somewhat *more* frequently, and "superiority" somewhat *less* frequently than did the nonstutterers. The subjects in both groups differed widely among themselves about what they perceived in the listeners' reactions and, for the most part, interpretations of listeners' reactions by both groups failed to correspond with the reactions admitted by the listeners themselves. Wingate and Hamre (1967) reported a similar study in which a group of 20 young adult stutterers and a matched control group were presented a movie of ten persons, shown sequentially, as in the Bloodstein study. These persons were identified to the subjects as having been filmed while listening to an individual speaker. Actually, these persons were not listening to anyone; they had simply been instructed to make occasional slight movements of the head and face. The subjects were asked to indicate, for each listener, whether the "unseen speaker" was a stutterer, a nonstutterer, or if it were not possible to tell. In each case subjects were also asked to rate the listener's reaction on a five-point scale of favorability of reaction. The results revealed that the identification and descriptions from stutterers were comparable in all respects to those of the nonstutterers. Both groups used each speaker identification category with comparable frequency, and their ratings of favorability of listener reaction did not differ.

A study by Silverman (1970) bears particularly on the presumed role of fear-of-stuttering in the genesis or exacerbation of stuttering. Silverman used the "Three Wishes" technique with 62 stuttering children, approximately 15 from each of grades two through five. (In the "Three Wishes" technique a youngster is asked to tell what he would ask for if he could have three wishes magically granted.) Only four of the wishes expressed by these children made any reference to speech, and of these two did not really suggest a wish for better speech. Consistent with what is regularly found among normal children, most of the wishes from these youngsters were for tangible things for themselves, with the older youngsters also wishing for tangible and intangible things for others.

FEAR AND THE CLINICIAN

Many therapists appear to have a fear of stuttering which surpasses that of most of the stutterers they treat, especially when one considers that the majority of stutterers who receive therapy are children.

An unfortunate number of speech therapists—particularly in the public schools, where the clientele is largely young children—are reluctant to work with stutterers. Often the therapist is either not sure of what to do or uncertain whether what is done will have a beneficial effect. Timidity based on such grounds is understandable in view of our uncertain knowledge of the nature of stuttering and the correct ways of treating it. The therapist's apprehension and tentativeness have emanated from psychological interpretations of stuttering; overtly or by implication, these views convey the message that stuttering—particularly in youngsters—represents a delicate condition which can develop unfortunate consequences if not handled carefully. Theories of psychological causation of stuttering do not really specify what these consequences might be. However, clinicians who have been impressed by all the supposed psychological complexities of the stutterer are prone to the apprehension that what they do might be harmful to the child's psychological adjustment. The fact that there is no evidence to supply substance for this fear remains beside the point.

Another complication springs from the belief that stuttering develops (becomes worse) as a result of psychological influences. This belief supports a fear that, unless early "simple" stuttering is handled with great care and finesse, it will exacerbate. Even more oppressive is the contention that the fluency disruptions identified as stuttering are really misperceived normal nonfluencies. This contention, often stated openly, is bulwarked by frequent references in the literature to "alleged" stuttering, "so-called" stuttering, "labelled as" stutterers, "said to be" stuttering, and the like. The impact of such beliefs supports the fear that one may *create* stuttering out of essentially normal speech—a formidable fear indeed! Again, the fact that there is no good evidence to justify such fears remains beside the point.

All these fears minimize the clinician's effectiveness by constricting flexibility and encouraging persistence in token management procedures which are questionable, unproven, and untestable. Thus, the clinician works at avoiding use of the "label" stuttering through circumlocution, euphemism, or subterfuge; yet for all we know, this is wasted effort (which has unfortunate by-products). Or, the therapist works diligently to "prevent the child's awareness" of stuttering (or disfluency) in the untestable assumption that this really makes a difference, and with the ingenuous presumption that awareness has not yet occurred, and that it is subject to control.

References

Adler, S. A test of stutterers' attitudes regarding humor about "The Handicapped." *South Speech J.*, **22**, 79–84, 1956.

Bloodstein, O. and Annette Bloodstein. Interpretations of facial reactions to stuttering. *J. Speech Hearing Dis.*, **20**, 148–155, 1955.

Brown, S. F. and H. C. Hull. A study of some social attitudes of a group of 59 stutterers. *J. Speech Dis.*, **7**, 323–324, 1942.

Brutten, E. J. Palmar sweat investigation of disfluency and expectancy adaptation. *J. Speech Hearing Res.*, **6**, 40–48, 1963.

Bryngelson, B. A study of the speech difficulties of thirteen stutterers. In Johnson, W. (Ed.), *Stuttering in Children and Adults*, Univ. of Minnesota Press, Minneapolis, 1955, Chapter 36.

———Voluntary stuttering. *Proc. Am. Speech Corr. Assn.*, **5**, 35–38, 1935.

Clevenger, T., Jr. A synthesis of experimental research in stage fright. *Quart. J. Speech*, **45**, 134–145, 1959.

Diven, K. Certain determinants in the conditioning of anxiety reactions. *J. Psychol.*, **3**, 291–308, 1937.

Dixon, Carmen C. Stuttering adaptation in relation to assumed level of anxiety. In Johnson, W. (Ed.), *Stuttering in Children and Adults*, Univ. of Minnesota Press, Minneapolis, 1955, Chapter 12.

Erickson, R. L. Assessing communication attitudes among stutterers. *J. Speech Hearing Res.*, **12**, 711–724, 1969.

Friedman, Gladys M. A test of attitude toward stuttering. In Johnson, W. (Ed.), *Stuttering in Children and Adults*, Univ. of Minnesota Press, Minneapolis, 1955, Chapter 25.

Gray, B. B. and E. J. Brutten. The relationship between anxiety, fatigue and spontaneous recovery in stuttering. *Behavior Research and Therapy*, **2**, 251–259, 1965.

Grubman, S. Loci of stuttering, grammatical function and position of selected one-syllable and two-syllable words used by stutterers and non-stutterers in isolation and in different types of sentences. Unpublished research, State University of New York at Buffalo, 1970.

Hahn, E. F. A study of the relationship between the social complexity of the oral reading situation and the severity of stuttering. *J. Speech Dis.*, **5**, 5–14, 1940.

Johnson, W. and R. Ammons. The construction and application of a test of attitude toward stuttering. *J. Speech Dis.*, **9**, 39–49, 1944.

———F. L. Darley, and D. C. Spriestersbach. *Diagnostic Methods in Speech Pathology*, New York, Harper & Row, 1952.

———and S. Ainsworth. Studies in the psychology of stuttering: X. Constancy of loci of expectancy of stuttering. *J. Speech Dis.*, **3**, 101–104, 1938.

———, J. R. Knott, and Mary J. Webster. Studies in the psychology of stuttering: II. A quantitative evaluation of expectation of stuttering in relation to the occurrence of stuttering. *J. Speech Dis.*, **2**, 20–22, 1937.

——— and Arlien Sinn. Studies in the psychology of stuttering: V. Frequency of stuttering with expectation of stuttering controlled. *J. Speech Dis.*, **2**, 98–100, 1937.

——— and A. Solomon. Studies in the psychology of stuttering: IV. A quantitative study of expectation of stuttering as a process involving a low degree of consciousness. *J. Speech Dis.*, **2**, 95–97, 1937.

Karmen, J. L. A comparison between generalized anxiety adjustment and adaptation of stuttering behavior. Doctoral dissertation, Univ. of Arizona, 1964.

Kline, D. F. An experimental study of the frequency of stuttering in relation to certain goal-activity drives in basic human behavior. (abstract) *Speech Monogr.*, **26**, 137, 1959.

Knabe, Judith M., Lois A. Nelson, and J. Williams. Some general characteristics of linguistic output: Stutterers versus non-stutterers. *J. Speech Hearing Dis.*, **31**, 178–182, 1966.

Knott, J. R. A study of stutterers' stuttering and non-stuttering experiences on the basis of pleasantness and unpleasantness. *Quart. J. Speech*, **21**, 328–331, 1935.

——, R. E. Correll, and J. N. Shepherd. Frequency analysis of electroencephalograms of stutterers and non-stutterers. *J. Speech Hearing Res.*, **2**, 74–80, 1959.

Knower, F. H. A study of speech attitudes and adjustments. *Speech Monogr.*, **5**, 130–203, 1938.

Lerman, J. W. and G. H. Shames. The effect of situational difficulty on stuttering. *J. Speech Hearing Res.*, **8**, 271–280, 1965.

Lingwall, J. B. Galvanic skin responses of stutterers and non-stutterers to isolated word stimuli. *Program of 43rd Annual Convention, Am. Sp. Hearing Assn.*, 90, 1967, (abstr.).

Martin, R. R. and S. K. Haroldson. The relationship between anticipation and consistency of stuttered words. *J. Speech Hearing Res.*, **10**, 323–327, 1967.

Maxwell, D. L. A palmar sweat investigation of stuttering adaptation under two levels of audience complexity. Master's thesis, Southern Illinois Univ., 1965.

Meltzer, H. Talkativeness in stuttering and non-stuttering children. *J. Genet. Psychol.*, **46**, 371–390, 1935.

Moore, W. E., G. A. Soderberg, and Donna Powell. Relations of stuttering in spontaneous speech to speech content and verbal output. *J. Speech Hearing Dis.*, **17**, 371–376, 1952.

Muma, J. R. and J. V. Frick. Fluent and disfluent speech by four-year-old children: Productivity and grammar. Paper presented at the annual convention, Am. Sp. Hearing Assn., Nov., 1967.

Peins, Maryann. Consistency effect in stuttering expectancy. *J. Speech Hearing Res.*, **4**, 397–398, 1961.

Phillips, M. Reticence: Pathology of the normal speaker. *Speech Monogr.*, **35**, 39–49, 1968.

Porter, Harriet von K. Studies in the psychology of stuttering. XIV: Stuttering phenomena in relation to size and personnel of audience. *J. Speech Dis.*, **4**, 323–333, 1939.

Razran, G. H. S. A quantitative study of meaning by a conditioned salivary technique (semantic conditioning). *Science*, **90**, 89–90, 1939.

Razdol'skii, V. A. State of speech of stammerers when alone. *Zhurnal Neuropatol. i Psikhiatr. im S. S. Korsakova*, **65**, 1717–1720, 1965.

Reiss, B. F. Genetic changes in semantic conditioning. *J. Exper. Psychol.*, **36**, 243–152, 1946.

———Semantic conditioning involving the galvanic skin reflex. *J. Exper. Psychol.*, **26**, 238–240, 1940.

Shaw, I. Speech fright in the elementary school, its relation to speech ability and its possible implication for speech readiness. Wayne State Univ., Detroit, 1966, Project No. S-936-63.

Sheehan, J. G., R. Hadley, and E. Gould. Impact of authority on stuttering. *J. Abn. Psychol.*, **72**, 290–293, 1967.

Shrum, W. F. A study of the speaking behavior of stutterers and non-stutterers by means of multichannel electromyography. *Program of 43rd Annual Convention, Am. Sp. Hearing Assn.* 90, 1967 (abstr.).

Siegel, G. M. and D. Haugen. Audience size and variations in stuttering behavior. *J. Speech Hearing Res.*, **7**, 383–388, 1964.

Silverman, F. H. Concern of elementary school stutterers about their stuttering. *J. Speech Hearing Dis.*, **35**, 361–363, 1970.

Staats, L. C., Jr. Sense of humor in stutterers and non-stutterers. In Johnson, W. (Ed.), *Stuttering in Children and Adults*, Univ. of Minnesota Press, Minneapolis, 1955, Chapter 24.

Tate, M. W. and W. L. Cullinan. Measurement of consistency in stuttering. *J. Speech Hearing Res.*, **5**, 272–283, 1962.

Trotter, W. D. and Margaret F. Bergmann. Stutterers' and non-stutterers' reaction to speech situations. *J. Speech Hearing Dis.*, **22**, 40–45, 1952.

Valyo, R. PGSR responses of stutterers and non-stutterers during periods of silence and verbalization. (abstract) *Asha*, **6**, 422, 1964.

Van Riper, C. and C. J. Hull. The quantitative measurement of the effect of certain situations on stuttering. In Johnson, W. (Ed.), *Stuttering in Children and Adults*, Univ. of Minnesota Press, Minneapolis, 1955, Chapter 3.

Wingate, M. E. Expectancy as basically a short-term process. *J. Speech Hearing Res.*, **18**, 31–42, 1975.

———Word availability and usage in stutterers and non-stutterers. Paper presented at the annual convention, Am. Sp. Hearing Assn., Nov., 1970.

——— and C. E. Hamre. Stutterers' projection of listener reaction. *J. Speech Hearing Res.*, **10**, 339–343, 1967.

Young, M. Audience size, perceived situational difficulty and stuttering frequency. *J. Speech Hearing Res.*, **8**, 401–407, 1965.

4

IDENTIFICATION OF STUTTERING

Particularly in the past 30 years a great deal of attention has been directed to the variation in "symptoms" among stutterers. Variation has been assumed to reflect differences of a functional or acquired nature and therefore corroborates the view that stuttering is the result of environmental factors. Regardless of the actual amount of variation to be found among stutterers, most observable differences are of secondary interest. We have not yet adequately identified the consistent, universal features of stuttering—which we have every legitimate reason to believe must exist, if for no other reason than that for centuries people have been able to identify stuttering.

One of the cardinal techniques of scientific inquiry is to observe, search for, and identify commonalities. Of course, differences may often be of great importance, but they can also be trivial, irrelevant, or immaterial. Usually, the relative values of differences do not become clear until the commonalities are reasonably well identified and understood.

The emphasis on variations of stuttering has been imbricated with the position that stuttering is continuous with normal speech. From this position, making a decision about whether or not speech is stuttered represents an arbitrary judgment, having an uncertain basis. The issue was drawn initially in respect to stuttering in children but has been extended to include stuttering at all ages. Essentially, the issue is whether one can reliably identify stuttering and consistently distinguish it from what would be considered as normal kinds of nonfluency.

Largely through the efforts of Wendell Johnson and his followers, and based on Johnson's "diagnosogenic" theory of stuttering, there appears to be rather widespread acceptance among professional people—predominantly in the United States—that it is difficult to discriminate stuttering from normal nonfluency. Moreover, a great deal of professional writing and research has been undertaken to support this contention and, indeed, a large proportion of this literature has been so interpreted.[1]

Speech therapists appear to have been more vulnerable to this notion than have less sophisticated people. This situation was the basis for West's (1957, p. 15) remark that " . . . everyone but the expert knows what stuttering is . . . ." However, research data strongly suggest that speech pathologists, too, can readily identify stuttering in spite of their inclinations to quibble about it, to introduce myriad qualifications, and to be continually distracted by presumed etiology or supposed contributing factors. The extent to which "the experts" do readily identify stuttering is revealed indirectly in the many research studies in which it is necessary to demonstrate reliability of judgments of stuttering. These data reveal very high levels of both intra- and inter-judge reliability. At the same time, in studies in which judgments of stuttering made by lay persons have been compared with those made by speech pathologists (Bar, 1968; Boehmler, 1958; Tuthill, 1946;) the lay judges agreed better among themselves than did the speech pathologists with each other. This suggests that speech pathologists tend to be more subjective in their judgments.

It might be objected that the claim of difficulty in distinguishing stuttering from normal nonfluency applies primarily to young children. It is frequently contended that the speech of the child considered to stutter is "not always to be distinguished" from the speech of the child not considered to stutter. But this argument is misleading on several dimensions.

First, it involves a generalizing statement in which the exception is implied to be the rule. To say that something is "not always to be distinguished" from something else implies only that the accuracy of discrimination is something less than 100 percent. However, it does not mean a level of accuracy substantially below 100 percent. Yet the phrase suggests that the discrimination occurs at almost a chance level. We do not know with certainty what the incidence of correct identification of stuttering is, but on the basis of considerable research (to be reviewed later in this chapter) we can be confident that the percentage of error is actually quite small.

Second, this argument ignores the matter of the speech sample obtained. Beyond the matter of possible rose-colored assessment, one must consider the fact that stutterers, particularly child stutterers, are not always stuttering—and they also evidence normal nonfluencies.

Third, to say that something is "not always to be distinguished" from something else does not mean that there is therefore no basis for making a distinction. Further, one cannot make the assumption that two things are similar simply because there may be certain obstacles to a complete differentiation between them.

Lastly, and here lies a contradiction, in comparative research involving children youngsters "identified as stuttering" are regularly assigned to the experimental group for contrast with the control group of normally speaking children, suggesting that the experimenters implicitly agree with the identification made.

The considerable effort that has been made to meld stuttering with normal nonfluency is motivated by the theoretical position that stuttering is a *degree* of nonfluency rather than a separate kind and that it develops out of what was originally a normal kind of fluency irregularity. While this interpretation is plausible, it cannot sustain two very basic demands of the scientific approach: one is refinement and circumspect use of terminology; the other is careful observation and analysis.

THE ESSENTIAL FEATURES OF STUTTERING

Distinguishing between stuttering and normal disfluency is of great practical, as well as theoretical, significance. A clinician should not be in the position of making a diagnostic appraisal and subsequent recommendations if he is not able to differentiate between stuttering and normal nonfluency. Making an appropriate distinction represents a professional obligation to the patient and his family—and, in the long run, to the profession itself.

In order to perform in a reliable manner, the therapist should know what stuttering "is" in at least the descriptive sense. It should be understood from the beginning that the essential and universal features of stuttering are *speech* features. In the plethora of stuttering literature there has been a tendency—inflated substantially in modern times—tc ignore or minimize the simple fact that in essence "stuttering" means a unique form of disfluent speech *and nothing else*. The speech features are the *necessary* and *sufficient* criteria for the identification of stuttering. All other considerations are subsidiary. If the speech features were eliminated from the catalogue of "symptoms" and "characteristics" found in so many discussions of stuttering, one would no longer be talking about stuttering. "Stuttering" means a particular kind of speech disfluency.

Linguistic Evidence

The structure and etymology of words for stuttering in different languages contain clues regarding its distinctive and identifiable characteristics. Our English word presents a particularly appropriate example. *Stutter* is derived from the German word *stossen*, which means "to knock or push." *Knock* and *push* will be recognized as equivalents of *clonic* and *tonic*, terms first suggested by Serre d'Alais in 1829 (Klingbeil, 1939) to describe the essential forms of stuttering and widely used until quite recent times. Since formerly these words were used frequently with the word *spasm*, which suggests a neurologic anomaly, and since the prevailing current attitude is to view stuttering as a variante of normal nonfluency and the product of learning, all three of these words—clonic, tonic, and spasm— have fallen into disfavor. Nevertheless, we are well reminded of the long-standing use of the terms clonic and tonic and the significance of their references.

The Russian word for stuttering is *zaikivatsa*, of which the root word *ikat* means "to hiccough." *Zaikivatsa* has the significance of repetitive hiccoughing, with emphasis on repetitiveness. In Finnish the word is *ankytys* and again the meaning of the word conveys the idea of repetition. The French *bégaiement* is derived from a Flemish word meaning "to chatter." The Spanish word for stuttering is *tartamudo*, in which *mudo* means "dumb" (unable to speak), and the prefix *tarta* suggests intermittency. The Nepalese *bha-ka-ú-nu* refers to a jumping or palpitating in speech. In the Tagalog *paútalútal* the root word *utal* means "stopping and hesitating."

These words also have an onomatopoeic character, that is, the form suggests the referent. This quality is found in the words for stuttering in most other major languages and in the languages of many smaller and less sophisticated cultures of Africa, Asia, the South Pacific (Morgenstern, 1953), and in the Pacific Northwest Coastal Indians (Lemert, 1952). Consider, for example, the Cowichan (Northwest Indian) *sutsuts* or *hus-sutsuts*, the Hausa (West African) *i'ina*, and the Tabiyang (New Guinea) *ngak-ngak*. Such findings extend into ancient history; an Egyptian hieroglyphic has been translated as "stuttering" not only because of the context in which it occurs but also because the transcription calls for a phonetic rendition as *nitit* (Calzia, 1941) or *nyetyet*.[2]

Examples of the metaphorical use of the word *stutter* also suggest the implicit recognition of its unique meaning. Thus, novelists and reporters speak of the "stuttering" of a machine gun or of a ticker-tape machine; sportcasters describe the "stutter-step" of a football player as he maneuvers around would-be tacklers; Kipling once described the "stuttering" of a laboring railroad locomotive.

Thus, in etymology, phonetic structure, and figure of speech we find compelling evidence of certain widely recognized distinctive features of stuttering. These designations clearly point primarily to a staccato kind of sound and secondly to a difficulty in making sound.

Keeping in mind this widespread, culturally independent, vernacular identification of the distinctive features of stuttering, let us turn to the substance of our analysis, which takes more technical sources as its point of departure.

Analysis of Disfluency: Basic Considerations

The descriptive words to be found in the professional literature on stuttering consist of the following: *repetitions*, *hesitations* (or *pauses*), *interjections*, *part-word repetitions*, *word repetitions*, *phrase repetitions*, *prolongations*,[3] *blocks* (or *blockings*), *broken words*,[3] *revisions*, and *incomplete phrases*.

It is a matter of first importance to draw attention to two of these words: *repetitions* and *hesitations*. Each of these words must be recognized as a general referent, that is, a class word which refers to a category containing discriminably different subcategories. Recognition of these subcategories is particularly significant, because they can be shown to be relevant to the identification of stuttering and to differentiating it from normal disfluency.

In the literature the word *hesitations* generally occurs less frequently than *repetitions*, although in many places the two words appear as an almost automatically occurring pair.[4] The more frequent use of the word *repetitions* reflects the extent to which "repetitions" are associated with the idea of stuttering. Some sources, particularly those of a research nature, do mention differences in repetitions on the dimension of length, but even in such cases there is a tendency to favor the general term in discussion and in interpretation of experimental findings. In some cases the differences among repetitions are stated, but their potential value and significance is implicitly denied.[5]

A similar problem is presented by the term *interjections*, which is mentioned less frequently than the other two. Somewhat more often there is some specification of type of interjection, but here too there is a tendency to use the general term.

The words *repetitions*, *hesitations*, and *interjections* are *class* terms and their use is a flagrant violation of the first demand of a scientific approach, namely, refined and circumspect terminology. Because these words are *general* referents, they obscure distinctions that are particularly relevant to the identification of stuttering.[6]

Analysis of Disfluency: Significant Features

We will consider first the categories of repetitions and hesitations. Their consistent and meaningful classification can serve as the basis for distinguishing stuttering from normal disfluency.

Repetitions.—Repetitions vary on several dimensions, of which length is the most obvious and very likely the most important. The original list of terms contains three items which designate variations in length of repetitions: *part-word repetitions*, *word repetitions*, and *phrase repetitions.*[7]

The latter term is the least troublesome of the three. "Phrase repetition" is unambiguous to the extent that it indicates the minimum length of its referent: a phrase repetition *must* be a repetition of two or more syllables, that is, of a syllable string.

The other two terms, however, are less determinate. The category of "word repetitions" is very ambiguous. Words vary in length and one does not know whether a "word repetition" refers to the repetition of a word having one, two, or five syllables. It is misleading to employ a category which includes units of varying size, particularly when there is reason to believe that differences in the size of the units may have discriminitave significance. For the moment, let us consider as example the two words "he" and "heater," which differ in length by only one syllabe. It is not very likely that repetition of the word "heater" would be identified as an instance of stuttering. Repetition of the word "he," on the other hand, may or may not be. The uncertainty is occasioned by the fact the "he" is a single-syllable word. In such cases the final distinction is made with the assistance of other criteria, to be discussed presently. In contrast, repetition of /hi/ ("he") as the first syllable of "heater" would almost cerainly be identified as an instance of stuttering. There is a meaningful distinction to be drawn between single-syllable words and words of more than one syllable: it is a distinction between repetition of a syllable and repetition of a syllable string.

The category of "part-word repetitions" seems reasonably straightforward, yet it only refers to something smaller than a "word." The nature of this "something" is not clear; a part of a word might be one of several things. In a word of several syllables, for instance, a part of the word might consist of two or more syllables, one syllable, a phoneme group, or a single phoneme. Again, the size of the unit (the "part") repeated is of considerable significance. Consider the word "television"

(/tɛləvĩʒən/ or /tɛləvĩʒn/). Repetition of /tɛləvĩʒ/, or /tɛləvĩ/, or /ləvĩʒ/, or /ləvĩʒn/ would hardly be considered a stutter. However, repetition of /t/ or of /tɛ/ almost certainly would be.[8] Again the distinction to be drawn is between repetitions of a syllable (or less) and repetitions of a syllable string.

Reclassification of repetitions.—The preceding analysis permits a simplified reclassification of repetitions on the basic dimension of length. One class includes repetitions of a syllable or less; the other includes repetitions involving more than one syllable.

Table 4:1 presents a comparison of the old and new systems of classification. As the table entry suggests, one-syllable words present a special case, which we will consider soon.

Elemental repetitions.—Repetitions the length of one syllable or less, described as "unitary" or "elemental" repetitions (meaning small units or elements), are the unique, distinctive form of repetition which characterize what is meant by "stuttering." This conclusion is supported by our knowledge of the structure and etymology of words for stuttering in different languages; it is consistent with metaphorical use of "stuttering" in our own language; it coincides with the meaning of the word *clonic*, which has been widely employed to designate the most frequently observed form of stuttering; and it is confirmed by a great deal of research.

Other features of these elemental repetitions increase the confidence with which they are identified as stutterings. One is the number of repetitions per repetition-instance. Thus: "he-heater" may be questionable, "he-he-he-heater" is not; "he-he went" may be uncertain, "he-he-he went" is much less so. A second aspect is the amount of effort involved. Audible or visible signs of undue effort, either in the repeated syllable or the one following it, reflect the abnormal character of the repetition. Thus: in "*he-he*ater" or "he-*he*ater"; and "*he-he-w*ent" or "he-he-*w*ent," the aspect of effort affords a distinctive additional cue. A third aspect takes into account the spacing of the repetitions and what occurs during the intervals between them: that is, whether what occurs during the interval indicates (a) difficulty in moving on to what should follow phonetically

Table 4:1 Comparison of syllable-length classification of repetitions with traditional classification

	TRADITIONAL		
Syllable-Length	*part-Word*	*Word*	*Phrase*
phoneme	x		
phoneme group	x		
syllable	x	x	
syllable string	x	x	x

or (b) pausing to reflect or to search for words. These aspects are essentially elaborations on the basic criterion of repetition length; the principal features are the elemental repetitions.

It should be added that certain of the elemental repetitions, while ordinarily audible, may be silent and detectable only visually; for example, repeated lip movements forming /b/ prior to saying "boy." Thus we should recognize *silent* as well as *audible elemental repetitions.* Our analysis would identify such repetitions as constituting one of the two types of disfluency which are the focal characteristics of stuttering.

One-syllable word repetitions present a special case, since such repetitions can also occur as normal disfluencies. The syllable-length criterion is thus not sufficient.[9] However, such matters do not materially affect the validity of the syllable-length classification approach. In the case of questionable one-syllable word repetitions the distinction as to whether it is stuttered or not is usually determined by the additional criteria reviewed above. Besides, it is difficult to imagine a case in which one-syllable word repetitions would be the only disfluencies evidenced. An appraisal is always made on the basis of a much broader spectrum of disfluencies.

Repetition of syllable strings.—This kind of repetition has little uniqueness or significance for our interest. Those which are distinctive (part-word syllable string repetitions) occur with such rarity as to be of little consequence. Repetitions of syllable strings, such as multisyllable words and phrases, are found in the speech of both stutterers and nonstutterers and it is very unlikely that they would be judged as stutterings in either case. There are instances, in the speech of stutterers, that this kind of repetition may be involved in a stuttering event. In such instances, however, they are not themselves identifiable as the stutter, even though associated with it. Such repetitions of syllable strings are identifiable as "verbal features" of stuttering, a matter to be discussed later.

Hesitations.—This term, and *pauses,* have been used traditionally to refer to silent intervals of unspecified length or character in the flow of speech. There is no reason to suspect that the length of a hesitation is of particular significance. However, it is certain that qualitative distinctions of very definite significance can be made within this category.

It is possible to specify four different kinds of hesitations. First are *voluntary* hesitations, in which a speaker decides to pause in order to emphasize a point, or because he is waiting for his auditor's attention, or because he expects to be interrupted. Such hesitations occur relatively often in the speech of all speakers and are perfectly normal occurrences. Second are *circumstantial* hesitations, caused by some distracting event which may be external to the speaker or arise from within himself. Thus, he may pause in his speech because of something he sees, hears, or feels, or because of some momentarily intruding thought or image. Again, such hesitations are a normal kind of occurrence. Third are *meditative* hesitations, in which the speaker pauses to reflect on his choice of words, or to recast the form of his expression, or to organize his approach in a different manner. Speakers vary in the extent to which they evidence such hesitations, but their occurrence is quite common. Fourth are *involuntary* hesitations, which occur for unknown reasons. This type differs from the others in that the speaker does not intend to pause but is unable to continue.

The first three types of hesitation are observed in everyone's speech, although their frequency varies from one individual to another, and in the same individual from time to time. Even when such hesitations occur with sufficient frequency that the person's speech is described as "hesitant" (either temporarily or characteristically), there is evidently no need for a specific term to indicate that these hesitations are somehow unique. They are not unique, because (a) they do not contain certain features which accompany the abnormal hesitations—as noted below; (b) they occur relatively frequently in the speech of all speakers; and (c) the circumstances giving rise to them are often apparent. These are *normal* hesitations.

The fourth type, the involuntary hesitations, are the *abnormal* hesitations. In actual usage they are denoted by the terms *block* or *blockings* which appropriately signify their unique character. This type of hesitation may be distinguished from the other three by one or more of the following features: (a) visual cues, occurring during or at the end of the pause, such as exaggerated or inappropriate oral or facial movements; (b) auditory cues which occur when the silence is eventually broken, such as excessive loudness of the ensuing sound or a prolongation or repetition of it; and, to some extent, (c) an inappropriate locus or occurrence of the pause—for example immediately before a very familiar word which should be readily "available" for use in the word sequence, or when the pause is an abrupt stop in a seemingly flowing utterance. For purposes of systematic classification we may designate these abnormal hesitations as *silent prolongations.*

Prolongations.—This term has been used traditionally to mean the extension of a sound beyond its appropriate duration, for example in saying "wwwwater." This fluency defect is rather easy to detect, primarily because linguistic constraints limit acceptable phoneme duration. Temporal length is thus the essential dimension for discriminating these audible prolongations. In addition, there are very often associated visual or auditory cues which, in indicating undue effort, give further evidence of abnormality.

Broken words.—This type of fluency disturbance is exemplified in the sentence, "I was g . . . (pause) . . . oing home." It seems clear that the inappropriate and unnatural "hesitation" marks this disfluency as a special instance of a silent prolongation occurring within a word rather than between words.

The preceding analysis suggests a second class of distinctive fluency irregularities, prolongations, which includes those disfluencies traditionally identified by that name and, in addition, "broken words," and the abnormal type of "hesitation." It is obvious that prolongations cannot involve more than one speech element; therefore, a "unitary" or "elemental" character is implicit. Prolongations, like the abnormal type of repetitions, also have silent and audible forms. Our analysis then identifies a class of *silent and audible (elemental) prolongations* as the other focal characteristic of stuttering. One is reminded here of the correspondence to the word *tonic.*

Interjections.—This word revives our concern about the use of general referents, for *interjections* is another class term. It refers to extraneous utterances in the flow of connected speech, such as sounds ("uh," "um"), words ("well," "okay"), or phrases ("lemme see," "excuse me"). In ordinary usage the word interjections is as confounding as *repetitions* and *hesitations,* since one can identify very different kinds of interjections.

Interjections may be considered as essentially sound-filled pauses, for they constitute a temporal interval in the flow of a speech sequence to which they are not integral. There exist subtypes similar to silent hesitations, namely, the normal voluntary, meditative, and circumstantial, and others which are not normal. The latter assume the proportions of elemental prolongations and repetitions. Finally, there are certain interjections which can be classified as *verbal features.*

Table 4:2 presents the analysis of interjections in outline form. Interjections of the "lengthy normal" type are among the most frequent in ordinary conversational speech, yet this is rarely recognized or acknowledged. An instance of a *voluntary* interjection would be: "I want you to watch . . . look here! . . . how this is done." A *meditative* interjection: "We'll have to . . .let's see now . . .swing this part around." A *circumstantial* interjection: "I'm trying to . . . excuse me . . . find my coat."

In Table 4:2 the neutral vowel "uh" (/ə/) appears as both a normal and an abnormal interjection. The normal "uh" is a simple and unremarkable occurrence. Probably all speakers use "uhs," some more regularly than others.[10] The frequency also varies with the situation. Especially when used very frequently the interjection may be noted because of its frequency, but not because of its quality. In contrast, the abnormal "uh" is noted because of its nature, regardless of its frequency. As indicated in the table, such interjections have the character of a prolongation or an elemental repetition. Also, other cues are often present—the visual and auditory cues of undue effort, or the occurrence of the interjection at an inappropriate place, for instance, at a grammatically unlikely locus or immediately prior to a very familiar word. Stuttered interjections, then, are identifiable as elemental repetitions and prolongations, the core features of stuttering.

Certain longer interjections may be involved in an instance of stuttering or may be used where a stutter might have occurred, but such interjections are not themselves denotable as the stuttering. In the professional idiom they are referred to as "starters"; in the present classification they are assigned to the category of "verbal features."[11]

Revisions and incomplete phrases.—These kinds of fluency irregularity represent changes in pronunciation, wording, grammatical structure, or content of what is said. They are to be observed, in varying degree, in all speakers. They are accepted generally as normal disfluencies, and there is no basis to consider them as uniquely related to stuttering. Some stutterers report occasionally revising what they were about to say, or not finishing it, in order to avoid difficulty, but the maneuver itself is not considered to be a stutter by either the stutterer or his auditor. On those occasions where a revision or incomplete phrase is used in this way they may be considered a verbal feature. Verbal features will be discussed in the next section.

To recapitulate, the essential features of stuttering are certain kinds of disfluencies: audible and silent elemental repetitions and prolongations. One or the other, or both, of these disfluency types are found in all cases of stuttering—they are the universal and distinctive features of

Table 4:2 Types of interjections

CLASSIFICATION	*DESCRIPTION*	
	Brief	*Lengthy*
Normal		
voluntary		(words of any length; phrases)
meditative	"uh," "um," "m"	
circumstantial	" " "	
Abnormal		
prolongation	"uhhhhhh"	(words of any length; phrases)
repetition	"uh-uh-uh"	
Verbal features		

stuttering. Other disfluency types can be either reduced to these features, assigned to an ancillary status, or identified as normal.

ACCESSORY FEATURES OF STUTTERING

Often one can observe in stuttering certain characteristics in addition to the speech anomalies themselves. In professional usage these characteristics are referred to as *secondary mannerisms*, following Bluemel's (1939) suggestion of differentiating primary[12] and secondary stuttering. Secondary mannerisms are assumed to be learned behaviors which are *temporally* second in appearance and reflect the stutterer's efforts to produce fluent speech.

Objectively, "secondary" should neither mean that these features necessarily occur secondly nor imply that they are learned. It is more correct to understand "secondary" to mean second in significance because these features are not universal in the observable symptom picture of stuttering. The term *accessory features* is employed here intentionally to avoid the usual implications of "secondary" as well as to assign these features their proper status.

While the identification of stuttering must certainly give consideration to such features, one must nevertheless emphasize: (1) that these are not essential characteristics of stuttering, and (2) that any preoccupation with these features which minimizes attention to the speech characteristics previously identified represents a distortion of the problem. Accessory features vary considerably in their expression; they are much more pronounced or extensive in some individuals than in others, and in many cases they are not in evidence. They do not invariably occur secondly in temporal sequence; in some cases they are present from the very outset of stuttering. While they appear to show some gross correlation with age, some young stutterers manifest them dramatically and some older stutterers are quite free of them.

Accessory features may be separated into three classes: (1) speech-related movements, (2) ancillary body movements, and (3) verbal features (cf. Table 4:3).

Speech-related movements.—This designation refers to those exaggerated or inappropriate movements of the peripheral speech mechanism which are concurrent with stuttering. Examples include pursing the lips, protruding the tongue, and clenching the teeth. They are movements localized in the area of the mouth which may or may not be consistent with the sound being attempted. They are the immediately localized features which are commonly taken to be indicators of struggle. While it is widely accepted that such characteristics are learned, it is by no means certain that they are. It remains very possible that they reflect nonspecific errors in articulatory execution, failures in synergy, lapses in fine motor control, or some other anomaly.

Ancillary body movements.—This category includes all other kinds of body activity that accompany difficulty in producing speech. Examples include eye blink, dilation of the nostrils, jerking the head, leaning forward, and clenching the fists. These features are ordinarily viewed as somewhat dramatic indications of struggle. They often give the appearance of being intentional maneuvers and thus are assumed to be learned reactions, but again the possibility remains that some of them may well represent "overflow" expression of a spasm, or they may reflect some other immediate origin similar to that suggested for the speech-related movements.

Verbal features.—Under this heading are classified verbal expressions of one to several words in length which occur immediately prior to a point where a stuttering might occur. As mentioned earlier, this category includes certain kinds of interjections, repetitions of phrases and words of more than one syllable, and even some single-unit word repetitions. Verbal features are notable in that they either appear at relatively inappropriate points in the context of a message, are unduly repetitive, are associated eventually with signs of struggle, or are followed by an obvi-

Table 4:3 Outline of stuttering

A. Speech Characteristics
   1. Audible/silent elemental repetitions and prolongations

B. Accessory Features
   1. Speech related movements
      a) compressed lips
      b) lingual posturing
      c) mouth held open
      d) holding breath
   2. Ancillary body movements
      a) blinking eyes
      b) dilating nostrils
      c) raising eyebrows
      d) grimacing
   3. Verbal features
      a) repetition of syllable strings
      b) interjections (longer than 1 syllable)

C. Associated Features
   1. Negative emotional state
   2. Positive emotional state

ous repetition or prolongation. Careful observation or questioning of the patient will reveal that the verbal features are not themselves instances of stuttering but rather that the stuttering involves the word immediately following. In those instances in which the immediately following word is initiated with a repetition or a prolongation, the locus of the stuttering is quite obvious. In some instances in which the actual stutter is very mild it may be difficult to detect; this is particularly true of minimal prolongations. In such cases speech-related or ancillary movements may supply additional cues. In some instances frank audible or visual cues are not apparent, but the undue repetition of a word or phrase, or the inappropriate site of an interjection, will identify the locus of the difficulty to which the verbal feature is an adjustment.

To clarify this description the following examples present a word repetition, a phrase repetition, and two interjections, each of which occurs at an inappropriate site—inappropriate because the following word is simple and familiar enough that it should be have produced readily in its proper sequence. Statements such as, "We had a good . . . good . . . good time," or "We had a good . . . had a good . . . had a good time" exemplify the repetitions. The same function is served by interjections in: "We had a good . . . well time" or "We had a good . . .lemme see time."[13] In all of these examples the actual point of difficulty involves the word "time." Both the stutterer and the speech pathologist recognize that what we have called "verbal features" are *not* instances of stuttering but rather that the stuttering, if it occurs, involves the word following the verbal feature. [It is for this reason that verbal features have been called "starters."]

Of the three categories of accessory features, verbal features are almost certainly the result of a learning process. They are evidently efforts to pass a point of difficulty which were at least originally quite intentional. In fact, some stutterers report volitional use of certain verbal features for this purpose. Some develop considerable skill in the use of "starters" of the interjection type. One stutterer had special finesse in such use of the words "well," "really," and "actually." Instances of their usage were often quite difficult to detect from tape recordings, although through careful attention one could discern inappropriate sites of occurrence and very brief associated silences which were passed over in casual listening. When listening to this patient in person such detectable episodes were frequently accompanied by very mild exraneous movements. When the patient was successful in the use of these interjections, he did not stutter.

ASSOCIATED FEATURES

In some cases of stuttering one may observe certain accompanying features of a more or less general or vague nature along with the features reviewed above. These associated features include indications or reports of excitement, tension, personal reactions, feelings, or attitudes. Many older stutterers give personal account of such features. Parents of younger stutterers may often report that the child stutters more when he is excited or apparently tense. While parents sometimes mention a youngster's negative feelings or personal reactions, these reports are frequently more interpretation than supportable fact. The nature and extent of such features show considerable variation, among older as well as younger stutterers, and their relationship to stuttering is not very well known; that is, whether they are reactive, causal, interactive, or simply concurrent. Development of a supportable hypothesis about their nature is part of the task of diagnostic assessment. Because of the long-standing preoccupation with these associated facets of stuttering, diagnostic evaluation has overemphasized ascribing a cause of the stuttering, and often some standard explanation is invoked routinely. The important matter of diagnostic appraisal will be considered in a later chapter.

EVIDENCE FROM THE RESEARCH

The overall concurrence between research findings and the analysis developed in the preceding sections can be summarized as follows.

1. The results of research addressed to associated features (cf. Chapters 2 and 3) have been contradictory, inconsistent, and equivocal, indicating that there is little of comprehensive significance in this area.

2. There is essentially no research dealing with the accessory features alone, indicating that they are not recognized as entities worth considering as separate phenomena.

3. In contrast, a very substantial amount of research has investigated speech characteristics of stuttering, and the results of this research have consistently pointed to the same conclusions. The following material reviews this evidence.

Disfluencies of Nonstutterers

A number of studies have investigated disfluencies in the speech of nonstuttering children. This work has been undertaken with an implicit reference to stuttering, that is, with stuttered speech as the ultimate object of comparison. It stands in some contrast, therefore, to another body of research on normal disfluency in which the matter is approached from a different frame of reference. This material will be mentioned later (p. 59).

Two studies by Davis (1939, 1940) are the sources most frequently cited in support of the contention that "repetitions" occur normally in the speech of young children. Davis studied several aspects of the speech and language of 62 preschool children, ages 2 to 5, and from her data concluded that *repetition*[14] is a part of the speech pattern of all children. However, her data actually reveal that children differ considerably not only in amount of repetition but also in kind. Word and phrase repetitions were not remarkable, but syllable repetitions were atypical.

At all ages among the children Davis studied, syllable repetitions occurred much less frequently than either word or phrase repetitions. The differential frequency of occurrence of these repetition types could be expressed as a ratio of 1:3:6—that is, for every syllable repetition there were three word repetitions and six phrase repetitions. Also, the number of repetitions per instance of repetition was more than twice as great for syllable repetitions as for word repetitions, and more than three times as great as for phrase repetitions. Almost half of the children showed *no* syllable repetition of two or more in extent (they did not repeat a syllable more than once in those instances when a syllable repetition occurred). In contrast, syllable repetitions stood out as the type in which more than half of the repetition instances fell in what Davis termed the "extreme extent range." It is of some interest that she found word and phrase repetitions to decrease with age, but not frequency of syllable repetitions.

The following quotations from Davis (1939) indicate the kind of repetitions which might be considered normal and those which are evidently abnormal.

> This material would tend to show that a child whose speech is such that approximately one *word* in four is a repeated *word*,[15] either in part or in whole in a word or phrase repetition, is not presenting any abnormality in speech, but is talking "normally."

However:

. . . in consideration of the instances of *syllable repetition* in terms of verbal output a very different picture was presented.

And later:

In consideration of all these measures it was found that the two which deal with the *instances of syllable repetition* and with the *number* of *repetitive syllables* used *in syllable repetition*, were the best measures for determining the children who deviated markedly from the group. In each of these measures the child who was termed "a stutterer" stands out dramatically from the balance of the group.

Davis' work, particularly her summary statements quoted above, point up emphatically the distinctiveness of syllable repetitions and their role in identifying stuttering.

Oxtoby (1943) made a statistical comparison between boys and girls on four repetition measures: syllable, word, phrase, and total repetitions. Among these the only difference which approached significance at the 10 percent level of confidence was that boys showed more syllable repetition than girls. Davis had also found more instance of syllable repetition in boys. The relevance of more syllable repetitions in boys is that there is considerably more stuttering in boys than girls.

Metraux (1950) described the speech characteristics of 207 young children on several dimensions, including repetitions. She reported that 18-month-old children repeat syllables or words more often than not. At 24 months there was occasional syllable repetition and use of "uh" before many remarks, but the most common characteristic was repetition of a word or phrase, sometimes with variation. Even at this young age there was much variation from child to child in amount and type of repetition.

At 30 months most of these children repeated a word or phrase occasionally; certain children continued this repetition "interminably" with increase in force, pitch, and volume. Such repetitions seemed to occur most often during the child's attempt to make personal-social contact, but they were also related to the child's "interest in repetition" and his demand for repetition from others. Metraux reported that some 30-month-old children evidenced what she called "developmental stuttering," identified as "first-word or syllable repetitions which frequently progresses to a mild tonic block that is easily broken." However, her findings emphasize that most children of this age show only occasional repetition of a beginning syllable and some instances of word repetition within a sentence. "Tonic blocking," she noted, was infrequent.

At 42 months of age repetitions (type unspecified) were reported to be more frequent than at other ages and also to have the "somewhat compulsive quality" noted at 30 months. The repetitions noticed at 42 months of age often seemed to occur when the child was asking for information or when apparently making a bid for attention or encouragement. The general rate of speech seemed to be faster in this age period, and "developmental stuttering" was again evident in some children, sometimes with breathing notably disturbed. However, she reported that " . . . more individual variations begin to appear with children whose tensional overflow affects the speech."

At 48 months of age most children were found to show little repetition except for an occasional phrase. But again, " . . . the child whose speech has been characterized by periods of developmental stuttering up to this time . . . may continue to have phases when repetition and blocking occur."

At 54 months of age children were reported to interject often at the beginning of a phrase, but seldom to repeat except for emphasis. Once more, however, the child who had evidenced speech blocking earlier was noted to be still likely to have occasional difficulty.

Metraux's article was not sufficiently explicit regarding the types of repetition observed, but it is certainly adequate to demonstrate that: (1) most children do not show the same kinds of repetition with comparable frequency, (2) regardless of type, repetitions are not common in the speech of young children, (3) syllable repetitions and "blocking" are very uncommon, and (4) only certain children exhibit "extremes in nonfluency," which are evidently characteristic of these children in that they persist over relatively long periods of time.

Branscom *et al.* (1955) summarized the findings of four studies on nonfluency in 193 nonstuttering preschool children from the ages of 2 to 6. Their report included the work of Davis and of Oxtoby. In their summary of the frequency of syllable, word, and phrase repetitions recorded in three of the studies which appraised speech behavior during free play, the values for the respective frequencies provide a ratio of approximately 1:2:3. That is, syllable repetitions occurred less than half as often as word repetitions and less than a third as often as phrase repetitions. These authors reported an insignificant correlation between syllable repetitions and phrase repetitions, indicating a lack of relationship between these two types. Word repetition correlated to some extent with both syllable repetition and phrase repetition, which may reflect the failure to consider the number of syllables in the word. One would not be surprised to find a correlation between repetition of syllables and words of one syllable, and between multisyllable word repetitions and phrase repetitions, but no correlation between the two latter and the two former repetition types.

A series of studies at Indiana University (Burstein, 1965; Helsabeck, 1965; Ortsey, 1964; Port, 1955) investigated the occurrence of disfluencies in the spontaneous speech of normally speaking young children. Analyses were made of 300-word speech samples from each of 40 children (20 males and 20 females) in preschool and first, second and fourth grades. These studies found that interjections were by far the most frequent type of disfluency and, in fact, accounted for almost half of the total disfluencies observed. The next two most frequently occurring disfluency types were revisions and word repetitions. In all four studies these three types of disfluency accounted for between 70 to 80 percent of all disfluencies observed. Part-word repetitions occupied either a low or intermediate rank; prolongations and broken words were the most infrequent disfluencies. Ortsey, who studied both first and second graders, noted that in almost all categories of repetition the repetitions were limited to one unit per instance; two repetitions per instance were rare; and three-unit repetitions never occurred.

Comparison of Stutterers and Nonstutterers

Studies comparing the speech characteristics of stutterers and nonstutterers have consistently yielded findings very similar to those just reviewed. Furthermore, these studies provide evidence regarding not only syllable repetitions but also the other distinctive feature of stuttering—prolongations.

In one of the earlier comparative studies Johnson (1942) obtained data on 46 stuttering and 46 nonstuttering children between the ages of 2 and 9. This investigation was concerned primarily with possible differences between the two groups on a number of developmental and case history variables. Very little detailed data was compiled in regard to the speech characteristics of the two groups, but a summary dealing with this aspect provides some evidence of differences between them:

> . . . it is sufficient to say that in approximately 92% of the (stuttering) cases the first phenomena that were diagnosed as stuttering were beyond doubt essentially effortless repetitions of words, phrases, or the first sounds or syllables of words. In other cases also these phenomena were, so far as could be determined, the predominating features, although there is some question as to whether, in these cases, diagnoses of stuttering were made before the child had begun to exhibit some degree of hypertonicity in connection with the repetition or before the

child had begun to exhibit such other reactions as prolongations of sounds, conspicuous pauses, etc.

This statement, while lacking clear specification, does indicate at least that features correlated with the distinction made between the stuttering and the nonstuttering children consisted of: prolongations (audible prolongations), conspicuous pauses (silent prolongations), and signs of undue effort concurrent with "repetitions."

Voelker (1944) compared the speech characteristics of 62 nonstuttering orphanage adolescents, ages 12 to 19, with those of seven stutterers of similar age. He reported a wide range of fluency in his normal group, with some individuals showing some kind of "break" every 2.3 words and others having a "break" only once every 12.5 words. He found a sex difference, with girls showing 20 percent fewer breaks, the boys being more subject to hesitation and repetition. However, he found that the average speaker had no syllable repetition per 100 words and less than one word or phrase repetition per 100 words. They also had very few other kinds of "breaks," although hesitations (10 per 100 words) and conspicuous pauses (3 to 6 per 100 words) were relatively prominent. His stutterers, on the other hand, showed a fluency break ranging from one every 1.2 words to one every 3.7 words. When compared to the normal speakers, the mean fluency rating of the stutterers was in the lowest decile; their scores on half the measures of nonfluency were subnormal. The stutterers were not equally nonfluent in all aspects of fluency. For example, while they were slightly above the average in number of conspicuous pauses, they did not have notably more hesitations than the normal speakers. However, the stutterers' speech was clearly characterized by excessive syllable and word repetitions and prolongations.

Egland (1955) investigated the occurrence of nonfluencies in a group of nonstuttering kindergarten children to which he compared similar observations from three preschool-age stutterers. Repetition of parts of words constituted the most common type of repetitious speech of both groups, yet the stutterers differed substantially from the nonstutterers. The stutterers showed a higher percentage of repetitions of all types; their repetitions consisted more prominently of sound and syllable repetitions, they had more repetition units per instance, and they evidenced very few phrase repetitions. Their speech samples also contained a high percentage of prolongations, whereas the samples from the nonstutterers had a greater percentage of what were called "stalls" ("ah," "um,").

In Johnson's major work (1959), he reported three separate studies which drew comparisons between nonstuttering children and children "regarded as stutterers." The combined samples contained 246 children in each group, ranging in age from approximately 2 to 14 years. In his treatment of the findings Johnson stressed the matter of "overlap" in disfluency in the two groups (all kinds of disfluencies were noted in the speech of both stutterers and nonstutterers). Actually there were some important differences. The stutterers evidenced significantly more syllable repetitions than the nonstutterers, who had significantly more phrase repetitions. Further, significantly more of the stuttering children evidenced prolongations, whereas significantly more nonstutterers had silent intervals, pauses (normal hesitations), or interjections (type unspecified, but evidently no prolongation or repetition types). All of these differences were significant at the .01 level of confidence.

Johnson's most recent report on a study of this type (1961) deals with adults, but it is included here because of the relevance of its content. In this study Johnson made comparisons between 100 stuttering and 100 nonstuttering college-age adults (50 males and 50 females in each group) on a number of measures of "disfluency." Special statistics were employed in treating the data because of the considerable skew in the distributions. This fact in itself provides a significant commentary on the "normality" of disfluencies. Even when all types of disfluency were considered together, nonstutterers were found to be "considerably less disfluent than the stutterers." When type of disfluency was taken into account, the results clearly revealed that the stutterers evidenced many more "part word repetitions" (sound and syllable repetitions) than the nonstutterers. The evidence regarding prolongations is not reported as clearly. Johnson expressed the comparison inversely and in terms of proportions, as follows:

> The proportions of both major groups presenting no broken words or prolonged sounds were sufficiently large to warrant the statement that approximately half of the stutterers were indistinguishable from most of the nonstutterers with respect to these types of disfluencies.[16]

Even when expressed in this manner, it seems clear that prolongations and broken words were much more characteristic of the stutterers; it is evident that these features were manifest in the speech of at least half of the stutterers and few of the nonstutterers. Further, the tabled data reveal that as an average for the three conditions of the study, the stuttering group showed 22 prolongations per 100 words, whereas among the nonstuttering group there were only 0.6 prolongations per 100 words; the stutterers averaged 12.2 broken words per 100 words but the nonstutterers only 0.6 per 100.

The two groups were said to show "extensive" overlap in interjections, although the data show the stutterers to evidence considerably more of them. These findings were not analyzed adequately, that is, no attempt was made to differentiate types of interjection. In particular, no notation was made of variants of the neutral vowel interjection ("uh"). The tabulation of these interjections made no distinction in terms of number of units (both "uh" and "uh, uh, uh" were counted as one instance of interjection) or in respect to such qualitative features as signs of undue effort.

Johnson also reported "extensive" overlap between the two groups in word repetitions, phrase repetitions, and incomplete phrases (stutterers slightly exceeded nonstutterers on all three of these disfluencies). The two groups were reported to show "virtually complete" overlap in respect to revisions. These findings accord well with the other material covered earlier.

Research aimed at determining the criteria by which stuttering is identified has produced results very similar to those reviewed above. Williams and Kent (1958) found that untrained judges consistently identified syllable repetitions and prolongations as "stuttered" and revisions as "normal." A study by Giolas and Williams (1958) yielded evidence that kindergarten and second grade children make similar appraisals. Boehmler (1958) found that both trained and untrained judges labeled sound and syllable repetitions as stuttered more often than revisions and interjections, and they did so regardless of the rated "severity of nonfluency" of the speech samples. Young (1961) found that the types of disfluency which correlate positively with ratings of stuttering severity are syllable or sound repetitions, sound prolongations, broken words, and words involving apparent or unusual stress or tension. Sander (1963) found that naive listeners were quite tolerant of single-unit syllable repetitions if they did not occur often, but judgments of "stuttering" were made more frequently as the incidence of these repetitions increased. In contrast, the occurrence of only a few double-unit syllable repetitions was sufficient to elicit judgments that the speech was stuttered. The present author (Wingate, 1972) has found evidence that judgments of stuttering made of written transcriptions of speech samples are highly correlated with the presence of single-syllable repetitions.

Careful reivew of the research relevant to the identification of stuttering thus gives consistent and definitive support to the analysis developed in this chapter. Certain kinds of disfluencies are invariable found to characterize the speech of stutterers. Also, in the most basic and comprehensive sense, it is in reference to those disfluencies that speech is identified as "stuttering." These disfluencies, denotable as elemental repetitions and prolongations, are the original and ultimate referents when speech is identified as "stuttered."

Other kinds of disfluency—normal disfluencies—are found in the speech of all speakers. Some of these disfluencies occur often, others appear only rarely. However, their normality is not dependent upon their frequency, but upon their character.

Contrary to what appears to be prevailing belief, normal speech is much more disfluent than ordinary awareness would suggest. Goldman-Eisler (1968) has stated the issue clearly in her findings from extensive study of spontaneous speech:

> Somehow the phenomenon of speech has become associated with images which suggest continuity in sound production. We speak of the even flow, of fluency in speech, of a flood of language, and many words relating to speech derive from descriptions of water in motion, such as "gush, spout, stream, torrent of speech, floodgates of speech, etc.
>
> The facts, however, show these images to be illusory; if we measure vocal continuity by the number of words uttered between two pauses, and call "phrase" the sequence uttered without break, we obtain a picture of fragmentation rather than of continuity.

The work of other authors confirms such evidence that normal spontaneous speech contains many disfluencies, most of which are not even noticed. Mahl (1956b), for instance, commented that " . . . the vast majority of the speech disturbances are 'unintended' and escape the awareness of both speakers and listeners, in spite of their very frequent occurrence." Tremendous amounts of disfluency occur in normal speech, yet these disfluencies go unnoticed, evidently because, being normal, they do not excite attention. It is not only the fact of normal disfluency, but the extent of it and its obscurity as well, which yield additional evidence that stuttering is a unique and discriminable kind of disfluency.

Too many students of stuttering seem unaware that disfluency has been studied by workers interested in normal speech. Disfluencies of normal speakers have been investigated for what they might reveal about language formulation and organization, cognitive function, and personality and intelligence (Bernstein, 1962; Blankenship and Kay, 1964; Boomer, 1965; Goldman-Eisler, 1958a, 1958b, 1958c, 1961, 1964; Lounsbury, 1954; Maclay and Osgood, 1959; Mahl, 1956a, 1956b). In these studies the terms used to identify the various kinds of disfluency are quite different from those in studies wherein stuttering determines the focus. For example, one finds identities such as: "word change," "false start," "filled pause," "incomplete sentence," "parenthetic remarks," and "vocal segregates." The reader should compare these words with the list on page 41 to appreciate the differences suggested. However, even among these studies, references to sound and syllable repetitions employ the term "stutter" (cf. Blankenship and Kay 1964; Mahl 1956a).

SUMMARY OF IDENTIFICATION ANALYSIS

The analysis developed in this chapter demonstrates that among the various kinds of speech disfluencies certain specific ones—audible or silent elemental repetitions and prolongations—are the essential features of stuttering. Occasional discriminations might be difficult (for instance, single-syllable-word repetitions), but this poses only a minor qualification in the overall analysis. As Stevens (1951, p. 33) has remarked, "No empirical class is ever water tight; we can always plague the taxonomist with the borderline case." However, as Stevens goes on to say, this fact does not vitiate a broadly supported system of classification.

The system of classification developed in this chapter does have broad support. It should serve as a reliable and effective frame of reference for identification of stuttering, particularly for diagnosis. Later we will see that, taking this analysis as the point of departure, the essence of stuttering can be identified in an even simpler way, which is particularly useful for stuttering therapy.

PRIMARY STUTTERING

"Primary stuttering" refers more to a concept than an observational reality. This is the basic reason that the term is surrounded by so much confusion, and why there is disagreement about its value and use. The term was suggested a number of years ago by Bluemel[17] (1932) as a point of departure from which the profession could reduce the number of stuttering theories on a rational basis and thereby proceed toward an understanding of the nature of stuttering. Bluemel believed that in order to do this the profession would have to resolve its " . . . confusion of the primary speech disorder with the various complications and emotional reactions that associate themselves with the later stage of the disturbance." He felt that all investigation of stuttering should recognize this distinction between the primary speech disorder and other facets of the problem, "otherwise our researches may merely add to the confusion that already confronts us."

Bluemel insisted that primary stuttering involves speech only: ". . . primary stammering is a speech disorder pure and simple . . ." He described this primary disorder as ". . . a simple disturbance in speech in which delay ensues between the commencement and completion of a word." He gave some illustration and examples of it:

> In primary stammering the disturbance is most frequently seen at the beginning of the sentence, and it commonly assumes the form of repetition of the first word of the sentence. The child says for instance, "I-I-I want that. Can-can-can I have it?" Often we hear repetition of initial consonants or initial syllables of words, and especially of the introductory words to sentences. The child says, "L-l-l-look at this. M-m-m-mother, what is it?

One should note (a) the emphasis on elemental repetitions, (b) the frequency of repetition per instance, and (c) that the word repetition examples given are single-syllable words. These items accord with the analysis made earlier in this chapter. Bluemel's remarks elsewhere in the article also allude to prolongations.

A study by Van Riper (1937) investigated individual variation in symptoms among 30 adult stutterers. While a considerable variety of (so-called "secondary") symptoms was observed, " . . . the clonic and tonic blocks alone were experienced by all." In reference to Bluemel's distinction of primary and secondary stuttering Van Riper commented, "It is interesting that the symptoms he termed primary are precisely those which we found to be common to all adult stutterers."

There are two essential points to be noted about the primary stuttering that Bluemel talked about. First, it is identified as a simple speech disturbance, nothing more. Nonetheless, it is a distinctive kind of disfluency (and furthermore, for Bluemel, unique to certain individuals who are prone to develop it). Second, primary stuttering is the first stage in the development of stuttering. Although Bluemel stated that primary stuttering may disappear, even several times in the course of a year or more, " . . . eventually the secondary stage of stammering is reached." The secondary stage develops when " . . . the child has become conscious of his defect, and attempts to control it and conceal it." The first point is consistent with most of the development in this chapter. The latter point is one with which we will shortly take issue.

Bluemel's concept of primary stuttering was not to have the effect he had hoped for it; it did not serve to reduce theoretic excesses or minimize confusion through research application. Nor did the profession adopt the concept as proposed. Instead, the identification of primary stuttering has been qualified to adapt the concept to one or another theoretical preconception. Most viewpoints seem able to accommodate that aspect of the concept of primary stuttering which suggests it is a stage of stuttering. However, differing viewpoints have found it necessary to make adjustments in that part of the concept which denotes what primary stuttering *is*. As a result, "primary stuttering" has existed as a term but its referent has been indeterminate and confounded.

This condition is clearly exemplified in a study by Glasner and Vermilyea (1953). Statements were obtained from 171 professional speech pathologists regarding how they defined primary stuttering. The authors reported that, overall, their results:

> . . . revealed a lack of agreement among qualified workers as to what is meant by "primary stuttering." In terms of speech, this survey indicates that "primary stuttering" could be anything from normal speech to obvious stuttering with awareness. Among those who mentioned behavior there was a wide range from "normal" to an "emotionally disturbed child." While most confined the age of "primary stuttering" to a preschool age group, several mentioned that the condition is known to persist into adulthood.

It is obvious that the term did not have a universal significance to the respondents in this study. At the same time, a review of the data reveals a core of agreement centering around certain kinds of disfluency commonly identified as stuttering—namely, repetitions, hesitations, and prolongations. The data are presented in Table 4:4.

Table 4:4 Summary of pertinent information relative to definitions of "primary stuttering" supplied by 171 speech pathologists (taken from data of Glasner and Vermilyea, 1953)

Essence of the Definition	*Percent of Total*	*Stuttering Acknowledged in the Statements of Definition*			*"Without Awareness" Qualification*
		Yes	*Uncertain*	*No*	
repetitions, hesitations, prolongations	36*	x			x
textbook definition (Bleumel or Van Riper)	12	x			x
no distinction made between primary and secondary	20	x			x
"a stage of stuttering"	11	x			x
developmental stage in speech learning	5		x		
excessive nonfluency reflecting emotional disturbance	2		x		
normal fluency	6			x	
refused to define	7	–	–	–	–

*This category combines groups 1 and 6 of the original data since the distinction made by the authors between these two groups was in respect to degree of emphasis.

Glasner and Vermilyea separated the speech pathologists' replies into several categories on the basis of content. The first column in Table 4:4 records the definition typifying each category; the second column indicates the percentage of replies falling in that category. The entries in the next three columns indicate whether the replies in each category associated "primary stuttering" with "stuttering" as a discriminable kind of disfluency. The entries reveal clearly that the vast majority of these respondents viewed "primary stuttering" in this way. Furthermore, 48 percent (the first two categories) make explicit use of the familiar denotative terms, and it seems reasonable to infer that at least an additional 31 percent (the next two categories) also had such features in mind.

The last column in the table indicates the extent to which the respondents in the study specified the qualification "without awareness" as a distinguishing feature of primary stuttering. Specific mention was made of "awareness" wherever the definition category accepted the idea of stuttering. The significance of the "awareness" qualification will be discussed shortly.

Objections to "Primary Stuttering"

"Primary stuttering" has been criticized essentially from two directions. The most vocal opposition has come from individuals who criticize the term for its "labeling potential." The basic contention here is that the term reifies something that does not actually exist. Proponents of this argument contend that all childhood disfluencies are normal and that to use a special name to refer to certain disfluencies (of certain children) is a practice that has serious consequences. First, the argument goes, use of a special term implies that one can discern differences in disfluencies from one child to another. Second, the difference thus "created" carries the implication of deviation. The term, then, is said to identify as abnormal a kind of speech that is essentially normal. Purportedly the "label" not only causes a distorted perception of disfluencies but, through its implication of abnormality, generates negative reactions which then do lead to an abnormal condition.

This criticism is dependent upon the argument that disfluencies identified as stuttering cannot be differentiated from other kinds of disfluencies. In view of the material presented earlier in this chapter this argument has no credibility as a general statement, and hence the criticism has no substance. Further, there is no evidence that the "label" has any negative impact.

A second line of criticism of "primary stuttering" is that one cannot reliably distinguish it from "secondary stuttering." Here there is no complaint with the basic identification of stuttering but simply that the criteria for distinguishing the two "stages" are either not adequately specified or not reliable. This criticism gets close to the basic fault in the concept of "primary stuttering" but only suggests it by implication.

The notion of "primary stuttering" cannot be considered in isolation from the idea of "secondary stuttering." If we begin with "secondary stuttering" and work back in the supposed developmental progression we can uncover the real difficulty in the concept of primary stuttering.

Supposedly secondary stuttering is identified on the basis of certain cues, other than the speech symptoms, which are observable in the stutterer's actions when he stutters. The cues, specified in only a very general fashion, are interpreted to reflect "struggle." The interpretation of "struggle" involves the assumption that these acts reflect a reaction to the

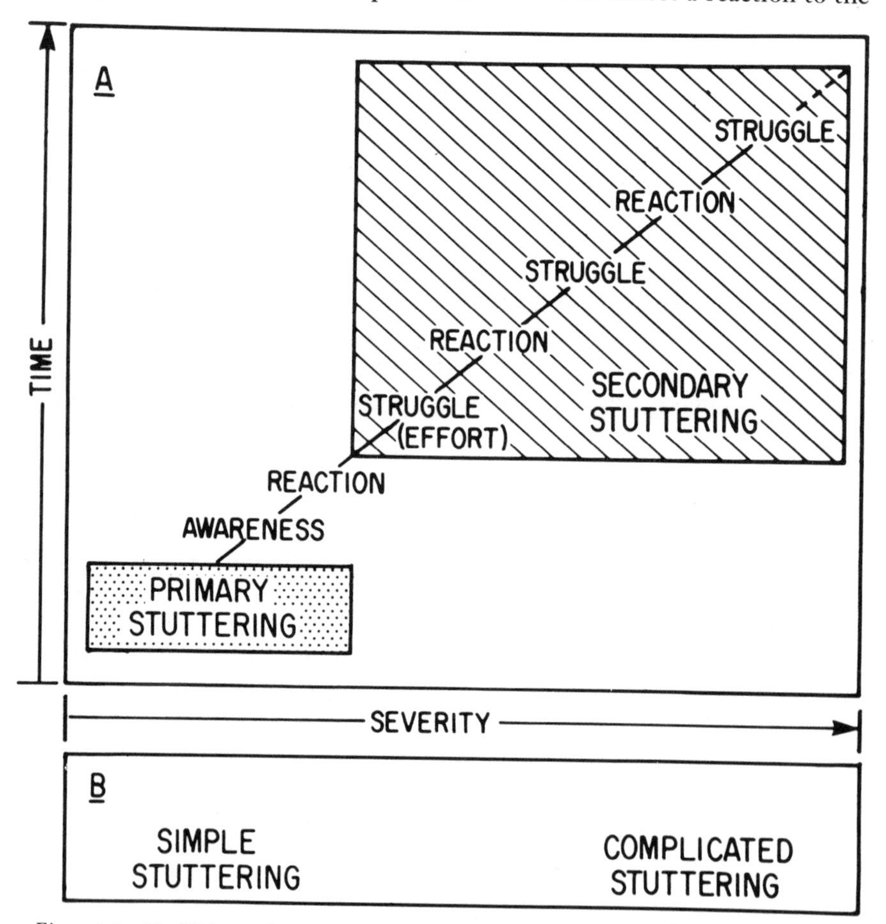

Figure 4:1 The "Primary-Secondary" progression scheme (A), and a more realistic alternative (B).

stuttering. Finally, this presumed reaction to the primary stuttering is supposedly a consequence of the child's becoming *aware* of his speech difficulty, that is, secondary stuttering develops after the child has become aware of his primary stuttering. Here we have the major problem: the matter of awareness.

The notion of awareness is a fault because it poses an insoluble problem to diagnosis, therapy, and theory. How can one determine whether another person is or is not aware of something? In particular, how can this be determined with the degree of certainty needed to make a differential diagnosis? Any determination of awareness based on other than the individual's testimony is nothing more than subjective judgment.

The differentiation between "primary stuttering" and "secondary stuttering" has to be made without asking the child, for fear of bringing it to his awareness. So, whether or not the child is aware is inferred from other information. Often the parents are asked for help, but this is only asking for more subjective judgment. Typically the decision is made from direct or reported observation of signs of effort—from which, then, interpretations must be made regarding the matters of "reaction" and "struggle." But what about the youngster who gives no sign of effort associated with his speech symptoms? Is he therefore unaware of them?

It is possible for someone to be well aware of an act which involves no sign of effort. In contrast, signs of effort in an act do not signal either an awareness of difficulty or a reaction to it. Nor do indications of effort indicate "struggle," particularly in any elaborated sense of the word. Consider the following examples. Most children use excessive pencil pressure while they are learning to write, and some also make extraneous movements, the most common being oral motions. Also, one frequently sees a child furrow his brow, tilt his head, or move lips, tongue, or jaw when cutting with scissors. In these instances one is justified in perceiving "effort," but not "struggle" in the sense used in respect to stuttering. In such circumstances, there also is little evidence of "awareness" or "reaction."[18]

The judgment of "awareness" of stuttering (or of "speech difficulty" or "disfluency") is thus very dubious. Clearly there will be some cases in which a judgment might be made with considerable confidence; for example, where verbal features occur as part of the instances of stuttering. It would also seem that awareness should accompany occurrences of the more dramatic accessory features. Still, however obvious an act may seem to be, one cannot be certain, from observation alone, that the individual is aware of it.[19]

The problem is most acute in cases where the accessory symptoms are relatively localized and mild in character, or where one observes little more than effort accompanying the speech features. In such cases a judgment of awareness is much more presumptive and much less defensible. Yet it is just such cases that make up the vast majority of instances in which the problem of differentiating "primary" from "secondary" stuttering arises. It should be obvious, then, why "primary stuttering" has presented so much of a problem and has been so unsatisfactory as a diagnostic category.

STAGES AND PHASES

A larger problem is posed by the idea of the *progression* of stuttering, that is, that stuttering gets worse. The notion of "primary-secondary" is only one expression of the conception that stuttering regularly or typically exacerbates through a chain of events that includes reaction, effort, and struggle (cf. Figure 4:1). The most defensible element in this particular scheme is the matter of "effort." Though admittedly a judgment, the perception of effort is based on observable cues, and there is little doubt that these cues could be scaled on a dimension of amount. Now it is reasonable to assume that effort is some function of the degree of difficulty involved in the execution of an activity. However, the signs of effort do not suggest anything else; they do not by any means indicate an emotional reaction to the difficulty, much less an emotional reaction mediated through an awareness of the difficulty. Nor do indications of effort necessarily signify "struggle" in the elaborated sense of the word.

The typical immediate adjustment any individual makes to an obstacle is to attempt to overcome it by the use of a little more force, which usually persists at least temporarily. Consider, for instance, the stuck drawer, the door that should be pulled instead of pushed, the pen whose ink does not flow at once, or the word not understood when first said. The young child is even more prone to act in this manner, and a more sophisticated form of adjustment may not develop for years.

Extraneous as well as excessive effort is elicited when the obstacle to performance consists of ineptness and lack of skill. Consider, again, the excessive pencil pressure and the extraneous oral and head movements children make while learning to print and write. When stuttering does worsen, it may indicate simply that the youngster has persisted in dealing ineffectively with an obstacle, rather than reflecting events hypothesized in this or similar models of stuttering progression.

Other models of stuttering progression (cf. Bloodstein, 1960a,

1960b, 1961; Brutten and Shoemaker, 1967) are essentially variations on the primary-secondary theme. Superficially they may seem to offer refinements, such as a greater number of phases, or more detailed cataloguing of features purported to characterize each phase, but basically they share the same limitations inherent in any progression concept.

Progression concepts depict stuttering as only worsening; there is no provision for those cases which show no appreciable change, nor those evidencing periodicity or fluctuation, nor those which ameliorate. The preponderant evidence indicates that a progression concept is possibly applicable to only a small proportion of cases of stuttering.

Progression schemes always link degree of severity to age level; that is, the stuttering is purportedly mild in early periods, becoming more severe at older age levels. But stuttering is not always mild at inception, nor is it uncommon to find mild stuttering at older age levels.

The unfortunate consequence of progression schemes is that they imply a known sequence of change believed to hold true for any given case of stuttering. This is an erroneous implication. It is not right to offer accounts of the "development of stuttering" which, at best, are plausible only for a minority of cases. In fact, we have absolutely no grounds for predicting either course or destination for any case of stuttering.

We should abandon the use of words with special and biasing connotations such as "primary," "secondary," "phase," "stage," and the like and instead stay closer to direct and verifiable observation. It would seem most appropriate to speak of stuttering as either "simple" or "complicated" and consider the particular features of each case individually. Referents for gradations of severity may be attached, as necessary, simply through the use of common adverbs expressing quantity. Where important, an appended phrase specifying the qualitative features would complete the individual picture. Such simplified identification cuts free of any regular connection to age level, temporal interval, indication of sequence, implication of change, or presumption of etiology. It also relieves adherence to faulty conceptions. Admittedly this is not a very sophisticated form of identification, but it is realistic.

Notes

1. For instance, Silverman and Williams (1967) refer to " . . . a series of investigations . . . which demonstrated that stutterings could not be reliably differentiated from other types of disfluencies in speech." Actually, a careful reading of the sources they cite suggests a quite different interpretation.

2. Personal correspondence from John A. Wilson, professor of Egyptology at the University of Chicago.

3. Williams *et al.* (1968) have reported a list in which *disrhythmic phonation* is evidently substituted for *prolongation* and *broken word*, and a category of *tension* is added. Such modifications are incorporated within the present analysis.

4. For instance, cf. Johnson (1959, p. 144), " . . . the ordinary repetitions and hesitations generally characteristic in varying measure of the speech of young children . . ."; or Sheehan (1958), " . . . the stage of hesitancy and syllable repetition through which nearly all children seem to pass."

5. For example, cf. Darley (1955, p. 138), ". . .repetition of a sound, syllable, word or phrase, speech phenomena well known to characterize the speech of normal young children."

6. It is strange that proponents of the "evaluational" theory, who have made so much issue of a presumed semantic problem in stuttering, have not only made no effort to deal with this matter, which is obviously a semantic problem, but instead have been instrumental in propagating it and providing it with apparent substance.

7. Some literature sources, discussing "repetitions" in young children, include even repetition of sentences and stories, or mention "interest in repetition," referring to the fact that children sometimes like to repeat certain expressions or enjoy hearing certain things repeated. Repetitions of such length or type hardly seem to have any relevance to the topic of disfluency, even in its broadest outlines.

8. The category "part-word repetitions" also does not indicate *which* part of the word is repeated. It is evidently well established that stuttered repetitions occur (a) primarily on the initial part of a word, (b) secondarily on the stressed part of a word if it is not also the initial part, but (c) not on the final part of a word. The matter of initial occurrence has been investigated less extensively than unit length, probably because it is so widely and regularly observed that it is taken for granted. (But see Brown, 1938; Hahn, 1942; Johnson and Brown, 1935; and Wingate, 1967.)

9. A potential syllable-length type of criterion might be affected by whether or not the word has a "bounded" ending. In the author's observation repetition of single-syllable words having a terminal consonant /e.g., /kip/) are less likely to be judged as stuttered than a comparable word with vowel termination (e.g., /ki/). It should be noted that the latter is more similar to an "elemental" part-word repetition. The matter deserves study.

10. Evidently the author is guilty of this from time to time, as reflected in the following episode. In 1968 I spoke at the luncheon of the California Speech and Hearing Association. During the question period someone asked me if I were, or had ever been, a stutterer; to which I responded negatively. Shortly

after the meeting I received an unsigned note through the message center which said, in part, "Probably you don't call yourself a stutterer. You don't need to. You did introduce well over 200 "uhs" in less than 10 minutes this morning." This is a clear example of the confusion in thinking that has developed in respect to the identification of stuttering. Certain kinds of "uh" are not criterial of stuttering, regardless of their frequency.

11. The following observation illustrates the distinction between a "starter" and a stutter. If a starter "works," we do not observe a stutter; if it is not successful, the stutter is evident.

12. The concept of primary stuttering will be considered later.

13. Note the qualitative difference between these interjections and those given as examples of normal interjections. Cf. p. 46.

14. This represents an outstanding example of the misleading use of the general term.

15. All underlinings are supplied by the present author. In these quotations, as elsewhere in the studies being reviewed here, the authors make no distinction between words of one syllable and words of more than one syllable.

16. The statement seems to convey a meaningful comparison, yet what it actually says is that if one were to consider only those individuals who *did not* evidence broken words or prolonged sounds one could not differentiate these individuals on the dimensions of broken words and prolonged sounds. The argument is circular and self-contained. If one compares two groups in terms of any chracteristic that is *not* manifested, obviously the groups will not differ in respect to that characteristic.

17. (a) In the United States, at least. Froeschels (1943) commented that Ssikorski, a German writer, had made a distinction of this type in 1891. (b) Note that Bluemel, being from England, used the word "stammering."

18. The author has substantiated this many times from youngsters' testimony obtained through direct questioning.

19. cf. pp. 25 regarding stutterers' awareness of their stutterings when alone. Further, any experienced clinician should recognize that stutterers are by no means aware of all their stutterings. Commonly the stutterer is poorly aware of what happens during his stuttering. As a matter of fact, as we shall see later, direction and control of awareness of stuttering is an important feature of effective therapy.

References

Bar, A. Effects of types of listener and listening instructions on the attention to manner and content of a stutterer's speech. *Program of 44th Annual Convention, Am. Sp. Hearing Assn.* 90, 1968 (abstr.).

Bernstein, B. Linguistic codes, hesitation phenomena and intelligence. *Language and Speech*, **5**, 31–46, 1962.

Blankenship, Jane and C. Kay. Hesitation phenomena in English speech: A study in distribution. *Word*, **20**, 360–373, 1964.

Bluemel, C. S. Primary and secondary stammering. *Proc. Am. Soc. for the Study of Speech Dis.*, 91–102, 1932. Also in *Quart. J. Sp.*, **18**, 187–200, 1932.

Bloodstein, O. The development of stuttering: I. Changes in nine basic features. *J. Speech Hearing Dis.*, **25**, 219–237, 1960a.

———The development of stuttering: II. Developmental phases. *J. Speech Hearing Dis.*, **25**, 366–376, 1960b.

———The development of stuttering: III. Theoretical and clinical implications. *J. Speech Hearing Dis.*, **26**, 67–80, 1961.

Boehmler, R. M. Listener responses to non-fluencies. *J. Speech Hearing Res.*, **1**, 132–141, 1958.

Boomer, D. S. Hesitation and grammatical encoding. *Language and Speech*, **8**, 148–58, 1965.

Branscom, Margaret E., Jeannette Hughes, and E. T. Oxtoby. Studies of non-fluency in the speech of preschool children. In Johnson, W. (Ed.), *Stuttering in Children and Adults*, Univ. of Minnesota, Minneapolis, 1955.

Brown, S. F. Stuttering with relation to word accent and word position. *J. Abn. Soc. Psychol.*, **33**, 112–120, 1938.

Brutten, E. and D. Shoemaker. *The Modification of Stuttering*, Prentice-Hall, Englewood Cliffs, 1967.

Burstein, Barbara. The loci of disfluencies in the spontaneous speech of normal speaking children in the first grade. M.A. thesis, Indiana Univ. 1965.

Calzia, G. Panconcelli. *Geschichtszahlen Der Phonetik, 3000 Jahre Phonetik*, Hamburg 11, Hanischer Gilden verlag, 1941.

d'Alais, Serre. In Klingbeil, G. M. The historical background of the modern speech clinic. *J. Speech Dis.*, **4**, 115–132, 1939.

Darley, F. L. The relationship of parental attitudes and adjustments to the development of stuttering. In Johnson, W. (Ed.), *Stuttering in Children and Adults*, Univ. of Minnesota Press, Minneapolis, 1955, Chapter 4.

Davis, Dorothy M. The relation of repetitions in the speech of young children to certain measures of language maturity and situational factors: Part I. *J. Speech Dis.*, **4**, 303–318, 1939.

———The relation of repetitions in the speech of young children to certain measures of language maturity and situational factors: Part II and Part III. *J. Speech Dis.*, **5**, 235–246, 1940.

Egland, G. O. Repetitions and prolongations in the speech of stuttering and nonstuttering children. In Johnson, W. (Ed.) *Stuttering in children and Adults*, Univ. of Minnesota Press, Minneapolis, 1955.

Froeschels, E. Survey of the early literature on stuttering, chiefly European. *Nervous Child*, **2**, 86–95, 1943.

Giolas, T. G. and D. E. Williams. Children's reaction to nonfluencies in adult speech. *J. Speech Hearing Res.*, **1**, 86–93, 1958.

Glasner, P. J. and F. D. Vermilyea. An investigation of the definition and uses of the diagnosis "primary stuttering." *J. Speech Hearing Dis.*, **18**, 161–167, 1953.

Goldman-Eisler, Frieda. Continuity of speech utterance, its determinants and its significance. *Language and Speech*, **4**, 220–231, 1961.

———Hesitation, information, and levels of speech production. In A.V.S. deReuck, and M. O'Connor (eds.), *Disorders of Language*, Little-Brown, Boston, 1964.

———*Psycholinguistics: Experiments in Spontaneous Speech*, Academic Press, New York, 1968.

———The predictability of words in context and the length of pauses in speech. *Language and Speech*, **1**, 226–231, 1958a.

———Speech analysis and mental processes. *Language and Speech*, **1**, 59–75, 1958b.

———Speech production and the predictability of words in context. *Quart. J. Exp. Psychol.*, **10**, 96–106, 1958c.

Hahn, E. F. A study of the relationship between stuttering occurrence and phonetic factors in oral reading. *J. Speech Dis.*, **7**, 143–151, 1942.

Helsabeck, Mary V. Types and loci of disfluencies in the spontaneous speech of normal speaking fourth grade children. M.A. thesis, Indiana Univ., 1965.

Johnson, W. A study of the onset and development of stuttering. *J. Speech Dis.*, **7**, 251–257, 1942.

———Measurements of oral reading and speaking rate and disfluency of adult male and female stutterers and nonstutterers. *J. Speech Hearing Dis., Monogr. Suppl.*, **7**, 1961.

———*et al. The Onset of Stuttering*, Univ. of Minnesota Press, Minneapolis, 1959.

———and S. F. Brown. Stuttering in relation to various speech sounds. *Quart. J. Speech*, **21**, 481–496, 1935.

Klingbeil, G. M. The historical background of the modern speech clinic. *J. Speech Hearing Dis.*, **4**, 115–132, 1939.

Lemert, E. M. Stuttering among the North Pacific coastal Indians. *Southwest J. Anthropol.*, **8**, 429–441, 1952.

Lounsbury, F. G. Pausal, juncture, and hesitation phenomena. In Osgood, C. E. and T. A. Sebeok (Eds.), *Psycholinguistics: A Survey of Theory and Research*, Waverly, Baltimore, 1954.

Maclay, H. and C. E. Osgood. Hesitation phenomena in spontaneous English speech. *Word*, **15**, 19–44, 1959.

Mahl, G. Disturbances and silences in the patient's speech in psychotherapy. *J. Abn. Soc. Psychol.*, **53**, 1–15, 1956a.

———"Normal" disturbances in spontaneous speech. Paper presented at American Psychological Assn. Convention, 1956b.

Metraux, Ruth W. Speech profiles of the preschool child, 18 to 54 months. *J. Speech Hearing Dis.*, **15**, 37–53, 1950.

Morgenstern, J. J. Psychological and social factors in children's stammering. Ph.D. dissertation, Univ. of Edinburgh, 1953.

Ortsey, Evelyn. Types of disfluencies in the spontaneous speech of normal speaking children in the first and second grades. M.A. thesis, Indiana Univ., 1964.

Oxtoby, E. T. A quantitative study of repetition in the speech of three-year-old children. Unpublished M.A. thesis, Univ. of Iowa, 1943.

Port, Karen B. Loci of disfluencies in the spontaneous speech of normal speaking preschool children. M.A. thesis, Indiana Univ., 1965.

Sheehan, J. G. Projective studies of stuttering. *J. Speech Hearing Dis.*, **23**, 18–25, 1958.

Silverman, F. and D. Williams. Loci of disfluencies in the speech of stutterers. *Perceptual and Motor Skills*, **24**, 1085–1086, 1967.

Stevens, S. S. Psychology and the science of science. In Marx, M. H. (Ed.), *Psychological Theory*, Macmillan, New York, 1955, Chapter 2, p. 33.

Tuthill, C. A quantitative study of extensional meaning with special reference to stuttering. *Speech Monogr.*, **13**, 81–98, 1946.

Van Riper, C. Effect of devices for minimizing stuttering on the creation of symptoms. *J. Abn. Soc. Psychol.*, **32**, 185–192, 1937.

Voelker, C. H. A preliminary investigation for a normative study of fluency, a clinical index to the severity of stuttering. *Am. J. Orthopsy.*, **14**, 285–294, 1944.

West, R., M. Ansberry, and Anna Carr. *The Rehabilitation of Speech*, 3rd ed., Harper, New York, 1957, p. 15.

Williams, D. E. and Louise R. Kent. Listener evaluations of speech interruptions. *J. Speech Hearing Res.*, **1**, 124–131, 1958.

Williams, D. E., F. H. Silverman, and J. A. Kools. Disfluency behavior of elementary stutterers and non-stutterers: The adaptation effect. *J. Speech Hearing Res.*, **11**, 622–630, 1968.

Wingate, M. E. Identification of stuttering from transcriptions of speech samples. Unpublished research, State Univ. of New York at Buffalo, 1972.

———Stuttering and word length. *J. Speech Hearing Res.*, **10**, 146–152, 1967.

Young, M. A. Predicting ratings of severity of stuttering. *J. Speech Hearing Dis., Monogr. Suppl.*, **7**, 31–54, 1961.

II

MITIGATION OF STUTTERING

5

REMISSION OF STUTTERING

A substantial number of stutterers do get over stuttering without therapeutic intervention. In spite of this and the fact that stuttering has been investigated and written about in the United States more than anywhere else, our textbooks and other sources usually pay little attention to remission.[1] When the subject is mentioned, the reference is typically brief and casual.

The American inclination to ignore this area is again undoubtedly a reflection of the theoretical climate which has been so pervasive in the past 30 years. With stuttering conceived as a self-generating emotional problem, or as "learned behavior" which is instated and maintained by mysterious processes of reinforcement, there is an inherent assumption that stuttering will not get better except through therapy. In effect, this position is required by any theoretical interpretation of stuttering which conceives it to be a psychological problem.

This situation is clearly reflected in sources on stuttering and the treatment of stuttering. Robinson (1964) paraphrases the prevalent thinking on this matter:

> Whatever may be its source, stuttering seldom remains static. It grows. And as it grows, it tends to change in form as well as in severity. Early patterns are replaced, obscured, or supplemented by more pronounced and abnormal behavior. Repetitions or prolongations become troublesome "blocks." Tremors may appear in certain oral structures. Word attempts may be interrupted and replaced with synonyms. Reattempts on words may be prefaced by noticeable pauses

during which a child can appear to be experiencing some sort of silent internal struggle. Some children become less talkative and occasionally may refuse to speak. Such changes signal the onset of the advanced stage of this disorder. They reveal much about the nature of stuttering and its impact on the speaker and the listener. (p. 47.)

Conceptions of stuttering built around the notion of "stages" or "phases" of progression obviously would tend to minimize the matter of remission. Thus, in a series of articles " . . . concerned with the changes which take place in stuttering as it grows from a phenomenon of early childhood into a disorder of adolescence and adulthood," Bloodstein (1960a, 1960b, 1961) devotes considerable space to a description of features purportedly characteristic of progressive "phases" in the development of stuttering, and to an account of their origin and development. While there is mention of individuals who do not follow this progression, the implication drawn is that such cases are exceptional.

Luper and Mulder (1964), who leaned heavily on the work of Johnson and Bloodstein, deal with the matter in similar fashion in their book on stuttering therapy for children. These authors make reference to reports of stuttering being "outgrown or cured" and acknowledge the possibility that some kinds of parental management " . . . may turn stuttering away as well as turn it on . . ." (p. 49.) However, their final statement on the matter of outgrown stuttering is that in such reported instances it is very likely that the child was not really stuttering to begin with. This explanation, also offered in other sources, does not dismiss the matter as neatly as it may seem. If it is true that making an issue of a child's disfluencies is instrumental in inducing stuttering, then it should make no difference whether or not the child was "really" stuttering. That is, whatever it was that such children evidenced in their speech it was *called* stuttering, and such "mislabeling" has been said to be sufficient to induce "real" stuttering. At least making this kind of issue about a child's disfluencies should be an "unfavorable critical evaluation" of it. If such mislabeling or the negative attitude presumably associated with it do in effect lead to stuttering, then these disfluencies, whatever their nature, should have worsened and become stuttering.

Brutten and Shoemaker (1967) conceive of the development of stuttering in the esoteric language of learning theory, and present the development of stuttering in three "stages." The inevitability of an increase in stuttering is retained in their formulation. The matter of recovery independent of the manipulation of environmental effects by a therapist does not receive consideration in their presentation.

The essential issue here is that stuttering remission has not received proper attention. To ignore, overlook, or minimize the fact of spontaneous remission or recovery attained independently of professional intervention is to disregard a great fund of information which is of import to both theory and therapy. It perpetuates constraints that limit and mislead, that obstruct progress toward a full understanding of stuttering, and that restrict the breadth and flexibility of therapeutic approach.

It is wrong to encourage the therapist to think only in terms of a disorder which gets worse unless treated. Many therapists become reluctant to work with stutterers for fear of doing the stutterer more harm than good. As discussed in Chapter 3, if stuttering does progress according to the formulations mentioned above, then, in terms of what we know about the effect of emotion, the stuttering child should become essentially mute within a few years. This certainly does not happen. Further, one can easily verify for oneself that it is *not* common for stuttering children to fear more and more words or situations, or to stutter more and more frequently, or to embellish their stuttering with increasingly numerous and complicated actions—those features which have come to be called "secondary mannerisms."

Inattention to the matter of spontaneous remission of stuttering is all the more surprising in view of the extent of relevant information available, much of which has existed for many years.[2] Evidently this information has been ignored because it is incompatible with the prevailing beliefs of the past few decades. Many widely held theoretical notions are contradicted by the information contained in reports of stuttering remission. Reasonably, what is known about remission should have significance for management, but it is rare to find any aspect of a therapy program which takes cognizance of recovery information. Treatment approaches are determined by theoretical concepts. A great deal of potentially worthwhile avenues of approach to modification of stuttering and suggestions for counseling thus have been eliminated autocratically by theoretical positions which determine what is good and what is bad in stuttering management.

We should be concerned not simply with the *fact* of remission but, more importantly, with what can be learned about factors and circumstances that contribute to remission. Such knowledge should be of value not only in dealing with the stutterer, but also in counseling parents and other persons concerned with helping him. Moreover, we need to consider what these findings indicate, even though indirectly, about the nature of stuttering. It must be remembered that the cause of stuttering is not known, despite several widely accepted theoretical notions to the contrary. The reader, having finished this chapter, will appreciate that many of the findings presented contradict a number of currently accepted ideas about stuttering.

The range of information on recovery varies from one source to another, since all of the investigations did not have identical objectives. Some studies were addressed directly to the issue of recovery, other sources yielded relevant information adventitiously. There were also certain differences in methodology. Consequently, some sources will yield considerably more information germane to stuttering remission.

A fair amount of the data was obtained through questionnaires, or from second parties, or was retrospective in nature. Appropriate cautions should therefore be exercised in the literal acceptance of any specific findings. However, we are most interested in the general picture yielded by the various sources both individually and as a whole. As therapists interested in the ingredients of recovery, we should be duly cognizant of recurring general or specific themes in these findings.

The possibility of bias is always present, of course, yet the information comes from many sources, and there is no reason to suspect that a similar bias should operate through all of them. In fact, the reader who is familiar with the names of personages in the field of stuttering will find contributions to the data on recovery from individuals representing divergent basic viewpoints about stuttering. In view of this it seems particularly appropriate to repeat that recurring findings merit special consideration.

STUDIES BEARING ON STUTTERING REMISSION

The evidence will be presented in a general chronological sequence, though organized first according to three approximate age-level groupings: (1) children of preschool and early grade level; (2) school-age children; and (3) young adults and adults.

Remission of Stuttering in Young Children

As a keynote to this section we might recall a statement made many years ago by Bryngelson that:

> . . . forty per cent of stuttering children need not worry a clinician, because before the age of eight, through general cerebral maturation assisted by developmental factors in the environment, stuttering subsides. In a few of these individuals there appears to be but slight remnants of an earlier severe type of stuttering. (Bryngelson, 1938.)

In a later publication (Bryngelson, 1943) he again mentioned the figure of a 40 percent recovery rate in reference to a review of 1492 cases seen at the University of Minnesota Speech Clinic.

At an earlier date Johnson (1934) had also noted that 30 to 40 percent of young stuttering children "outgrew" stuttering by the time they were 8 or 9 years of age.

Much later Johnson (1955) reported the findings of a study[3] " . . . designed to yield information concerning the characteristics of stuttering at its onset, and to explore the problem of the changes that occur as stuttering develops through its early stages into its more advanced phases." Although he indicated an interest in the "conditions surrounding the onset, aggravation, alleviation and disappearance of the disorder," he devoted much more attention to factors possibly related to onset and aggravation than to amelioration. Subsequent references to this work have repeated this emphasis.

The design of the study involved a matched control group of nonstuttering children in order to make comparisons of the conditions which, if different in the two groups, might have some explanatory significance. For present purposes we are interested only in the stuttering youngsters.[4]

The stuttering group consisted of 46 children, 33 boys and 13 girls, having a median age of 4 years 2 months at the time the study was begun.[5] It was considered desirable to study children in whom stuttering was of recent origin. For 75 percent of these youngsters the interval between reported age of onset and time of initial interview was less than a year; the median interval was five and a half months. The median age of stuttering onset was 3 years; for 75 percent of the youngsters stuttering onset was reported to have occurred prior to age 3 years 2 months.

These children were followed over varying periods of time during the course of the study, which extended for about five years. The median length of the observation period per child was 30 months. Seventy-five percent of the children were followed for at least six months.

Assessments of the speech status of these 46 youngsters at the time of first interview and at the end of the study are shown in Table 5:1. At the end of the study, 39 cases were judged to have shown improvement, six to have shown no important change, and only one to be worse. These figures are based on the assessment of the "judges"—presumably several of the investigators participating in the study. The judges disagreed in only three cases, which is the reason for the "Indefinite" category.

These data indicate that 85 percent of these stuttering children had shown improvement, and that 72 percent of them could be considered to have recovered during the period of approximately two and a half years that they were under observation. Since all but three of these children were age 5 or less at the time of initial interview, it is evident that most recovered before 8 years of age. Reportedly, the recovery occurred gradually.

None of these children received any direct professional attention. Johnson implied that the favorable outcome was due to parent counseling, in which they were advised to regard their youngsters as capable of normal speech, to lower their standards for speech and behavior generally, making it easier for the child to feel success and approval. However, Johnson provided no evidence that the parents were in any way influenced by these counseling efforts. Also, no mention was made of reasons the parents themselves might have given for the improvement in their children's speech.

A study by Glasner and Rosenthal (1957) was designed primarily to investigate certain theoretical issues particularly focal to evaluational theory. The study was undertaken to learn something about the occurrence of nonfluency in young children and its relation to parental thinking and attitudes about nonfluencies. The more important questions raised in the study were: the incidence of parental diagnosis of stuttering in preschool children, the criteria used by parents in their identification of stuttering, the purported times of stuttering, and the effect of parental treatment on the child and the course of his stuttering.

Information was obtained through questionnaire interview of parents registering their children for school entrance in 25 of the 60 schools in Anne Arundel County, Maryland. The schools were distributed between rural and urban centers. The children in question were all being registered for the first grade; they were at least 5 years of age but not yet 7. Standardized information was obtained about 996 children, 551 boys and 445 girls.

The investigators were careful in their questioning about stuttering. Parents were first asked if their child had ever gone through a period of

Table 5:1 Nature of childrens speech at beginning and at end of study (From Johnson, 1955, Table 8.)

Nature of Speech	*Beginning of Study**	*End of Study**
Severe stuttering	6	1
Average stuttering	28	11
Mild stuttering	12	1
Nearly normal	0	5
Indefinite	0	3
Normal	0	25
Total	46	46

*Figures indicate number of cases.

repeating words or sounds to excess, hesitating or being unable to get words out, or holding onto words longer than they thought was normal.[6] If the parents responded affirmatively, they were asked to describe and imitate what they meant by hesitation, repetition, and holding onto words. They were then asked if the youngster had ever gone through a period of stuttering, or if he ever stammered or stuttered. Again the parent was asked to give a description or imitation of the child's speech. Parents were also asked what they thought caused the stuttering, what they did about it, and whether the child was still stuttering.

One hundred and fifty-three parents said their child had stuttered at some time. This amounts to 15.4 percent of the total population sample, a figure which was found to be the same irrespective of the investigator or locale. The authors noted a direct relationship between the number of disfluency types (hesitation, repetition, prolongation) reported by the parents and the frequency with which they called it stuttering. The term was used in 94 percent of cases evidencing all disfluency types, in 65 percent of cases manifesting two types, but in only 29 percent of cases where only one type was observed.

The authors stated that all of the parents in the study gave evidence of being concerned about the problem. The degree of concern seemed to reflect how severe the parent thought the stuttering was. The authors evidently found the reported levels of concern to be justified, saying that their data " . . . do not indicate either undue anxiety or misperception in the judgments of these parents." They went on to point out that if one were to contend that these parents had high standards of fluency, as evidenced in their concern about their children's speech, it must also be recognized that more than half of them later completely reversed the "diagnosis," saying that their child had stopped stuttering. It did not seem judicious to the authors to suppose that in these cases the parents had simply lowered their standards of fluency, but rather more likely that observable changes in the children's nonfluency had occurred and that the parents' judgments were simply a reflection of such changes.

Of the 153 children reported to have stuttered for some time, 105 were said to have improved. Twenty-two of these children were stuttering only occasionally at that time; 83 were said to have stopped stuttering. This represents a 54 percent recovery rate. The authors found a positive relationship between incidence of recovery and the extent of the reported disfluency. Of the youngsters reported to have only one disfluency type, 51 percent had stopped stuttering, as compared to a 35 percent recovery rate for those with two or three disfluency types. This difference was statistically significant.

The authors grouped parental responses to the stuttering into three categories: (1) active correction, (2) minimizing the problem, and (3) seeking professional help.

Some of the *active correction* measures reported by parents include: "told him to speak more slowly and to take his time", "made him repeat", "made him stop and start over", "said the words for him", "reminded him not to stutter", "told him to speak more softly", "got angry", "corrected him", and "emphasized the sound of proper speech".

The category of *minimizing the problem* included such things as: "ignored it", "did nothing", "paid no attention to it", "gave him a little more attention", "just waited", and "nothing, just tried to have patience".

In 101, or 65 percent, of the cases parental response to the stuttering involved some active correction measure (see Table 5:2). In spite of the fact that the majority of these parents did things that most speech therapists would advise them not to do (for fear of inducing some complication of the stuttering), not one of the children was reported to have gotten worse. To the contrary, 64 percent of the youngsters treated in this fashion improved, 48 percent of them being reported to have recovered.

Casual inspection of Table 5:2 might suggest that the parental responses which were intended to minimize the problem were associated with a better rate of improvement (i.e., only eight of 47 still stuttering, with six stuttering only occasionally and 33 no longer stuttering). However, Table 5:2 omits an important variable. It was also found that parents were more inclined to employ active correction measures with those youngsters who evidenced the apparently more serious problem. The recovery rate among youngsters having only one disfluency type was significantly better than among those having more than one. Therefore, the seemingly higher rate of recovery among those youngsters whose parents reportedly minimized the problem is an artifact. Most likely the actual relationship expressed by these data is that recovery rate was higher among those youngsters who had a mild problem.

Table 5:2 Incidence of stuttering recovery in relation to how parents reported dealing with the stuttering (From Glasner and Rosenthal, 1957, Table 3.)

Parental Reaction	*Still Stuttering*	*Still Stutters Occasionally*	*Not Stuttering*	*Total*
Active correction	36	17	48	101
Minimizing	8	6	33	47
Seek professional help	1	1	2	4
Total	45	24	83	152*

*Information was incomplete for one subject.

Although we are not able, from these data, to assess adequately the relationship between severity of stuttering, type of parental intervention, and eventual outcome, it is certainly clear that parental efforts at active correction did not have a negative effect on stuttering. To the contrary, one would have to conclude that either stuttering improved in spite of parental corrections or that improvement was induced by them.

Results very similar to those of Glasner and Rosenthal, whose subjects were all Caucasian, were reported by Kelly and Frick (1966) in a comparable study of Negro children. The information was obtained through questionnaire interview of mothers of 197 children between 4 and 7 years of age. Thirty-nine (19 percent) of the total sample had been diagnosed as stutterers. Although many of these youngsters had been actively corrected by their parents, over half of them were no longer stuttering at the time of the interview.

In *The Onset of Stuttering*, Johnson *et al* (1959) presented the accumulated findings of three investigations of early stuttering which were concerned particularly with factors possibly significant in its inception and development. Most of the book is devoted to what the authors call "Study III," an extension and elaboration of two earlier works,[7] the pertinent results of which were covered earlier in this chapter.

In Study III parents of 150 "allegedly stuttering" children (experimental group) and 150 "allegedly nonstuttering" children (control group) participated in a comprehensive interview designed to elicit information thought to be relevant to their children's early stuttering (for the experimental group) or disfluency (for the control group). The two groups of children were matched for age, sex, and socioeconomic level. In both groups the children ranged in age from about 2½ to 7 years at the time of the investigation, their mean age being approximately 5 years.

Our interest here is limited essentially to the experimental group children and what happened in respect to their stuttering. The essential criterion for inclusion of a youngster in the experimental group was that the parents considered the child to be stuttering.[8] Evidently other people concurred in this diagnosis: the children were obtained through the clinical facilities of three midwestern universities, and most of the children had been referred to these clinics by speech clinicians, physicians, child welfare workers, special education teachers, and other school personnel. Further, the investigators themselves evidently did not disagree with the diagnosis.

The investigation was undertaken within a relatively short time after the child was first thought to be stuttering. The interval between reported age of onset and time of initial interview ranged from one to 39 months, the average interval being about 18 months.

On the average these children were 3½ years old when the stuttering was first noted. The authors state that few parents were able to remember the first instances of what they had regarded as their child's stuttering, yet nearly all gave accounts of " . . . something that they had noticed in their youngster's speaking . . ." (p. 133) over varying periods of time. According to the parents' descriptions, as recorded in the extensive tables of Study III, this "something" could be identified very realistically as stuttering. That is, what the parents reported to be characteristic of the speech of these children is consistent with well-documented identifications of the essential features of stuttering (see Chapter 4).

While the parents did attend to this "something," and also identified it as *stuttering*, the authors report that, "On the whole . . . they (the parents) did not consider it to be 'a problem' until about five months later, on the average." (p. 124.) At the same time, most of the parents reacted to it in an active manner, which certainly must have called the youngster's attention to the speech anomaly. Namely:

> . . . two thirds of the fathers and three fourths of the mothers indicated that something had been said to the child about what was referred to as his stuttering, and of these, about three fourths reported that something had been said either immediately or soon—that is, within one month. These persons had made a great variety of comments to the child . . . the most common of which were suggestions that he slow down, take it easy, and stop and start over. Such comments or suggestions were said to have been made as often as from five times a day to twenty-five times a month in roughly one third of the cases in the experimental group. (p. 149.)

Further, approximately one out of six fathers and one out of three mothers indicated that the child had been told that he was thought to have a speech defect or difficulty; yet, according to these parents, most of the children had not appeared to be bothered by this.

Follow-up information was obtained from parents of 118 of the experimental group children approximately two and a half years after the initial interview. At this time the average age of these youngsters would have been about 7½. Table 5:3 reveals that 36 percent of these youngsters can be considered to have recovered, that is, they were reported to have "No Problem" at the time of the follow-up evaluation. While it might be objected that these figures represent only parental judgment, it should be recalled that parental judgment of the *presence* of stuttering was the essential criterion for originally accepting these youngsters in the experimental group. The parental judgments regarding recovery were corroborated by the interviewers who had occasion to make a judgment about the speech of 50 of these youngsters at the time of follow-up. In

Table 5:3 Speech ratings made by parents of 118 of the stuttering youngsters at the time of follow-up evaluation (Adapted from Johnson et al., 1959, Table 57.)

Ratings	*Number of Cases*	*Percent of Total*
No problem	43	36.4
Much better	48	40.7
Somewhat better	13	11.0
Total improved	104	88.1
About the same	10	8.5
Somewhat worse	3	2.5
Much worse	1	0.8

fact, the interviewers made a more favorable evaluation of the children's speech than did the parents (see Table 5:4).

Contrary to the supposedly typical "development" (worsening) of stuttering, Table 5:3 indicates that fully 88 percent of this large number of young stutterers had shown at least some improvement within a period of about two and a half years. In 77 percent the improvement was substantial. In contrast, only four of the 118 cases were said to have gotten worse; this represents less than 4 percent of the total. The possible reasons for this improvement are not very well identified. Evidently the parents were not questioned routinely about their views in the matter (but see Table 5:5). The authors account for the improvement shown by these children as due to the counseling given the parents during the interview at the time of the initial assessment. They state:

> . . . the counseling that had been done and the experience of the interview and subsequent effects must have occasioned generally substantial changes in the relevant aspects of the thinking of most of the experimental group parents. (p. 174.)

Table 5:4 Speech ratings of the 50 stuttering youngsters as evaluated by both interviewers and mothers at the time of follow-up (Adapted from Johnson et al., 1959, Table 59.)

Ratings	*Interviewers*	*Mothers*
Normal speech	46	17
Still stuttering		
very mild	3	9
mild	1	15
average		5
moderately severe		4

This claim seems grossly presumptive,[9] particularly in view of the authors' description of the counseling afforded:

> . . . in general, counseling at the time of the original interview was restricted to that which could be done in the limited time available during the one day devoted in each case to the interview and related testing. It was of necessity, therefore, rather brief. . . . (p. 173.)

Further, parents of the "No Problem" group (the 43 children reported as recovered at the time of follow-up) and parents of the "Problem" group (those still stuttering) gave generally similar accounts of the recommendations made to them at the time of the original interview. At the same time, their testimony on such matters was "brief or fragmentary, vague, and undeveloped." Also, about 20 percent of the "No Problem" group parents and 27 percent of the "Problem" group parents had received, subsequent to the first interview, advice from other sources: doctors, teachers, public school speech therapists, psychologists, other clinics, and a few psychiatrists. The majority of those who had obtained this additional advice said they had followed it "either very thoroughly or fairly well." It does not seem realistic to look to such vague, indirect, and jumbled information for a sensible account of sources of improvement in these children's speech.

Table 5:5 Reasons given for the status of their child's speech at the time of follow-up interview by parents of 90 youngsters originally identified as stuttering (From Johnson et al., 1959.)*

Reasons Given	*"Problem" Group (Still Stuttering)*			*"No Problem" Group (Recovered)*
	Worse	*No Change*	*Better*	
Don't know	3	7	15	8
Child outgrew it				7
Child more mature			11	6
Child more confident				3
Parents ignored stuttering				4†
Child given more attention and chance to talk				3†
Less parental criticism				5†
Parental attitude improved				3†
Better parent-child relations			10†	
Poor parent-child relations	1†	1†		
Mother "very busy"		1†		
Father had heart attack		1		
Stronger habit	1			
Totals	5	10	36	39

*This table was compiled from narrative information reported on page 174 of *The Onset of Stuttering*. Evidently this kind of information was not obtained from parents of all youngsters at the time of follow-up; the tabled data represent only 76 percent of the cases participating in follow-up evaluation.

†Entries reflecting possible parental influence.

In contrast, it should be instructive to consider the reasons given by the parents themselves to account for the status of their child's speech at the time of the follow-up. Evidently this kind of information was not sought consistently by the interviewers. It receives very brief mention in the report and is incomplete in terms of numbers of cases as well as in potential detail. Pertinent statements were obtained from parents of 90 youngsters; the data are presented in Table 5:5.

Seventy-five of these children had shown improvement; 36 were said to be "better" and 39 were reported to have recovered. The answer most frequently given by their parents as explanation for the improvement was "don't know." The second most frequently stated reason was that the child was more mature. The meaning of "mature" is unclear; the original data give no more than this, and it is therefore left for us to assume that the parents must have meant a general maturity including both psychological and physiological changes. In only a third of the cases showing improvement did the parents suggest that the improvement was in some way influenced by what they did.

Stuttering Remission Among School-Age Children

A report by Bryne in 1931 is probably the earliest systematic attempt to assess the subsequent status of a large number of stutterers. From an initial population of 1,000 stutterers who had been seen in the speech therapy program of the Minneapolis public schools, Bryne was able to collect adequate information about 315 cases through questionnaires answered by parents, teachers, speech therapists and the former patients themselves. Most of the cases had been seen for therapy during kindergarten and the first three grades; 80 percent of them were still in school at the time of the inquiry. The length of time following dismissal from therapy ranged from one to 12 years; over 95 percent had been dismissed more than two years previously; over 73 percent had not been in therapy for over four years. The reliability of severity ratings was carefully checked by sampling and comparative methods.

A summary of Bryne's findings is presented in Table 5:6. At the time of inquiry 84 percent of the total number of cases were reported to be either no longer stuttering ("cleared") or to be better than when dismissed from therapy. Thirty-two percent of the total were reported to have recovered (no longer stuttering). It is especially instructive to note the very small number of cases who were reported to have gotten worse (only 4.4 percent of the total). It is equally relevant that in another 11 percent of the total group the stuttering reportedly remained the same.

The cases had been dismissed from therapy after varying degrees of

Table 5:6 Direction and degree of change in stuttering for 315 cases studied by Bryne (From Bryne, 1931, Table VI.)

SPEECH STATUS AT DISMISSAL FROM THERAPY		CONDITION OF SPEECH AT TIME OF INQUIRY							
		"HELD"		*STUTTER OCCAS.*		*SAME AS BEFORE THERAPY*		*WORSE*	
Condition of Speech	*Number of Cases*	*No.*	*per-cent*	*No.*	*per-cent*	*No.*	*per-cent*	*No.*	*per-cent*
Arrested (Cured)	83	36	43.4	42	50.6			5	6.0
		CLEARED		*BETTER*		*SAME*		*WORSE*	
Greatly Improved	31	9	29.0	11	35.5	7	22.6	4	12.9
Improved	149	44	29.5	82	55.0	20	13.3	4	12.9
Slightly Improved	36	12	33.3	20	58.4	3	8.3	4	2.2
Not Improved	16	1	6.3	9	56.3	5	31.3	1	6.2
Subtotal	232	66		122	38.8	35		9	
Total	315	102	32.2	164	52.0	35	11.2	14	4.4

rated improvement, from "Not Improved" to "Arrested" (cured). It will be seen from Table 5:6 that all of the cases dismissed as arrested did not "hold" (did not maintain the status of "arrested" stuttering). However, most of these cases (94 percent) either did "hold" or experienced recurrence of stuttering "...only occasionally under stress." Special attention is due those cases considered only "Slightly Improved" when dismissed from therapy: of these, 33 percent were reported to have stopped stuttering at the time of the inquiry, and an additional 58 percent had continued to make improvement.

Lest the reported improvement following therapy be interpreted as having stemmed in some direct or indirect way from the therapy experience (whether or not evidenced during the course of therapy), it is of particular interest to consider the statements given by the former patients regarding the reason for their improvement.

A rather wide variety of explanations was given to account for the amelioration of stuttering (see Table 5:7). The largest single proportion (22.9 percent) attributed their improvement to "relaxation." Equivalent numbers (14.6 and 14.3 percent respectively) reported improvement due to "speaking more deliberately" and becoming "better adjusted socially." The next largest categories are "don't know" (12.4 percent) and "no help" (11.4 percent). The remaining categories of notable size are "reading aloud" (7.9 percent) and "training received in speech class" (6.9 percent).

It seems reasonable to combine the categories of "don't know" and

Table 5:7 Reasons for speech improvement given by subjects in Bryne study (From Bryne, 1931, Table VII.)

Reason for Improvement	*IN SCHOOL*	*NOT IN SCHOOL* Em-ployed	Unem-ployed	*Total*	*Percent*
Relaxation	56	8	8	72	22.9
Became better adjusted socially	35	4	7	46	14.6
Speaking more deliberately	40	1	4	45	14.3
Doesn't know	33	2	4	39	12.4
No help	31	1	4	36	11.4
Reading aloud	21	1	3	25	7.9
Training received in speech Class	16	3	3	22	6.9
Deep breathing	1	4	2	7	2.2
Outgrown defect	3	1	1	5	1.6
Dramatization	2		2	4	1.3
Practice stuttering	4			4	1.3
Stopping to think	2	1	1	4	1.3
Shifting hands	3			3	.9
Tie-up with writing	1			1	.3
Good posture	1			1	.3
Health habits	1			1	.3
Total	250	26	39	315	100.0

"no help" and, as well, to include the category of "outgrown defect," since these three headings can justifiably be understood to have a similar connotation. That is, the individuals in these groups evidently could not specify anything to which they would attribute their improvement. It may be said, then, that the largest proportion of cases (25 percent) gave no reason for the amelioration of their stuttering.

The influence of therapy is indeterminable. Bryne reported that until two years prior to the time of inquiry the therapy approach in that school system had been entirely through mental hygiene; subsequently, methods based on cerebral dominance theory were added. It seems possible that improvement credited to "relaxation" and "better social adjustment" could have reflected an outcome of the therapy exposure. At the same time, only about 7 percent of the cases credited their improvement to their therapy experience. Furthermore, Bryne indicated that the therapists carried exceptionally heavy case loads, which clearly suggests that individual cases received proportionately little attention. If a mental hygiene approach were the mainstay of the therapy, one could justifiably question the extent to which therapy could have had an effect, in that a mental hygiene approach usually requires considerable time to produce results.

Bryne's findings indicate that continued improvement following discharge from therapy was related to improvement during therapy. This could indicate that therapy had a beneficial effect which persisted beyond the time of active involvement. On the other hand, those who improved (during and after therapy experience) might have improved regardless of their exposure to therapy. That is, the relationship between improvement and therapy may have been simply coincidental. In contrast, Bryne reported that improvement was closely related to the patient's claims of having made efforts to improve. She considered these findings reliable.

Two other matters deserve mention. First, the majority of these individuals, though improved, still stuttered to some degree in some circumstances. Most of them (79 percent) indicated that their stuttering was mostly likely to occur when they were "excited." Only 15 percent mentioned that current stuttering was associated with fear; 7 percent said it was likely to occur when they became angry.

The second item of interest involves a question Bryne asked these subjects about "inward" stutter: "Do you ever feel inwardly that you might stutter but do not do so." Over half of the cases (53 percent) responded affirmatively. Although Bryne questioned whether all cases were able to introspect with sufficient accuracy to make this a reliable finding, there is certainly some value to the fact that the responses were not routinely negative. Such findings have considerable bearing on the individual's perceptions of his speech characteristics and speaking tendencies, and the influence of such perceptions upon his speaking performance. For instance, they indicate that the threat of imminent stuttering is not necessarily followed by actual stuttering; they also indicate that individuals can recognize themselves as persons who have such tendencies, which though residual might erupt as actualities again, and yet not be so affected that the problem is renewed.

In 1936 Milisen and Johnson reported certain findings on recovery from stuttering which were obtained as part of a more extended study. These investigators began with an initial population of 8,000 school children who represented the enrollment in the entire school system of Council Bluffs, Iowa, from kindergarten through twelfth grade. From this overall population the authors identified 116 current stutterers and 85 former or "cured" cases.

Information about these individuals was gained through personal interview and case history analysis. Regarding the current and former stutterers as a group, the reported average age of onset of stuttering was 3 years: 70 percent had begun to stutter at or before 3 years, 36 percent began to stutter at approximately 18 months of age. The authors did not give actual figures regarding duration of stuttering or age range at recovery but did say that practically all of the former stutterers outgrew the disorder by the time they were 8 years old.

The Council Bluffs school system did not have a speech therapist at that time and most of these subjects had never been to a speech clinic. Further, the only advice they received about stuttering was obtained from the family physician and, with rare exceptions, " . . . any advice obtained was negligible." Thus, as the authors stated, " . . . these cases have not had clinical assistance in outgrowing their stuttering."

Thirty-two of the former stutterers were selected for more careful study. In all cases the authors' observations of the speech of these persons led them to agree with the individuals themselves that their speech was normal in character. However, some of the cases mentioned that they might infrequently stutter slightly under high nervous tension.

The majority of the recovered stutterers[10] offered some explanation for their recovery, and the authors included brief summary statements of these individual reports. Extracting the essential "reason for recovery" from these separate statements yields the following compilation: 7 subjects credited talking more slowly; 5 said change of handedness; 4 claimed some form of medical aid (1 for enlarged thyroid, 2 received worm medicine, 1 had tonsils removed); 1 joined a debating team; 1 reported that a general nervous condition cleared up; and another made a practice of "singing" her words.

One of the entries included in the category of "talking more slowly" represents a program of retraining which one of the recovered stutterers developed independently of any professional guidance. The "rules" of his program are as follows:

1. Talk very slowly at first until you are sure of yourself.

2. Try to divert your mind to something else when you are talking, for example, playing with a pencil or piece of paper.

3. Try to keep the speech in rhythmic form of some kind by keeping the body in motion, for example, tapping the foot or moving the fingers in a set rhythm. The activity must not attract attention.

4. If confused, stop entirely until you get straightened out and then start in again.

5. Just keep in mind that you stutter and it will help you to be careful.

6. Choose the words that are especially hard for you and practice them until you are sure of yourself.

On the basis of all the data the authors concluded that the factors most apparently related to disappearance of stuttering were: a slow rate of speaking, general improvement of physical condition, and change of handedness.

A subsequent study by Milisen (1936) yielded further information regarding recovery from stuttering among school-age children. The primary purpose of this study was to compare, on several measures of "special abilities and disabilities," school-age stutterers, former stutterers, articulation cases, and children with normal speech. A second purpose was to obtain general statistics about speech defects in a school population.

The groups selected for study were located through questionnaire survey, involving parents and teachers, of the school population of three towns in west central Pennsylvania. The original population consisted of 22,455 pupils[11] in grades 1 through 12. Milisen reported that 741 children, or approximately 3.3 percent of this population, had been identified as stutterers, either at that time or for some time in the past.

Of the total group who had been identified as stutterers, 32 percent were former, or recovered, stutterers. For these youngsters the average age of onset of stuttering was reported to be 3 years 8 months. The average duration of the stuttering was 2 years and 9 months. Recovery occurred " . . . before or during the school life of the children . . ." with the average age of disappearance of the stuttering being 6 years 9 months. Ninety-nine percent overcame their stuttering before or during the age of 14.

Milisen did not inquire into the possible reasons for the recovery but did indicate that the stuttering disappeared " . . . without any remedial work."

Andrews and Harris (1964) reported certain information about young stutterers discovered during the course of a large-scale longitudinal study of childhood diseases and disorders in Newcastle on Tyne, England. These children were followed from birth until they reached 16 years of age, with various kinds of assessments made at periodic intervals during that time. Health visitors, who saw the children regularly, reported the children who evidenced speech defects or abnormalities. These children were then seen by speech therapists, who also examined a random sample of one in ten children in the total population.

Within a population of 1,000 children, 43 were identified as stuttering during the 16-year period. Age of stuttering onset ranged from 2 to 10 years, the median age being 4 years (see Figure 5:1). Thirty-four of the children (79 percent) recovered; half of them remitted by age 5, the other half by age 12. Stuttering duration ranged from six months to nine and a half years. However, both median and modal durations were six months; nine children stuttered for a year, and only five stuttered longer than two years.

Of 25 children who began to stutter before age 5, 16 stuttered no longer than six months. While this might suggest some positive correlation between age of onset and duration, it will be noted that relatively brief periods of duration were also reported for 12 who had later onset ages.

Andrews and Harris did not discuss possible reasons for recovery in these youngsters. They implied a maturational factor for the children who recovered by age 5 (most of whom stuttered no longer than six months), referring to them as "developmental stutterers." They did not mention any influences that might have affected the remainder of the recovering children, who they identified as "benign stutterers." Actually, they made reference to all cases of remission as being "spontaneous" and did say that in no instance could it be claimed that the remission was induced by treatment.

Dickson (1965) investigated the incidence and remission of stuttering in 393 children attending kindergarten through ninth grade (the elementary school) at the State University College at Buffalo. The data for this study were obtained from questionnaires distributed to the parents of the youngsters.

Analysis of this material revealed that 42 of the children (slightly over 10 percent) were considered to stutter at the time or to have stuttered for some length of time in their earlier development. The age of onset of the stuttering was reported to range between 18 months and 12 years, with the majority (approximately 66 percent) beginning by 4 years of age. In slightly over a third of the cases the parents reported they

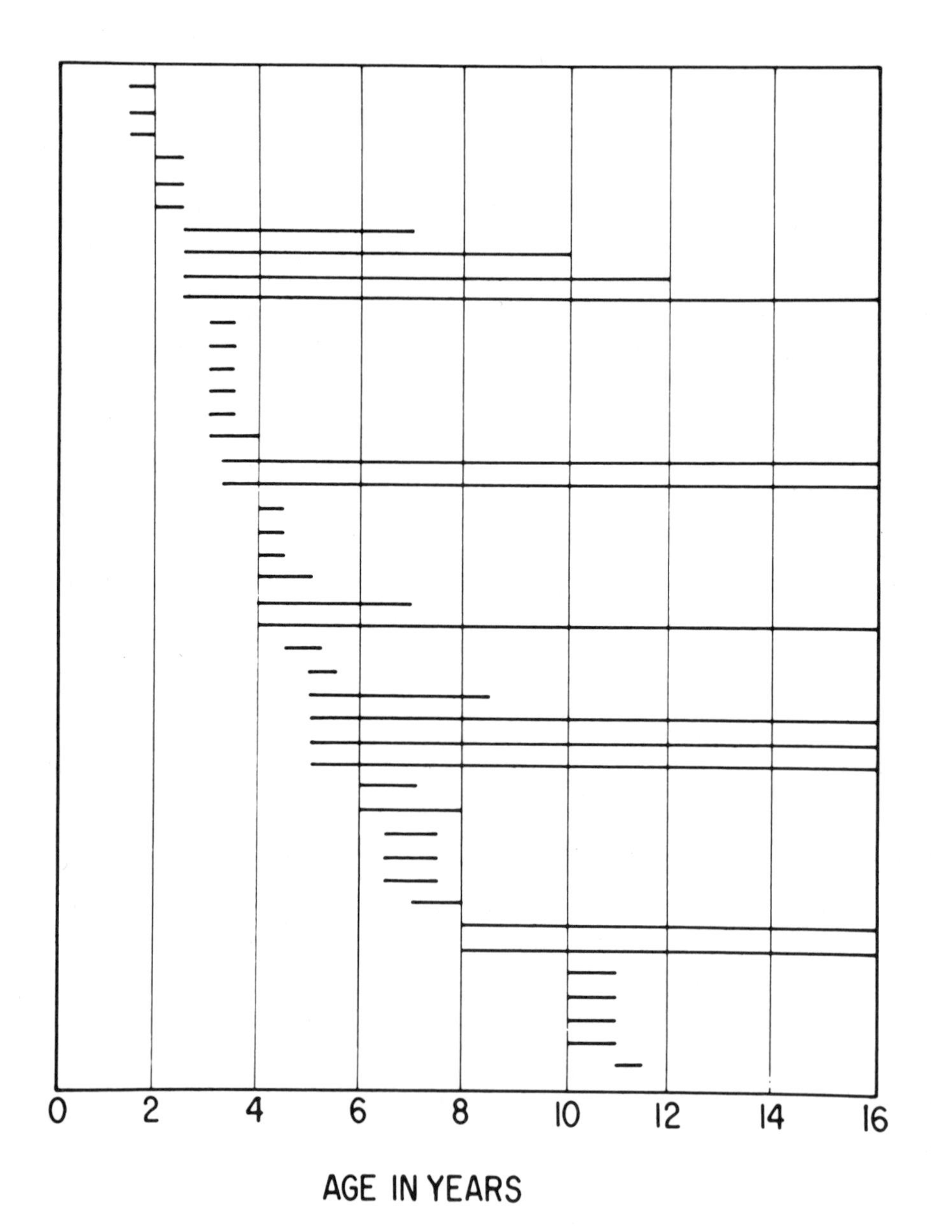

Figure 5:1 Onset and duration of stuttering in 43 cases (From Andrews and Harris, The Syndrome of Stuttering, 1964. By permission, S.I.M.P./Heinemann Medical, London)

believed the child knew he was having trouble speaking at the time it began or very soon thereafter.

Twenty-four of these children, or 51 percent, were reported to have experienced spontaneous remission. In a substantial majority of these cases (78 percent) the stuttering persisted at least six months; approximately 24 percent of them stuttered four years or longer. Four of the children were said to still have rare reoccurrences of their stuttering. Of the 18 cases reported to be still stuttering, not one parent reported the child's speech as having got worse.

Evidence of at least some amount of parental concern about the problem was reflected in the fact that 60 percent of the parents consulted some professional source (physician, teacher, speech therapist) regarding the stuttering. Further, parents were not personally passive or indirect in their own response to the problem. In 65 percent of the cases parents admonished the child as to what he should do not to stutter. The percentages of parents reporting use of several different suggestions are presented in Table 5:8. It is not known to what extent such suggestions were of benefit in the matter of recovery, but obviously they did not preclude it.

In a second study of similar nature Dickson obtained data from questionnaires distributed to the parents of 3,923 children in all the elementary and junior high schools in a suburban Buffalo, New York, community considered to be heterogenous in socioeconomic levels. Close to 10 percent of the children in each grade from kindergarten through ninth grade were considered by their parents to stutter or to have stuttered at some time in their development. Of the total of 369 children thus identified, 196 (53 percent) were reported to have recovered from stuttering independent of speech therapy.

The age of stuttering onset reported for the recovered youngsters ranged between 18 months and 10 years. Approximately half had begun to stutter by 3 years of age; 85 percent had begun by age 5. Seventy-one percent of these youngsters had recovered by 6 years of age; 83 percent were no longer stuttering by age 8. In the large majority of cases (70 percent) the symptoms did not persist for longer than two years. However, during this time the stuttering evidently was not minimal. For instance, parents of 48 percent of the children reported that the child experienced blocks in which it seemed hard to get the word out, or they noted "long pauses," or that the child was "taking a breath." In 46 percent of the cases the parents believed the child was aware of these features of the stuttering.

Parents of 65 percent of the youngsters who recovered admonished the child with some form of suggestion regarding what to do to minimize the stuttering. They types of correction advocated are presented in Table 5:8. Again, "slow down" and "think before you speak" occur prominently among the kinds of advice given. We do not know whether the stuttering remission was in some way due to, or positively influenced by, these suggestions, but we can be quite certain that at least they did not make the stuttering worse.

Stuttering Recovery Reported by Young Adults

Patricia Johnson (1951) studied 23 former stutterers, all but one of whom were college students between the ages of 17 and 31. These individuals gave adequate indication of having once been stutterers, as revealed in their recall of their former symptoms. Most of the subjects could not state a definite age of onset of stuttering, but each could recall having begun to stutter prior to a certain age. For most of them this was before age 8. Twelve rated their stuttering as having been mild, ten as "average," and one as severe. They could also recall their feelings about stuttering. Five said they had been relatively indifferent to it, but the other 18 reported having had varying kinds of personal reactions. These reactions included being annoyed, worried, embarrassed, ashamed, bothered, impatient, or feeling inferior, handicapped, or challenged. At the time of the inquiry, the majority of subjects still used terms such as "inferiority" and "handicap" to refer to their past stuttering.

Most of the subjects had experienced reactions from other people as well—parents, teachers and, to some extent, peers. References made by these subjects to the reactions of others, particularly parents and teachers, gave the author reason to describe these reactions as " . . . an active, not a passive, influence in the majority of instances . . ." and one which " . . . constituted a critical source in these persons' environment."

Table 5:8 Types of parental advice and percentage of remitting cases in which each was used (as reported by Dickson, 1965, 1967).

	PERCENTAGE OF USE	
1965 Study	*1967 Study*	
Type of advice	*(24 cases)*	*(196 cases)*
"Slow down"	43	51
"Think before you speak"	26	25
"Start over"	22	17
"Take a breath"	5	13
Other	2	0

Parental reactions varied. Six persons indicated that their parents did not think the stuttering was particularly important. However, the other 17 reported that their parents had thought of the stuttering as a handicap, several of them conveying the attitude that it was a mark of inferiority or a disgrace. Although many of the parents were said to have looked upon the stuttering as "a part of growing up," they were all concerned about it and gave their stuttering children advice regarding what to do to minimize it. Teachers also gave advice. The suggestion made most frequently by both parents and teachers was to "speak slowly and think."

These reactions evidently did not greatly affect the social adjustment of most of these individuals during the time they were stuttering. Sixteen reported that they had liked doing things with people and that they participated in various extracurricular school activities including student government, debate or acting, the school paper, athletics, music, and other socially involved interests. While 17 subjects indicated that their stuttering had affected their willingness to volunteer in class, only five said it had influenced their choice of vocation.

All of these individuals, to their own satisfaction and evidently to general appearances, had recovered from their stuttering.[12] At the same time, 15 of the 23 reported some residual tendency to stutter, which was said to be most likely to occur when they were excited or tired.

Although the subjects could report age of onset only approximately, they were more certain about age of recovery. Seven said they recovered by age 10; half of them recovered during adolescence; and four reported recovery at age 25 (see Table 5:9). Accepting the reported approximate age of onset as a minimal estimate, the duration of stuttering ranged from at least one to 15 years, with an average duration of approximately five and a half years. All but two reported their recovery as gradual.[13]

Table 5:9 Age at stuttering onset and at recovery as reported by 23 former stutterers (From Patricia Johnson, 1951.)

	AGE AT RECOVERY								
AGE AT ONSET	*8*	*9*	*10*	*11*	*12*	*13*	*14*	*15*	*25*
5	2								
6	1		1						
7		1	1			1		2	
8		1				3		2	
9									
10								1	1
11								1	1
12								1	1
13									1
14								1	

The reasons given for the recovery are listed in Table 5:10. Four subjects could offer no explanation. Two of seven subjects who had had speech therapy felt it had been responsible for their recovery; three others felt it had contributed. Five subjects attributed their recovery to speaking slowly and thinking before speaking; five more said this had helped. One person credited his recovery to "increased maturation and understanding"; another thought it was due mostly to his becoming more active socially. Except for "don't know," each of these reasons was also mentioned in conjunction with certain others. It is of special interest that the 15 subjects reporting a residual tendency to stutter indicated that they think they dealt with such recurrences by making an effort to speak slowly and think.

Wingate (1964) obtained information from 50 recovered stutterers, 32 males and 18 females, who ranged in age from 17 to 54, with the average age of the group being 34. All reported having stuttered for at least two years, most of them for five years or more. Although all of the subjects considered themselves to be "recovered," only half described their speech as that of a normally fluent individual. The other half said that they still had residual tendencies to stutter. The usual description given was that some minimal and transitory stuttering might reappear under conditions of particular stress, but that it could be controlled readily. They added that these tendencies present no problem in communication or in their personal adjustment. They indicated that they were regarded as normal speakers by their friends and acquaintances, and that most people evidently were not aware that they might occasionally "really" stutter.

The reported age of stuttering onset ranged from age 2 to 13,[14] but most of the subjects (25 males and 14 females) indicated they had started to stutter by 8 years of age. The median was 5 years for the males and 6 years for the females. As in the Patricia Johnson study, actual onset may well have occurred at a considerably earlier age than was reported.

Eight of the subjects rated their former stuttering as mild; 20 said it

Table 5:10 Reasons given for recovery by 23 former stutterers (From Patricia Johnson, 1951.)

REASON GIVEN	*TIMES*	
	Alone	*With other reason*
Don't know	4	
Slow down to think	5	5
Speech therapy	2	3
Increased maturation	1	9
More active	1	2

had been moderate; 22 reported it as severe. All but five said that they had had a negative reaction to their stuttering, most often mentioning such feelings as embarrassment, fear or shame. All reported their stuttering to vary with differing circumstances; all but six indicated that there were some situations in which they did not stutter at all.

They were not asked about the reactions of others, but inquiry was made about the psychological atmosphere in the home, since many people seem to think that unfavorable conditions in the home at least contribute to the persistence of stuttering. Forty percent of the subjects indicated that they had perceived their home atmosphere as unfavorable. Most often the reports described conditions which probably were not markedly adverse, such as tension, bickering, or excessive strictness. At the same time, eleven individuals described circumstances of a potentially more disrupting nature, such as alcoholism or a persistent atmosphere of parental hostility.

Recovery was reported from age 9 to age 40, though only three indicated recovery after 26 (see Table 5:11). Recovery age for females was scattered widely over this age range. Most (25) of the males, however, reported recovery between the ages of 13 and 20, or roughly the years of adolescence. All subjects but one reported the recovery as a gradual process.

The average duration of stuttering was 11.7 years for males and 12.2 years for females. Generally speaking, the later the onset of stuttering, the shorter its duration. This relationship was more evident for males than females, as reflected in correlation coefficients of −.69 and −.31 respectively.

Forty-four percent of these subjects had not received any therapy for their stuttering; the rest had had professional help of some kind (Table 5:12). Three kinds of professional assistance were described: symptomatic therapy, which was the most frequently obtained, supportive counseling, and psychotherapy. Symptomatic therapy refers to speech therapy focusing on the speech problem; supportive counseling refers to therapy undertaken with a speech therapist emphasizing the individual's attitudes and reactions involved with his speech; psychotherapy refers to psychological therapy in which the focus was the individual himself rather than the speech problem.

Most of those who received therapy reported having derived some benefit from it, yet only seven said that therapy was the important factor in their recovery; five had had symptomatic speech therapy and two had psychotherapy.

Table 5:13 identifies the major and secondary factors which these subjects said were responsible for their recovery. Again, one finds a not-

Table 5:11 Age at stuttering onset in relation to age at recovery as reported by 50 former stutterers (From Wingate, 1964.)

Age at Onset	*6*	*7*	*8*	*9*	*10*	*11*	*12*	*13*	*14*	*15*	*16*	*17*	*18*	*19*	*20*	*21*	*22*	*23*	*24*	*25*	*26*	*36*	*40*
Males																							
2								2		1		1											
3				1		1							1					1					
4									1				1	1	1	1					1		
5											2	1		1									
6													2		1								
7										1	1				1								1
8																							
9										1													
10									2		1			1									
11																							
12									1														
13																	1						
Females																							
2	1																			1		1	
3								1															
4					1												1			1	1		
5																							
6														1									
7				1							1		1								1		
8							1																
9																							
10													1										
11																		1					
12																							1
13																							
20																				1			

Table 5:12 Type of assistance obtained and reported benefit, as listed by 50 recovered stutterers (From Wingate, 1964.)

	Assistance		Benefit*			
			MALES		FEMALES	
	MALES	FEMALES	Yes	No	Yes	No
None	11	9				
Lay suggestions only†		2			2	
Symptomatic therapy	15	4	13	2	1	3
Supportive counseling	4	1			1	
Symptomatic and supportive		1			1	
Psychotherapy	2	1	1		1	

*Number of persons indicating that the reported assistance was at least of some benefit to them.
†Fifty-two percent of those reporting professional help also indicated they had received "lay" advice or suggestions.

Table 5:13 Factors identified by 50 former stutterers as responsible for their recovery (From Wingate, 1964.)

FACTOR	STATED AS PRIMARY FACTOR		STATED AS SECONDARY FACTOR*	
	Males	Females	Males	Females
Don't know	4	1		
Attitude change:				
Self	7	3	1	1
Speech	4	2	3	1
Both	2	2		
Practice:				
Speaking	4	4	3	1
Methods	4	1		
Speech therapy	5	0	3	1
Environmental change	1	3	5	3
Relaxation	0	1	2	1
Psychotherapy	1	1		

*Figures for the secondary factors do not represent number of cases; more than half of the subjects did not mention a secondary factor whereas several mentioned two.

able percentage who could offer no explanation. Among those who did account for the change, most gave reasons representing either a change in attitude or intentionally undertaking a direct attack on the speech problem.

Change in attitude was directed in some cases toward self-appraisal, as expressed in such statemements as "an acceptance of myself, an increasing awareness of my capabilities and limitations" or, "loss of feeling of inferiority with increase in age and accomplishments." In other cases the attitude change was focused on the speech problem itself. For some it took the form of desensitization, such as, "the fact that I admitted openly I stuttered and didn't try to pretend I didn't," or "just talking about it and not being ashamed of it." For others the attitude change was expressed simply as a resolve to do something about the stuttering, for example, "the knowledge that my father's youngest sister had overcome stuttering and the support this aunt gave me to persevere toward the same end," or "being able to feel that I could conquer it and that it need not continue to make me a social misfit."

Purposefully working on speech improvement tended to follow one of two emphases. One was to make a special effort to gain speaking experience, such as, "having to speak before groups through debate and public speaking in school, and of having to prepare and practice presentation," or "practice and a lot of speaking to gain self-confidence." The other was the use of certain methods of control, such as "learning to deal with the mechanical aspects of speech, especially when I knew a difficult sound was coming up," or "breath control and learning to relax before speaking or reading out loud."

A number of these subjects attributed their recovery to actions which are quite contradictory to currently held beliefs regarding what is necessary for amelioration of stuttering. For instance: "People bringing it to my attention and not listening to me because of my stuttering. I wanted my parents to like me, so I tried very hard to please them by not stuttering, especially my father who could not accept any imperfection,"; or, "dramatic training"; or "learning a foreign language, which gave me a chance to breathe correctly and slowly pronounce the words." Several mentioned "speaking more slowly," and some reported the persistent use of certain unusual techniques, such as, "reading the Bible out loud nightly may have taught me how to speak and breathe properly," or "the use of key words to get started and knowing what to avoid as trouble areas," or "speaking the difficult words aloud to myself alone shortly after the difficulty so I could remember the words."

For most of these subjects recovery was not a passive process, and there are many clear assertions of commitment and application. The obvious implication is that personal motivation was one important factor common to efforts of many of these subjects.

Shearer and Williams (1965) screened recovered stutterers from students examined at the time of college entrance. Since these authors were interested only in self-recovery, they selected from this original group[15] 58 individuals (43 males and 15 females) who had never received professional help for their stuttering. These individuals were between 17 and 20 years of age at the time of the interview.

All reported having stuttered "at an early age" and could recall the approximate ages of onset and recovery. Recollection was sufficiently clear that 86 percent of the subjects were able to describe the specific characteristics of their stuttering patterns.

The subjects also could recall reactions to their stuttering. Fifty-eight percent remembered some personal embarrassment or discomfort associated with the stuttering; 29 percent reported that a parent, teacher, or peer had called attention to it.

Age at time of recovery covered a fairly wide range, from 5 to 17 years of age. Recoveries occurred at every age level but were proportionately higher in the adolescent years (see Table 5:14). Every one of the subjects reported recovery to have been a gradual process.

All of these individuals considered themselves to be normal speakers subsequent to the date of recovery and reported that the people with whom they associated also thought of them as normal speakers. At the same time, 64 percent said that they still might stutter occasionally (see Table 5:14). Shearer and Williams noted a relationship between this re-

Table 5:14 Age of self-recovery and residual stuttering tendency reported by 58 recovered stutterers (From Shearer and Williams, 1965, Tables 1 and 2.)

AGE AT RECOVERY	NUMBER OF CASES	NUMBER OF CASES REPORTING RESIDUAL STUTTERING TENDENCY	
		Less than once per month	More than once per month
5	5		
6	2		
7	4		
8	5		
9	4	19	7
10	3		
11	3		
12	3		
13	7		
14	5		
15	8	6	26
16	7		
17	3		

sidual tendency to stutter and stated age of recovery: those recovering after age 13 reported some remaining tendency to stutter more often than did those who recovered prior to age 13.

Among the several reasons given by these subjects to account for their recovery, "speaking more slowly" was mentioned most often—by 69 percent of the subjects. Speaking more slowly was frequently mentioned in conjunction with one of several other reasons. Almost half of the subjects (43 percent) reported that "thinking before speaking" was a factor in their recovery. Other factors, mentioned less often, were: achieving greater self-confidence (26 percent), becoming more aware of the problem (22 percent), speaking more deliberately (20 percent), and relaxing (19 percent).

Sheehan and Martyn (1970) also reported on recovered stutterers obtained by screening students at the time of college entrance. This report incorporates material presented in two earlier publications (Sheehan and Martyn, 1966; Martyn and Sheehan, 1968). To avoid duplication of the findings, and since the authors' treatment of the information varies somewhat in the three reports, we will attempt to summarize the relevant information from each of the reports.[16]

The last report (Sheehan and Martyn, 1970) indicated that the total contact population consisted of 5,138 students screened during registration periods at three California universities. The investigators discovered 147 individuals who claimed to have stuttered at some time in their lives. Reportedly, 116 of these persons had recovered, a recovery ratio of 78 percent in this particular sample.

Information regarding stuttering and recovery was obtained through structured individual interviews. Evidently only 101 of the recovered stutterers participated in this process. The age range at the time of interview extended from 17 to 56, the average age being 24. Asked to estimate the severity of their stuttering at its worst, 58 reported it to have been mild, 35 said moderate, and eight severe. Neither the extent of this "worst" period nor the total duration of the stuttering was reported. Age at stuttering onset and span of duration were not reported, although one of the earlier reports (see below) gave data on age at the time of recovery.

A substantial majority of these recovered stutterers had not received speech therapy, including persons who said their stuttering had been moderate or severe; that is, recovery without therapy was not limited to individuals with mild stuttering. At the same time, recovery was related to reported level of severity: 87 percent of all identified stutterers in the mild category, 75 percent of the moderate, and 50 percent of the severe. This relationship was said to be statistically significant. Therapy experience was reported more frequently by those who said their stuttering had been moderate or severe: those individuals perceived as having more of a problem were more likely to have received therapy. However, no statistical relationship was found between recovery and therapeutic intervention. Moreover, most of those who had had therapy did not report having obtained very substantial benefit from it. The authors indicated that recovery for these individuals had been a gradual process, but they did not supply pertinent data.

Data on age of recovery were mentioned only in the second report (Martyn and Sheehan, 1968). This information, included in Table 5:17, involves 48 cases, approximately half the number on which discussion in the summary report is based. It should be noted that over half of these individuals reported recovery after puberty.

Information on the former stutterers' own views as to what was responsible for their recovery was contained in the first and second reports. The findings, reflecting statements made by 80 persons, are reproduced in Table 5:15. Unfortunately, the information is confounded by the manner of presentation[17] and inconsistency in categorization. Nevertheless, this material is consistent with the relevant findings in other studies which have dealt more systematically with this information. That is, one also finds here substantial testimony to the efficacy of such measures as "slowing down" and "practice in speaking." There is also indication that at least a fair number of individuals could give no reason for their recovery.

Cooper (1972) reported a study in which the student population in the junior and senior high schools of Tuscaloosa, Alabama, was screened. From a total population of 5,054 students the investigators identified 187 individuals who reported a history of stuttering. Of these,

Table 5:15 Reason for recovery given by 80 former stutterers as reported by Sheehan and Martyn (1966) and Martyn and Sheehan (1968)

1966 REPORT N = 32 Reason Given	*Individuals*	*1968 REPORT N = 48* Reason Given	*Individuals*
Don't know or other*	12	Don't know	4
		Other*	13
Slowing Down and Relaxing	11	Self Therapy†	30
Speaking More and Improved Self-Concept	8		
Speech Therapy	1	Speech Therapy	1

*The meaning of "other" is not explained by the authors
†This category includes: talking more, slowing down, taking speech courses.

119 were still stuttering and 68 had recovered, yielding a recovery ratio of 36 percent.

Information was obtained through individual interviews. Asked to estimate the severity of their stuttering at its worst, 46 percent reported that it had been mild, 36 percent said moderate, and 17 percent severe. As in the Sheehan and Martyn report, the extent of this "worst" period was not determined. Rate of recovery was related to reported level of severity; among all the stutterers recovery was achieved by 49 percent of the mild stutterers, 40 percent of the moderate, and 30 percent of the severe. This relationship was reported to be not statistically significant.

Fifty-two (76 percent) of the recovered stutterers had not had treatment. This included persons representing all severity levels, although those reporting severe stuttering were more likely to have received therapy. However, therapy evidently had little effect: statistical analysis indicated no significant relationship between therapy and recovery when level of severity was held constant.

Cooper did not report such other data as ages of onset and recovery, or what the subjects thought was responsible for their recovery. He mentioned that recovery had been gradual in these subjects, but gave no specific data.

SUMMARY AND DISCUSSION OF "RECOVERY" FINDINGS

The foregoing material presents a picture of stuttering considerably different from the image that has been widely accepted for many years. The evidence accumulated here would seem to require a substantial reorientation in the ways in which we have come to think and talk about stuttering and demands a considerable readjustment in our conceptions of the management of stuttering—both in regard to direct therapy with the patient and in counseling of those who are close to and interested in him.

It is good to be reminded that much of this evidence is in rough form. Certain portions of the data lack precision and many of the values are approximations. At the same time, not all of the studies involve recollection and estimate. Studies employing more direct procedures and current appraisal yielded findings that are consistent with the results from studies which were retrospective. In toto, these data are adequate to convey certain undeniable realities. In particular, some findings recur so consistently that one cannot fail to heed their impact and significance. Table 5:16 attempts a summary of the more extensively documented findings. There are other features, however, that should not be ignored and which we will mention presently.

The Progression of Stuttering

The most impressive feature of the data from these studies is the overwhelming evidence that stuttering does not by any means typically "develop" or "grow." Quite to the contrary, the evidence consistently indicates that it is actually rather rare for stuttering to get worse. Moreover, the considerable available data indicate that it is not even common for stuttering to remain the same over the course of years. Most often, it would appear, stuttering improves. In fact, in a very substantial number of cases it improves to the extent that the individual can be considered to have "recovered," an appraisal shared by the patient, his family, and associates. The extent of recovery is best reflected in the overall average computed in Table 5:16. This figure indicates a ratio of recovery, relative to total identified stutterers, of 42 percent. Only two of the 12 values depart notably from this average figure.[18]

The Value of Therapy

A second highly impressive and consistent finding is that professional therapy is by no means necessary or sufficient to recovery from stuttering. Most of these persons did not have professional assistance, yet they achieved a goal that too frequently eludes many therapists. Additionally, among individuals who did have formal assistance the extent of the therapy was evidently minimal. This may be a partial explanation for the finding that very few persons thought the therapy was responsible for their recovery. Yet this does not account adequately for the compelling impression that, for the most part, therapy was of limited benefit. There must have been among these hundreds of cases many individuals who received substantial professional assistance; yet while some say they were helped by therapy, it is rare to find testimony that therapy provided the resolution of the problem.

Similarly, professionally based parental counseling is obviously not necessary to the amelioration of stuttering. In the vast majority of the many cases covered in these studies there is little evidence of effort at, or opportunity for, parental counseling. Although there is, within these reports, some claim that parental counseling influenced a favorable out-

Table 5:16 Summary of pertinent information from reports of stuttering recovery.

SOURCE	AGE RANGE AT TIME OF INTERVIEW	SIZE OF REFERENCE POPULATION	TOTAL STUTTERERS IDENTIFIED	PERCENT STUTTERING PREVALENCE	RECOVERED STUTTERERS	
					Number	Percent
Kelly and Frick	4- 7	197	39	19.8	20	51
Glasner & Rosenthal	5- 7	996	153	15.4	83	54
Johnson, W. (1955)	5-11		46		25	54
Johnson, W. (1959)	5-10		150†		43	36
Dickson, I. (1965)	5-14	393	42	10.7	24	57
Dickson, II. (1967)	5-14	3923	369	9.4	196	53
Andrews & Harris	2-16	1000	43	4.3	34	79
Milisen & Johnson	5-17	7452	201	2.7	85	42
Milisen	6-18	22455*	741	3.3	227	32
Cooper	12-18	5054	187	3.8	68	36
Bryne	6-20		315		102	32
Shearer	17-20				58	
Johnson, Patricia	17-31				23	
Wingate	17-54				50	
Sheehan & Martyn	17-56	5138	147	2.9	116	78
Totals			2433		1023‡	42

*Estimated from the authors' figures.
†The follow-up group consisted of 118 of these subjects.
‡Excluding those having no "total stutterers" figure.

Table 5:16 (Cont.)

PERCENT IDENTIFIED STUTTERERS WHO WERE			NO. OF RECOVERED STUTTERERS WHO		PERCENT RECOVERED STUTTERERS REPORTING		REPORT OF		
Improved§	*Same*	*Worse*	*Rec'd therapy*	*Credit therapy*	*Don't know*	*Residual tendency*	*Active correction*	*Slow down*	*Gradual recovery*
15	33	0	0				x	x	
16	29	0	0				x	x	
30	13	2	0						x
51	7	3	0		35		x	x	x
	43	0				17	x	x	x
		0					x	x	x
			0						
			0		40	x	x	x	
							x		
			16				x		x
52	11	4	102	7	25	85		x	
			0			64	x	x	x
			7	2	17	69	x	x	x
			28	7	10	50	x	x	x
			35	2	16		x	x	x

§In addition to those recovered.

come of the stuttering in some instances, there is actually no reasonable evidence that such was the case even for this small number. We are faced with the realization that if parental influence was in some way beneficial, it operated independently of someone with professional training.

Parental Intervention

In contrast to the lack of evidence that stuttering was beneficially influenced by professional counseling, there is substantial evidence that those things which parents are likely to do "naturally" are not as harmful as we have been led to believe.

For some time it has been widely accepted that parental suggestions to the child that he slow down, or think before he speaks, or stop and start over will only aggravate the problem. The extensive material reviewed here contradicts this contention. Evidently such admonitions do not necessarily have a deleterious effect on stuttering—even with children who are quite young. Further, there is evidence that corrective measures of an even more "active" nature—extending even to physical punishment—do not regularly have a negative effect on stuttering.

That parental intervention does not typically exacerbate stuttering is in itself a finding of great value, for this alone should occasion a fundamental reorientation in attitude toward management. However, one must also wonder whether this finding means that the reported parental intervention simply had no negative effect on the problem. Should we not consider that it might have done some good, especially in view of the fact that most of these children recovered? This possibility is enhanced by the finding that many of the recovered stutterers credited their recovery to "slowing down."

The Effect of Awareness

Awareness of stuttering is a matter closely related to the topic of parental intervention. The majority of these recovered stutterers had been aware of their stuttering; not only those who gave personal recollections of their stuttering, but also many youngsters for whom the relevant information was reported by someone else.

The implication from the findings regarding awareness is the same as those for parental intervention—it does not necessarily lead to unfortunate consequences. In fact, it is clear that awareness of stuttering does not regularly lead to a negative reaction to it. In particular, awareness of stuttering does not typically elicit any specific kind of negative reaction, such as fear. Although fear has long occupied a prominent place in explanations of stuttering, it does not figure noticeably in the findings of these studies. Even where evidence for it was specifically sought (for example, in the Patricia Johnson study), we find that it is by no means ubiquitous. Further, even where present, its relation to stuttering is not clear; twelve of Patricia Johnson's (1951) subjects reported recovery from stuttering before they lost their fear of it, and in the remaining cases there is no reason to believe that fear augmented the stuttering.

More importantly, however, there is evidence that even when negative feeling does become involved in the problem, it does not necessarily lead to its exacerbation. A negative reaction may have relatively little effect on the stuttering; on the other hand it may well serve as a motivation to do something about the problem.

Much of this material would seem to force acknowledgement that in many cases awareness of stuttering is clearly associated with a favorable outcome. Undoubtedly something more than awareness is required, but we must not lose sight of the real possibility that awareness can have a beneficial influence on stuttering. At least we can be assured that there is little justification for the alarmed preoccupation with preventing a child's awareness of stuttering which has characterized approaches to management for so many years.

Some Technical Matters

Stuttering has been called a disorder of childhood because in almost all cases stuttering begins during the early childhood years. These recovery findings add a new dimension to the identification of stuttering as a disorder of childhood, namely, that stuttering is a disorder *manifested* largely during the years of childhood. This would seem to be the broad inference to be derived from the data as presented in Table 5:17. However, because of differing design and organization, it is unfortunately not possible to combine data from all of the studies for purposes of computation. It is for this reason that the pertinent information from these studies has been separated into three categories, Group A includes those studies which: (a) dealt with subject groups having a lower age limit of 5 or less; (b) lend themselves to ordering recovery data for the first two age-level headings; and (c) indicate the size of a reference group of all identified stutterers. Group B includes those studies which: (a) indicate the size of the total stuttering sample; but (b) do not indicate recovery age other than by implication from the upper age limit of the sample studied. Group C includes those studies which: (a) did not have the reference figures of a total stutterer sample size; (b) dealt with adolescents

Table 5:17 Age at time of recovery from stuttering as reported in the studies reviewed.

SOURCE	AGE RANGE	TOTAL IDENTIFIED STUTTERERS	NUMBER OF RECOVERED STUTTERERS	Reported age at recovery					
				by 8	9-14	15-18	19-22	23-26	27†
A									
Kelly and Frick	4- 7	39	20	20					
Glasner and Rosenthal	5- 7	153	83	83					
Johnson, W. (1955)	5-11	46	25	18	7				
Johnson, W. (1959)	5-10	118	43	43					
Andrews and Harris	2-16	43	34	26	8				
Milisen and Johnson	5-17	201	85	80†	5†				
Subtotals		500	290	270	20				
B									
Dickson I (1965)	5-14	42	24		24				
Dickson II (1967)	5-14	369	196		196				
Milisen	6-18	741	227		227				
Cooper	12-14	103	31	31					
	15-18	84	37			37			
Subtotals		1339	515		478	37			
C									
Shearer	17-20		58	16	25	17			
Johnson, P.	17-31		23	3	8	8		4	
Wingate	17-54		50	1	12	16	10	8	3
Martyn and Sheehan	17-56		48	6†	17†	10	13	1	1
Subtotals			179	26	62	51	23	13	4

*Many of the youngsters in these studies must have recovered before age 8. For instance, Milisen reported that the average age at recovery for his 227 subjects was 6 years 9 months.

†Estimated from the authors' figures.

and adults; and (c) gave specific information regarding reported age at recovery.

The data of Table 5:17 yield a fair corroboration of the early estimates made by Johnson (1934) and Bryngelson (1938) that from 35 to 40 percent of stuttering youngsters no longer stutter by 8 years of age. The figures in the table indicate that 54 percent of the children represented by the studies in group "A" alone recovered by age 8. It is more than likely that the studies in group "B" would have yielded similar findings had ages of recovery been tabulated. It is practically certain, for instance, that a majority of Milisen's 227 subjects recovered by age 8, since he reported the average age at recovery to be 6 years 9 months. It is also very likely that at least a fair number of the 251 cases represented in the reports of Cooper and Dickson actually recovered by age 8.

One can say with somewhat greater confidence that the data indicate an overall recovery rate of approximately 43 percent by age 14. However, this value also may be low, since in four of the studies in Group A, which encompass a total of 356 youngsters originally identified as stutterers, the age range did not extend beyond 11.

The pattern of reported recovery age seems to be in some measure a function of the age range studied. It appears that as the age range increases one finds recovery extending into older age levels. One also finds proportionately less frequent report of recovery at the younger age levels. The latter feature might well reflect distortion due to recollection; it also might suggest that some cases of early stuttering and remission are forgotten. In sum, there is reason to suspect that the overall figure for rate of recovery may be well above the composite value of 42 percent computed from those studies reviewed here which permit such combination.

The provisional inference from this material is, then, that the bulk of stuttering recovery takes place in childhood, a sizable amount occurs in adolescence, and a lesser amount in adulthood. It is particularly noteworthy to find so much recovery during adolescence, an era in development that is generally believed to be a period of considerable psychosocial stress. Evidently these purported stresses are not generally of such impact on stutterers that they preclude stuttering remission. Recovery beyond adolescence seems less probable, yet it evidently does happen. Indirect corroboration of such findings is suggested by the results of a survey conducted by Shames and Beams (1952). They reported a definite downward trend in the number of stutterers found in older age groups.

The severity judgments reported in this material are probably the most equivocal of the data considered. Research (e.g., Aron, 1967; Cullinan, Prather, and Williams, 1963; Naylor, R. V., 1953) has shown that judgment of stuttering severity is not a simple matter, and that self-judgments of severity do not regularly correspond well with judgments made by an observer. The problem is undoubtedly magnified when judgments are retrospective. On the other hand, use of a three-point scale (as was the case in almost all of these studies) modifies the reservation to some extent.

However, we need not be so concerned here with the precision of the severity judgments, nor even their individual validity. Our interest centers more in whether these reports, on the whole, are credible in the sense that these recovered stutterers represented a range of severity. Once again, the studies are consistent in reporting recovery for individuals reporting all three severity levels. Evidently there is also an adequate representation of individuals at each level of severity; that is, there is not a highly disproportionate number of cases reporting mild stuttering. This feature assumes particular significance in view of the fact that stutterers often underestimate the severity of their stuttering.

We should not overlook the suggestion from these data that frequency of recovery is related to severity level, being more likely in cases reporting lesser severity. Such a relationship would be consistent with commonsense expectation. However, it is not solidly established by the findings, even if they are accepted at face value. The important finding is that level of severity does not necessarily limit the expectation of recovery in any particular case.

In all reports making mention of the length of time involved in recovery the process was reported as gradual. Some reports did not record specific data on the matter, and the implication was that recovery occurred gradually in all cases. Among those reports making a specific statement of this information (P. Johnson, 1951; Shearer, 1965; Wingate, 1964), the claim of rapid recovery was made very rarely. The significance of gradual recovery for an understanding of stuttering and its remission is presently a matter of conjecture. However, it would seem to suggest rather strongly the operation of maturational factors. Of course, it might also reflect that a good deal of time is required for an individual to learn his techniques of coping with the problem. But at least this finding provides valuable information for management purposes: therapist, patient, and parent can be better prepared for realistic expectations in regard to the course of improvement.

In many cases recovery may not amount to "cure" in the ordinary sense. For most people "cure" appears to signify a complete return to, or attainment of, normality, with no trace of the malady. This would seem to be the aspiration of many stutterers, or families of stutterers, who seek help, yet it seems a likely prospect that many of them will retain some vestige of the disorder. Report of residual stuttering tendencies was mentioned regularly in those publications which considered the matter (see Table 5:16).

Apparently much of the information about residual tendencies was obtained in studies reporting a large proportion of recoveries after age 12. The three studies which gave specific information on both residual tendencies and ages of recovery were those of Patricia Johnson (1951), Shearer (1965), and Wingate (1964). If the recovery figures for these three studies are combined, 70 percent of the recoveries occurred after age 12. In all three studies the incidence of reported residual tendencies is quite high. At the same time, an indeterminate amount of residual tendency must also occur in many cases of earlier remission: Dickson (1965) reported a 17 percent frequency of residual tendency in his subjects, whose ages ranged from 5 to 14 years. Also, childhood recoveries made up a substantial proportion of the cases reported by Bryne (1931) and Milisen and Johnson (1936), both of whom reported residual tendencies.

The evidence of residual tendency does not qualify the matter of recovery in the sense of raising the question as to whether these individuals have "really" recovered. The typical finding about residual tendencies is that they are vestiges of former stuttering—they are covert or very minimal aspects of stutterings, known only to the former stutterer himself. They are potential stutterings that rarely become manifest, at least in readily recognizable form. Usually they were said to occur in association with episodes of emotional arousal, notably excitement. The significance of residual tendencies lies in its value for realistic counseling of the stutterer and those close to him. We will return to this in a later chapter.

Some Practical Matters

The data from these studies most likely to elicit controversy are those which pertain to the reasons given by these individuals for their recovery, because they are so clearly contrary to what should have been found if current beliefs about stuttering are accurate.

In all studies where statements were obtained regarding what was thought to be the reason for recovery, a sizable proportion of the respondents indicated that they did not know, or that the problem was outgrown. Such replies were given by from 10 to 40 percent of individuals in six studies (cf. Table 5:17), which represent a combined sample of 330 recovered stutterers. Similar reasons probably would have been given for a substantial number of the recoveries among the cases reported by Andrews (1964), Dickson (1965, 1967), Glasner and Rosenthal (1957), Johnson (1955), and Kelly and Frick (1966) since these studies all dealt with younger children who had not had therapy.

The currently favored theories, based on complexities of the individual's psychology and the influences of his environment, are not only confounded by the fact of unassisted recovery but are particularly embarrassed by recovered stutterers' reports that they do not know why they recovered. That is, if stuttering is adequately accounted for as an expression of psychological pressures within or upon the individual, then recovery should demonstrably be associated with relief of those pressures. Of course, it is possible for protagonists of psychological theories to contend that the appropriate relief occurred without the individual's awareness. For most cases—at least those old enough to make the report personally—this claim would quite clearly be unreasonable; for the remainder such an explanation would still be pure speculation. A much less devious, and more realistic and defensible, explanation of the "don't know" and similar explanations of recovery is that they reflect a maturational process.

The more substantive reasons for recovery are also very likely to meet with objection from sources within the profession, since they contradict well-entrenched notions about what is worthwhile, what is useless, and what is damaging to the amelioration of stuttering.

The reasons for recovery reported in these studies represent for the most part naive testimony. Yet there is no good reason why the testimony of these persons is any less credible, reliable, or valid than that of any other stutterer, or stutterer's therapist, who has offered the account of his personal experience. In fact, one might reasonably contend that in the field of stuttering naive testimony has more inherent credibility, since it is not likely to be contaminated by some predilection based on sophistication.

Of course, testimony should always be recognized as an individual statement, representing only the individual who gives it. But the import of testimony increases in proportion to the extent to which the same message recurs—if obtained separately and independently. We cannot overlook such patterns of testimony if we are seriously intent on developing a realistic approach to the management of stuttering. We should also interrelate it with other information that bears meaningfully on the amelioration of stuttering. We will defer the latter objective until a subsequent chapter. For the moment, let us consider several items which deserve our attention because of their recurrence in the testimony of these recovered stutterers.

For a long time the idea of suggesting to a stutterer that he slow down has been either dismissed off-handedly as useless or repudiated as actually harmful. As noted earlier, many of the youngsters covered in these studies had been admonished to slow down, and, although no evidence was available that this had a beneficial effect, it obviously did not do harm. It becomes even more illuminating, then, to find among these studies of recovery such frequent report that "slowing down" (or some variant of it) was given as either the principal or a contributing reason for recovery (cf. Table 5:16).

Perhaps the technique of slowing down has found disfavor within the profession because it is just too obvious and too commonplace; it has no aura of special process, no pedigree of scientific derivation, no suggestion of esoteric knowledge. However this may be, it seems clear that one source of the premature denial of its value has been the claim made by some stutterers that they have tried it unsuccessfully. The widespread acceptance of such testimony has been abetted by a failure to inquire of these individuals how long and with what diligence the technique was tried. The implication here is that those who claimed no success with the technique may have put forth minimal effort. It is also unfortunate that contrary testimony has been either not available or not considered.

Another item encountered with impressive frequency among the stated reasons for recovery is one that might best be summarized as "practice in speaking." This does not mean the kind of speaking activity that is incorporated in such procedures as voluntary stuttering, modified stuttering, or "go ahead and talk even though you stutter." It consisted rather of directing attention to the process of speaking, of exercising a certain deliberateness, of making an effort to develop a "feel" for the acts and sequence of events that constitute speaking. It also included taking advantage of, or creating, opportunities to provide themselves with these experiences.

One should appreciate that there is a kind of interrelationship between the activites of slowing down and deliberateness. There is also an interlacing of these two procedures with a third feature that appears to stand out in the findings of these recovery studies—motivation.

In a fair number of cases stuttering remission was a relatively passive process; for instance, in the recovery of the many children for whom no stated reason for recovery was given, and for those older individuals who could not state a reason. On the other hand, it is clear that a substantial number of these recovered stutterers committed themselves in some measure to an active role. The value of motivation and involvement is not a novel contribution to the treatment of stuttering, but its significance is underscored by its recurrence in these findings.

Of the several major points that have been derived from analysis of these recovery data the features having the most immediate relevance to actual "treatment" (remediation of the problem) are those of slowing down, practice in speaking, and personal motivation. The following section will present three case illustrations of their use.

Three Illustrations

The cases to be presented here were purposefully selected to represent different sources and different times, portraying individuals in different personal circumstances and with seemingly different ways of approaching the same objective—recovery from stuttering. The common thread in the three examples is that their recovery was based on the same three principles: slowing down, deliberateness, and motivation.

Example number one.—The first case is one selected from my personal experience, largely because of the uniqueness of his story and the method he described. This man was 66 years old at the time of the interview; the appointment had been arranged after I learned, through a chain of several acquaintances, that he was a former stutterer who had never had therapy. Mr. B's speech at the time of the interview seemed well within normal limits; in listening to him I would have had no reason for suspecting that he might be a stutterer. At times he seemed to speak "haltingly" but I doubt that I would have noticed this if I had not known beforehand that he was a former stutterer. Also, I got no confirmation that these instances represented potential stutterings.

Mr. B. claimed to have been a severe stutterer as a child and in his youth; he said that he had had particular trouble with words beginning with /s/, especially the word "seven." He remembered it vividly because even after he considered himself recovered he occasionally felt incipient stuttering tendencies, again especially on /s/ words and on "seven." He demonstrated what could happen if he did not heed a prescience of difficulty and neglected to use his method of control. What he intentionally allowed himself to do in one instance of saying the word "seven" was very convincing as a stuttering event. He said that actual occurrences of such tendencies were infrequent and sporadic.

Mr. B. said that he stuttered until he was about 25 years old. Between completion of his schooling and service in the United States Army in World War I he worked at several jobs that did not require much speaking. He was drafted into the Army in spite of his stuttering, and assigned to duties that did not depend upon speaking—for instance, he drew K.P. instead of guard duty (where he might need to challenge intruders or summon the corporal of the guard). He was sent overseas and into combat, where he was used effectively as a sapper, another job not requiring verbal communication.

A few years after his discharge from the service he happened to be in downtown Portland, Oregon. Being unfamiliar with the city he needed to ask directions. He approached a man at a street corner and asked for directions. He recalled that the man, middle-aged and kindly looking, listened to his query but instead of answering it immediately took hold of his arm and said something like, "Young man, I used to stutter as badly as you do, but I found a way to overcome it." The stranger went on to relate that he was an attorney who regularly spoke a good deal to individuals and groups, including trying cases in court. He then described his method for overcoming stuttering—a very simple one. The method called for making a "dry run" on any word which one sensed might create difficulty. The "dry run" consisted of a three-stage progression in saying a troublesome word, with progression to the next step undertaken if one felt comfortable about the previous one. The first step was an unvoiced imitation of the word—carefully making only the articulatory gestures; the next step was to gently whisper the word; and the final step was to say the word easily and deliberately with voicing.[19] Each stage could be abandoned as soon as one felt he did not need to use it but with freedom to use it whenever it seemed necessary. The objective was to use each stage only as long as it was needed.

The advocate made one stipulation—that the method must be practiced faithfully until mastered, indicating that from his experience it would be at least a year and a half before one could expect to talk without signs of stuttering.

Mr. B. said he was so impressed by the sincerity of his street-corner mentor that he decided to use the method. He persisted with it although during the first several months he seemed to be plodding yet making little progress. Gradually, though not continuously, he found himself able to omit the first step. After a few more months he could more often leave out the second stage also. Eventually he could use the third stage almost exclusively. He said that it was almost two years before he reached the point that he could move through a threatened difficulty by careful speaking and without the use of the "dry run" stages. He added that he felt this had had a generally good effect on his speech, not just dealing with his stutterings.

Example number two.—The second example is not as dramatic as the first one, nor does it reveal quite so obviously the principles set forth earlier. Still, it seems clear that practice in speaking must have been a formidable force in this person's recovery, with careful speaking and motivation intimately involved. This case was reported by Heltman in 1941; the report is reproduced here in its entirety.[20]

J. C. (boy), seven year old stutterer, tonic spasms of the muscles of the jaw, with a right side downward thrust, mouth open, high, weak vocal tone, no inflection. Had four months instruction beginning February, 1923, two half-hour lessons weekly. No apparent improvement June 1st. Boy went away to camp for the summer. No professional or casual contact with this case again until 1928 when he was 12 years old.

I saw him standing on a corner and engaged him in conversation. I discovered there was no trace of his former stuttering disorder. I did not see him again until he was a senior in high school in 1933, when he called on me professionally to get aid for the disorder which had again made its appearance during the latter half of his third year, and remained during the first half of his senior year. Both clonic and tonic spasms of the musculature of the neck and jaw as well as the tongue marked the extreme symptoms. His excuse for returning, however, was to receive some coaching for an oratorical contest in which he was scheduled to take part. He had memorized a speech that had obviously been coached in a rather bombastic style of delivery by some person who was considerably older. In reciting his speech to me he was able to get through it without a single stuttering symptom. In the meantime, every attempt at conversation was a failure because of the seriousness of the stuttering symptoms. In this particular contest he succeeded in winning the city championship, the state championship, and was given third place in the national in Washington. The stuttering remained. That was the last contact I had with him until two weeks ago, when I saw him again in a chance meeting in the city. We visited for ten minutes, during which time he showed no trace of stuttering symptoms. His voice is flexible and pleasant. He is well-poised and speaks with a rhythm in his speech that is as natural as one would find in the cultured speech of anyone who has never been afflicted with stuttering. During the conversation he told me that after he had seen me the last time, and incidentally, after the series of contests, he had gone to college to take his bachelor's degree, still stuttering very seriously. In college, however, he became interested in debating, entered into the activity wholeheartedly and, as he stated it, never had any trouble after that. It will be four years next June since he completed his bachelor's work.

In this connection may I call attention to a statement I made ten years ago in my mimeographed notes for my beginning course in Speech Re-education: "For those cases for which we have specific records of recovery with no relapses over periods of eight years or longer, there appears to have been in every case, after the treatment, participation in speech activities such as debating and contest speaking while in school, and considerable group and platform speaking for those who have finished school and have gone out into adult life." This, I believe, is the cue to the solution of the perseveration problem in the successful treatment of stuttering.[21]

In this case we do not have the individual's testimony regarding what he thought was responsible for his recovery. However, the account is clear-cut in its emphasis on speaking experience and the attendant implication of extensive practice in careful speaking. Further, the report has special value in view of Heltman's observations that continued practice in formal speaking is important to long-term gains in attenuation of stuttering.

Example number three.—The third case illustration is from a much earlier time. It is provided in the story of Cotton Mather, related by Bormann (1969). Cotton Mather was a figure of considerable stature in colonial America. He is probably best known as a Puritan minister, but he was also a significant figure in early American medicine, and an influential writer on many secular issues.

Cotton Mather's progenitors were eminent in the church, and he aspired to follow them in this calling. However, he stuttered, and presumably for this reason he began to study medicine instead of initially preparing for the ministry. While pursuing his studies at Harvard an incident occurred which led to his recovery from stuttering, a "deliverance" for which he and his father had prayed for a long time. The matter is recorded in a section on stuttering which is part of a long medical treatise completed by Mather in 1724.

Mather does not present the matter openly as being a personal account but, as Bormann indicates, the identity of the case example is only thinly disguised. According to what is recorded in Mather's " . . . Advice to Stammerers," his recovery followed upon the counsel of a Harvard tutor that he should speak more deliberately. As reproduced in Bormann (1969, pp. 459–460) the tutor advised Mather:

> *My Friend,* I now visit you for Nothing, but only to talk with you about the *Infirmity* in your *Speech,* and offer you my Advice about it; because I suppose tis a Thing that greatly troubles you. What I advise you do, is, to seek a Cure for it, in the Method of *Deliberation.* Did you ever know any one *stammer* in singing of the *Psalms?*

The schoolmaster then demonstrated the method while reciting from Homer. He continued with his advice as follows:

> While you go to *snatch* at Words, and are too *quick* at bringing of them out, you'll be *stop'd* a thousand Times in a Day. But first use yourself to a very *deliberate* Way of *Speaking*; a *Drawling* that shall be little short of *Singing.* Even this *Drawling* will be better than *Stammering*; especially if what you speak, be well worth our waiting for.
>
> This *deliberate* Way of Speaking will also give you a great Command of pertinent *Thoughts*; yea, and if you find a Word likely to be too hard for you, there will be Time for you to think of substituting another that won't be so.[22] By this *Deliberation* you will be accustomed anon to speak so much without the *indecent Haesitations*, that you'l always be in a Way of it; yea, the *Organs* of your *Speech* will be so habituated unto *Right-Speaking*, that you will by Degrees, and sooner

than you imagine, grow able to *speak as fast again*, as you did when the Law of *Deliberation* first of all began to govern you. Tho' my Advice is, beware of *speaking too fast*, as long as you live.

It is not known how much time was required to satisfactorily implement this advice, but the record states that the young man "soon" became a preacher to great congregations. He continued to preach for over forty years, evidently without manifestiations of his former stuttering.

Mather's " . . . Advice to Stammerers" contains a good deal of sermonizing, including, as one might expect, assertions of the value of prayer. He also makes a brief reference to pharmaceutical aids. But he returns to emphasize the method that brought relief of his stuttering:

Deliberation; I say it again, *Deliberation*; I say it once more: *Deliberation*, was the Thing that Heaven gave this happy Success unto.

The intent in presenting these three illustrative cases[23] is to focus attention on the matters of motivation, slowing down, and something we have called "practice in speaking" (which incorporates speaking with attention to the actions of speaking and implementing these actions regularly).

It may seem superfluous to make much of a point about the matter of motivation, since this is evidently recognized as important by all approaches to stuttering therapy. However, one is well reminded of the focal value of motivation, since its significance is easily obscured when a therapist attempts, and expects, to do something "for" or "to" a patient.

I wished to emphasize slowing down, not only because it is mentioned so frequently in the reports of these recovered stutterers, but also because it has been so arbitrarily dismissed by the profession as useless or actually deleterious. The evidence we have accumulated in this chapter strongly suggests the contrary. Moreover, "slowing down" articulates well with certain other effects that ameliorate stuttering, which we will consider later. "Slowing down" also makes sense as part of an integrated approach to therapy, which is also to be considered later.

Emphasis was directed to "practice in speaking" for several reasons: (a) the extent to which it is mentioned by these recovered stutterers; (b) its unique position in extant systems of therapy (many incorporate it partially or in some form; some advocate it, though by different names; others repudiate it); (c) the fact that it interrelates well with "slowing down"; and (d) it also makes sense within the integrated approach to be discussed later.

One last point should be made about "slowing down" and "practice in speaking." Both of them direct attention and actions toward working at producing essentially normal speech. The attack on the problem of generating normal speech is straightforward. This stands in contrast to the widespread tendency in extant stuttering therapies to be preoccupied with stutterings and ways of dealing with them.

Notes

1. In contrast, certain professional sources outside the United States have openly recognized the matter of remission and treat it as one of the facts of the disorder (e.g., Ward, 1941; Morley, 1957; Andrews and Harris, 1964).

2. It is of particular interest that data regarding recovery has been available in sources whose objective was to demonstrate that stuttering "develops" (cf. Johnson, 1955, 1959) and that many subsequent references to these works have considered only the matter of the "development" of stuttering therein reported and have completely ignored the data relating to remission.

3. The study was actually done in 1938–39. An abstracted version of it was published in the *Journal of Speech Disorders* in 1942 (pp. 251–257) with the title, "The onset and early development of stuttering."

4. Except for a passing interest in the six children of the control group who were later found to have had a history of stuttering. Johnson decided not to exclude these children from the control group on the grounds that this would have implied, "Once a stutterer, always a stutterer." The validity of this position need not concern us here, but we can at least point to six more cases of spontaneous remission of stuttering in young children.

5. The age range was 2 years 2 months to 9 years 3 months, but only three youngsters were over five years of age.

6. The reader should note that what is being denoted in these questions corresponds closely to the results of the analysis developed in the preceding chapter.

7. One of these ,identified in the book as "Study I," is Johnson's "The onset and development of stuttering," which was discussed earlier. The other, called "Study II," was Darley's "The relationship of parental attitudes and adjustments to the development of stuttering," which appeared as Chapter 4 in *Stuttering in Children and Adults*.

8. There were four other criteria: (a) Caucasian, (b) no gross sensory or motor impairment, (c) duration of stuttering not over 36 months, and (d) the child must have lived in the home since six months of age.

9. The claim is extended in the popularized version of this work which is presented in *Stuttering and What You Can Do About It*.

10. The authors state that 17 of the 32 individuals reported possible reasons for the disappearance of their stuttering and listed these reasons along with the number of times each was mentioned, as follows: 12 indicated that their parents

made them stop and repeat words and phrases on which they were having trouble; 5 stated that the stuttering cleared following a change in handedness due either to teaching or injury; 4 reported that stuttering disappeared following an improvement in general physical condition; 3 said that a chiropractor initiated more normal speech; 1 said stuttering disappeared immediately after his lingual frenum was clipped; 1 said his mother spanked him every time he stuttered and made him talk more slowly; 1 attributed his cure to a definite retraining program which he devised himself. Since the tally of these reasons totals 27, some subjects must have listed more than one reason.

In addition, the authors recorded a summary statement of the reason for improvement given by individual subjects. Presumably these brief summaries refer to the same individuals for whom the above list was compiled, yet there are 19 summary statements. Since each of the latter is identified by a subject number, it seems safe to assume that 19 is the correct value to identify the number of subjects giving a reason for recovery. It is for this reason that the list presented in the text is based on this information. It should, of course, be considered jointly with the reasons listed in this footnote.

Proceeding on the assumption that 19 is the correct number of cases who gave some explanation of their recovery, the actual number of cases who could give no clue to their recovery becomes 13, or 40 percent of those who recovered.

11. Milisen reported only the sizes of his selected groups and the percentages of the population they represented. The figure for the total population which is given here was computed from those values.

12. In interview one person was noted to evidence occasional lip tremors and another was described as having an eyelid flutter, poor eye contact, frequent use of "a-a-a," and unusual amounts of hesitation.

13. One of the two who reported a more sudden recovery said he had stuttered for three years, between ages 5 and 8. He said that his stuttering "stopped when I learned the trick of stomach breathing and talking slowly."

14. Except for one female who reported starting to stutter at 20 years of age. She said she had a vague memory of previously having been a "nonfluent speaker" but that it was never brought to her attention until her senior year in college when a friend pointed it out to her. After this it became a problem, from which she reported recovery at age 25. This is an atypical case. It is reminiscent of other cases of very late onset who, upon careful case history exploration, are found to have had an earlier episode (or episodes) of frank stuttering.

15. The authors did not indicate how many former stutterers they discovered by this procedure, but mentioned that between one and two percent of the entering students said they had stuttered as a child.

16. It is difficult to summarize these reports adequately. Not only are there such obstacles as lack of consistency in organization and the use of varying numbers of cases in statistical assessments, but it seems that much potentially worthwhile information is omitted or obscured.

17. Several of the classifications are double-headed, and the meaning of "Other" is not made clear by the authors.

18. The divergent values are those derived from Andrews and Harris (1964) and from Sheehan and Martyn (1970). The Andrews and Harris figure might be reconciled with the others by eliminating, in their sample, the 15 cases in which stuttering lasted for six months in the age period under 3½ years. One might guess that stuttering episodes of this duration and at this age level could well be the sort of thing readily forgotten. They would never show up, therefore, in

studies involving personal recollection; they might also be forgotten by parents of children at the kindergarten level. Omitting these cases from the Andrews and Harris computation results in a recovery ratio of 44 percent.

At least two factors might have contributed to the apparently inflated value in the Sheehan and Martyn report. Their figures are the only ones that involve a substantial adult population; other studies (Shames and Beams, 1952; Wingate, 1964) suggest that recovery continues to take place into adulthood. Also, their population was not representative of the general population, probably on several dimensions, but at least in respect to level of mental ability, which may well be of significance in "spontaneous" recovery.

19. Although moving slowly is not verbalized here, performance of the method clearly demonstrates that slowing down is definitely involved.

20. Reprinted by permission from the *Journal of Speech and Hearing Disorders*.

21. Of special interest here is the report of an initial period of remission with subsequent reappearance of the stuttering. In my experience this phenomenon occurs more frequently than has been reported in the literature; in some cases it may happen three or four times. It appears to be one form in which gradualness of recovery finds expression.

22. In current times the suggestion that the stutterer should substitute an easier word for a more difficult one would be decried by most therapists as "avoidance," which, it is claimed, only perpetuates the difficulty—presumably through reinforcement of the act and the associated fear. However, I have known a number of stutterers who successfully employed word avoidance (with varying frequency) and who clearly did not suffer as a result of it. A well-known and respected colleague, Spencer Brown (1972), acknowledges using word-avoidance himself, believes it is an "almost universal practice among stutterers," and openly advocates its use.

23. There are many other cases whose personal accounts of recovery highlight the principles emphasized in these three illustrations. For instance, cf. Aten, 1972; Agnello, 1972; Betz, 1968; Freund, 1972; Neely, 1972; and Starbuck, 1972.

References

Agnello, J. G. Change: Potential qualities become actualities. In Hood, S. B. (Ed.), *To The Stutterer*, Speech Foundation of America, Memphis, Publ. #9, 1972.

Andrews, G. and Mary Harris. *The Syndrome of Stuttering*, Heineman, London, 1964 (Chapter 3, The Natural History of Stuttering).

Aron, Myrtle L. The relationship between measurements of stuttering behavior. *J. South African Logopedic Society*, **14**, 15–34, 1967.

Aten, J. L. Overcoming fear and tension in stuttering. In Hood, S. B. (Ed.), *To The Stutterer*, Speech Foundation of America, Memphis, Publ. #9, 1972.

Betz, D. W. Recovery from stuttering: Some factors related to acquisition of normal fluency in one individual. *Program of 44th Annual Convention, Am. Sp. Hearing Assn.* 119, 1968 (abstr.).

Bloodstein, O. The development of stuttering: I Changes in nine basic features. *J. Speech Hearing Dis.*, **25**, 219–237, 1960a.

———The development of stuttering: II Developmental phases. *J. Speech Hearing Dis.*, **25**, 366–376, 1960b.

———The development of stuttering: III Theoretical and clinical implications. *J. Speech Hearing Dis.*, **26**, 67–80, 1961.

Bormann, E. G. Ephphatha, or some advice to stammerers. *J. Speech Hearing Research*, **12**, 453–461, 1969.

Brown, S. F. From one stutterer to another. In Hood, S. B. (Ed.), *To The Stutterer*, Speech Foundation of America, Memphis, Publ. #9, 1972.

Brutten, E. and D. Shoemaker. *The Modification of Stuttering*, Prentice-Hall, Englewood Cliffs, 1967.

Bryne, May E. A follow up study of one thousand cases of stutterers from the Minneapolis Public Schools. *Proc. Am. Soc. Study Dis. Speech*, 1931.

Bryngelson, B. Prognosis in stuttering. *J. Speech Disorders*, **3**, 121–123, 1938.

———Stuttering and personality development. *Nervous Child*, **2**, 162–166, 1943.

Cooper, E. B. Recovery from stuttering in a Junior and Senior High School population. *J. Speech Hearing Research*, **15**, 632–638, 1972.

Cullinan, W. L., E. M. Prather, and D. E. Williams. Comparison of procedures for scaling the severity of stuttering. *J. Speech Hearing Research*, **6**, 187–194, 1963.

Dickson, S. Incipient stuttering and spontaneous remission of stuttered speech. ASHA, **12**, **74**, 1967 (abstr.).

———Incipient stuttering symptoms and spontaneous remission of stuttered speech. ASHA, **10**, 371, 1965 (abstr.).

Freund, H. Self-improvement after unsuccessful treatments. In Hood, S. B. (Ed.), *To The Stutterer*, Speech Foundation of America, Memphis, Publ. #9, 1972.

Glasner, P. J. and D. Rosenthal. Parental diagnosis of stuttering in young children. *J. Speech Hearing Dis.*, **22**, 288–295, 1957.

Heltman, H. J. History of recurrent stuttering and recovery in a twenty-five year old post graduate college student. *J. Speech Hearing Dis.*, **6**, 49–50, 1941.

Johnson, Patricia A. An exploratory study of certain aspects of the speech histories of 23 former stutterers. Unpub. M.A. thesis, Univ. of Pittsburgh, 1951.

Johnson, W. A study of the onset and development of stuttering. In Johnson, W. and R. R. Leutenegger (Eds.), *Stuttering in Children and Adults*, Univ. of Minnesota Press, Minneapolis, 1955.

———*Stuttering and What You Can Do About It*. Univ. of Minnesota Press, Minneapolis, 1961.

———Stuttering in the preschool child. *State Univ. Iowa Child Welfare Pamphlet* #37, 1934.

———The onset and early development of stuttering. *J. Speech Dis.*, **8**, 251–257, 1942.

———and Associates. *The Onset of Stuttering*. Univ. of Minnesota Press, Minneapolis, 1959.

Kelly, S. M. and J. V. Frick. Diagnosis of stuttering in young Negro children. ASHA, 11, 62, 1966 (abstr.).

Luper, H. L. and R. L. Mulder. *Stuttering: Therapy for Children*, Prentice-Hall, Englewood Cliffs, 1964.

Martyn, Margaret M. and J. G. Sheehan. Onset of stuttering and recovery. *Behav. Res. Ther.*, **6**, 295–307, 1968.

Milisen, R. A comparative study of stutterers, former stutterers, changed handedness normal speakers and articulation cases. *Proc. Am. Speech Hearing Assn.*, **6**, 168–177, 1936.

———and W. Johnson. A comparative study of stutterers, former stutterers and normal speakers whose handedness has been changed. *Arch. Sp.*, **1**, 61–86, 1936.

Morley, Muriel E. *The Development and Disorders of Speech in Childhood*, E. and S. Livingstone, London, 1957.

Naylor, R. V. A comparative study of methods of estimating the severity of stuttering. *J. Speech Hearing Dis.*, **18**, 30–37, 1953.

Neely, Margaret M. Suggestions for self-therapy for stutterers. In Hood, S. B. (Ed.), *To The Stutterer*, Speech Foundation of America, Memphis, Publ. #9, 1972.

Robinson, F. B. *Introduction to Stuttering*, Prentice-Hall, Englewood Cliffs, 1964.

Shames, G. H. and H. L. Beams. Incidence of stuttering in older age groups. *J. Speech Hearing Dis.*, **21**, 313–316, 1952.

Shearer, W. M. and J. D. Williams. Self-recovery from stuttering. *J. Speech Hearing Dis.*, **30**, 288–290, 1965.

Sheehan, J. G. and Margaret M. Martyn. Spontaneous recovery from stuttering. *J. Speech Hearing Research*, **9**, 121–135, 1966.

———Stuttering and its disappearance. *J. Speech Hearing Research*, **13**, 279–289, 1970.

Starbuck, H. B. Do-it-yourself kit for stutterers. In Hood, S. B. (Ed.), *To The Stutterer*, Speech Foundation of America, Memphis, Publ. #9, 1972.

Ward, Kingdon. *Stammering*. Hamish Hamilton, London, 1941.

Wingate, M. E. Recovery from stuttering. *J. Speech Hearing Dis.*, **29**, 312–321, 1964.

6

THE COMMERCIAL VENTURE

The foundations of speech pathology as a discipline were laid in the early part of this century by such men as Scripture, Blanton, Makuen, Kenyon, and Fletcher, whose work was an expression of a long-developing interest in this special area of human function. By the end of the second decade of this century the increasing identity of a professional specialty was marked by a growth in publication of scientifically based studies and in the development of special courses in universities. These movements culminated in the establishment of the national professional association[1] in the middle '20s.

In the subsequent fifty years the profession has grown remarkably, and with this rapid expansion has come the development of areas of specialty within the discipline, each with its accumulating literature. Stuttering has always been a prominent area of interest within the profession, as reflected in the fact that in our journal, articles on stuttering have been consistently far more numerous than articles dealing with any other single area (see Paden, 1970, pp. 34–35).

For most people trained in the field the awareness of stuttering treatment ordinarily extends roughly to a time when the profession had become well established (the middle 1930s), and is associated primarily with familiar names in the profession's brief history. Most people in the profession tend to think of stuttering therapy as being conducted only by speech pathologists, or practitioners in such peripheral disciplines as clinical psychology, since within this span of time most of the work with stutterers has been done by persons trained in these fields.

However, during the early years of the development of the profession, as well as in the times before its origin, stuttering was dealt with by other vocational specialists, whose attentions to the disorder seemed appropriate and pertinent at the time. Stuttering has been treated by physicians, teachers of singing, speech and voice tutors, instructors in drama, elocutionists, and educators, who were all trained in their own particular field. In addition, there were certain self-styled "speech specialists" whose credentials ranged from suspicious to plausible.

The latter type of practitioner appears sporadically in the history of stuttering therapy. Klingbeil (1939) refers to several who operated during the 18th and 19th centuries. There were many to be found in the early part of this century; in fact, the heyday of this kind of "speech specialist" dawned and passed during a period of some 40 to 50 years spanning the turn of the century. This era, which reached its zenith in the first two decades of this century, saw the establishment of numerous "Stammering Institutes" or "Schools for Stammerers and Stutterers."

Apparently some such schools existed in Europe, but they were most numerous in the United States (possibly a reflection of our emphasis on free enterprise). Their numbers declined steadily as the 20th century unfolded, particularly as our profession developed in size and influence. Nonetheless, an itinerant, advertising "therapist" evidently toured this country as recently as 1966[2] (see Figure 6:1), and the private school that had achieved the greatest notoriety (*see below*) was still in operation as late as 1959.

When mentioned in professional discourse or literature these schools are referred to as "the commercial schools" of stuttering therapy. That is, they were "selling" a service and engaged in certain activities common to such endeavor: they advertised, made claims regarding the value of their "product," and offered guarantees. Most of these schools were residential: students roomed and boarded there while pursuing their goal of attaining fluency.

Each of the schools touted its own "method," with the claim, or heavy implication, that its method was the only one of its kind and, in most cases, certain to produce results. Attempts were made to keep the methods secret, such efforts amounting in some cases to requiring of incoming students that they make a pledge not to reveal the method once they left the school. In actuality, it appears that many of the methods were quite similar, consisting of a core technique around which certain other features were built. The core technique of those schools achieving the greatest prominence was the use of rhythm.

Attendance at one of the schools was said to have been expensive, with payment of tuition reportedly due in advance. An estimate of the expense can be made from a 1911 announcement from the Bogue Institute, which offered the complete course at a special reduced rate of $125.

From within the profession the view of the commercial schools has typically been a jaundiced one, the reaction vigorous, and the appraisal caustic. There was objection to the unprofessional attitude reflected not only in the fact of advertising but also in respect to the expansive claims made. There was concern about the image of speech correction that might be conveyed to the public. The atmosphere of secrecy was deplored as both unprofessional and suggesting trickery. The methods were denigrated as unscientific, simplistic, and superficial, founded in ignorance, and likely to be eventually deleterious in effect. Under-

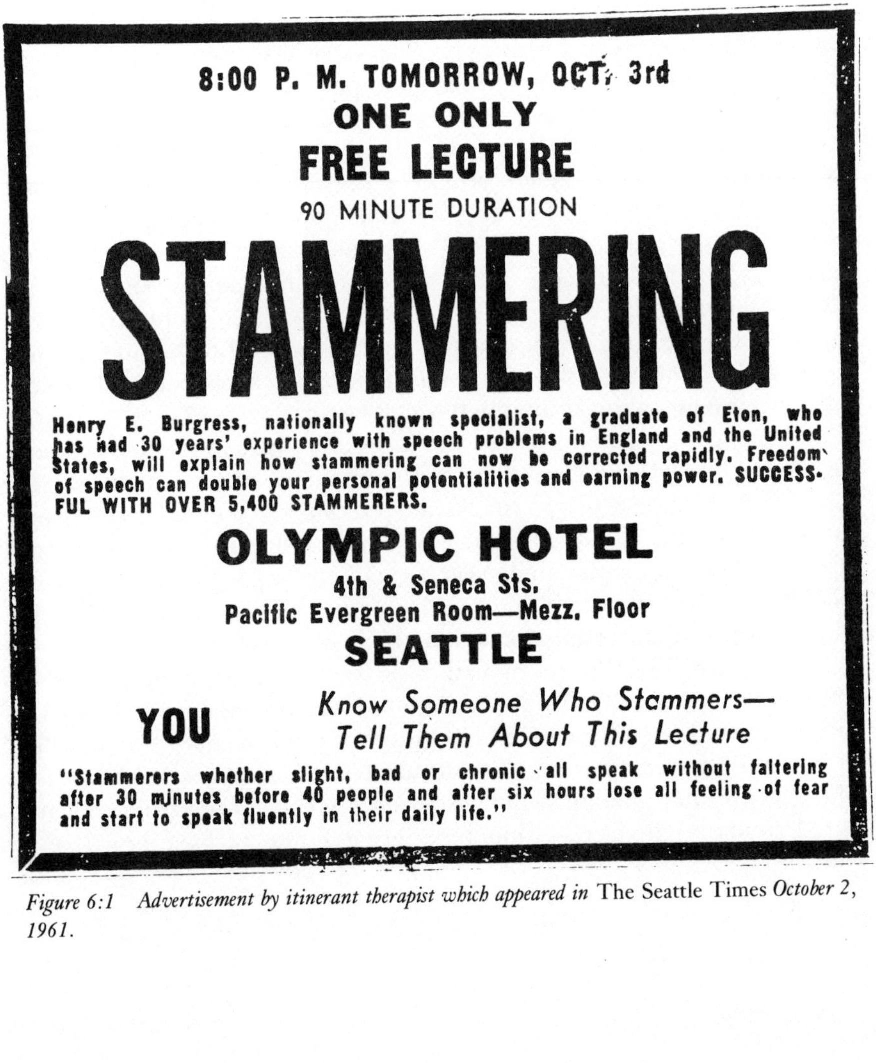

8:00 P. M. TOMORROW, OCT. 3rd

ONE ONLY

FREE LECTURE

90 MINUTE DURATION

STAMMERING

Henry E. Burgress, nationally known specialist, a graduate of Eton, who has had 30 years' experience with speech problems in England and the United States, will explain how stammering can now be corrected rapidly. Freedom of speech can double your personal potentialities and earning power. SUCCESSFUL WITH OVER 5,400 STAMMERERS.

OLYMPIC HOTEL

4th & Seneca Sts.

Pacific Evergreen Room—Mezz. Floor

SEATTLE

YOU *Know Someone Who Stammers— Tell Them About This Lecture*

"Stammerers whether slight, bad or chronic all speak without faltering after 30 minutes before 40 people and after six hours lose all feeling of fear and start to speak fluently in their daily life."

Figure 6:1 Advertisement by itinerant therapist which appeared in The Seattle Times *October 2, 1961.*

standably, the matter of guaranteed cure aroused the most strenuous complaint.

All of these reactions were intensified by the reports received from some stutterers who had attended the schools and who were dissatisfied with their experience. Often these former students would report that they had achieved fluency while attending the school and that this new-found fluency had persisted for some indefinite period following their return home, but that eventually they found themselves stuttering again. Sometimes the report of recurrent stuttering was embellished with the claim that it was then "worse than ever."

Reaction within the profession developed into the position that the proprietors of the commercial schools were unscrupulous charlatans, using worthless methods, who preyed on public ignorance and took advantage of hapless and trusting unfortunates.

In retrospect the negative judgment of the commercial schools seems to have been excessive, although certain aspects of the reaction were probably justified in some measure. A principal complaint about the schools was that the directors were untrained people who had little education, at least in respect to speech disorders. However, one must emphasize that while this might arouse reservation it does not necessarily justify condemnation. After all, the development of modern medicine has not contravened or invalidated all of the home remedies. At least in some cases it has only been able to provide an adequate, or a better, explanation for their effectiveness. It would have been more fitting, and more defensible, had the profession adopted an attitude of inquiry toward the treatment methods of the commercial schools and undertaken objective investigation of the methods.

Making a gaurantee of cure was a different matter. Here education in the field could have been very relevant; that is, professionally trained personnel could be expected to take the position that a cure for stuttering is sufficiently unlikely that making a guarantee of cure is highly unwarranted. Moreover, a guarantee was particularly improper in view of the reports of relapses, which one could well assume had been brought to the attention of the proprietors of the schools as well as to members of our profession. Further, even with a guarantee qualified by a money-back provision, there remains a violation of the professional ethic that a patient should not be led to expect a result that might not be attainable.

Certainly the directors of these schools made expansive claims for the effect of their methods. But professionally trained practitioners have acted similarly. In fact, within very recent times we have heard very extravagant claims for the efficacy of behavior modification approaches to stuttering therapy (e.g., Goldiamond, 1966, 1971).

An appraisal of the schools' efforts to maintain secrecy requires something of an adjustment in point of view. The schools were secretive about their methods for several reasons. The most likely reason seems to be that the methods were relatively simple and therefore easy to copy. These people were in business, and secrecy was important to the protection of their business interests. Most professions are operated as a business; protection of business interests is simply accomplished in more subtle ways than was possible for the commercial schools.

The reaction of our profession to the high fees reportedly charged by the commercial schools can also be understood to reflect its academic provincialism. Charging high fees is not unprofessional; in fact it is commonplace in most professions. And the fees are for services rendered, not for results achieved.

There is no attempt here to exonerate the commercial schools. One cannot help gaining the impression from samples of their literature that there was a considerable element of opportunism and drumming. But even if the reactions and appraisal made by our profession were fully justified on most of the grounds mentioned above, the absolute and rigid repudiation of the methods was unfortunate and premature.

The outright rejection of the methods of the commercial schools as superficial and valueless did in itself reflect a lack of scientific attitude. It precluded an adequate pursuit of two very important questions: first, how does the method achieve its effect, even though it may be temporary; second, are the results only temporary in all instances—or are the cases who report relapse an unrepresentative, though vocal, sample?

The latter question evidently was never asked, though it should have been. It is still a good question, and an adequate answer would still be of great value. The former question was dispatched with a facile, unreflective and ingenuous answer: the effect was said to be due to suggestion and distraction. There are several crucial points to be made about distraction, which we will defer to a later time (see page 187). At the moment it is enough to say that distraction explains nothing in this context; the notion is simply inappropriate.

The methods used by the commercial schools deserve some attention from anyone seriously interested in the treatment of stuttering, not only out of historical interest but, more importantly, because of the possibility that there is something to be learned from them.

TWO OF A KIND

For several reasons we will give some consideration to two of the commercial schools: the Bogue Institute for Stammerers, which was located in Indianapolis, Indiana, and the Lewis School for Stammerers, situated in Detroit, Michigan. These two schools were among the most widely known and, I think it accurate to say, the most notorious from the point of view of our profession. The Bogue Institute has probably received the lion's share of opprobrium. The two schools had many features in common: active advertising, expansive claims, the offer of cure, and type of method.

The Bogue Institute

The Bogue Institute was founded in 1901 by Benjamin N. Bogue. The descriptive advertisement reproduced in Figure 6:2 appeared in a book by Bogue (1927)[3] in which he chronicled the events leading to the development of his method. The book contains indirect as well as direct advertising, with certain sections stoutly acclaiming the efficacy of the system. Bogue also published a little periodical, called "The Emancipator"[4] which evidently was regularly loaded with appeal, exhortation, and inducement to stutterers to resolve their problem at the Bogue Institute. From time to time circulars such as the one reproduced in Figure 6:4 were sent out, evidently with the same objective.

While Bogue's book contains more than a thread of pretension and flamboyance, one also finds a quality of sincerity and genuine conviction. It seems that Bogue was not an uneducated man; evidently he had at least attended college, and his book contains evidence that he was reasonably knowledgeable about stuttering.[5] He claimed to have made a study of speech disorders and relevant topics such as anatomy and physiology, and to have read widely about stuttering. References made in the book to persons such as Alexander G. Bell and W. B. Swift provide suggestive corroboration. Even more persuasive is the information conveyed to me indirectly that Mr. Bogue had quite an extensive personal library of publications dealing with speech disorders.

Benjamin Bogue was a stutterer himself (as were a number of those who established such schools). His father, grandfather, and at least 14 other blood relatives stuttered, and he accepted quite matter-of-factly that his stuttering was an inherited condition.

It is appropriate to note that Bogue's story of his success is saturated with an air of persistence and determination. He reports having tried

THE BOGUE INSTITUTE

INDIANAPOLIS, INDIANA

AN INSTITUTION for the successful treatment of stammering, stuttering and kindred forms of defective speech. Training is based on scientific recoordination of brain and speech. No drugs, electricity, hypnotism or medicines employed. Bogue Unit Method used exclusively. Best of home care and comfort are to be found in the dormitories which are maintained under the supervision of and in connection with the Institute.

In continuous operation for more than twenty-six years under the personal direction of the founder.

BENJAMIN NATHANIEL BOGUE

President and Principal

Figure 6:2 Typical advertisement of the Bogue Institute. This one appeared in Bogue's book, Stammering, Its Cause and Cure.

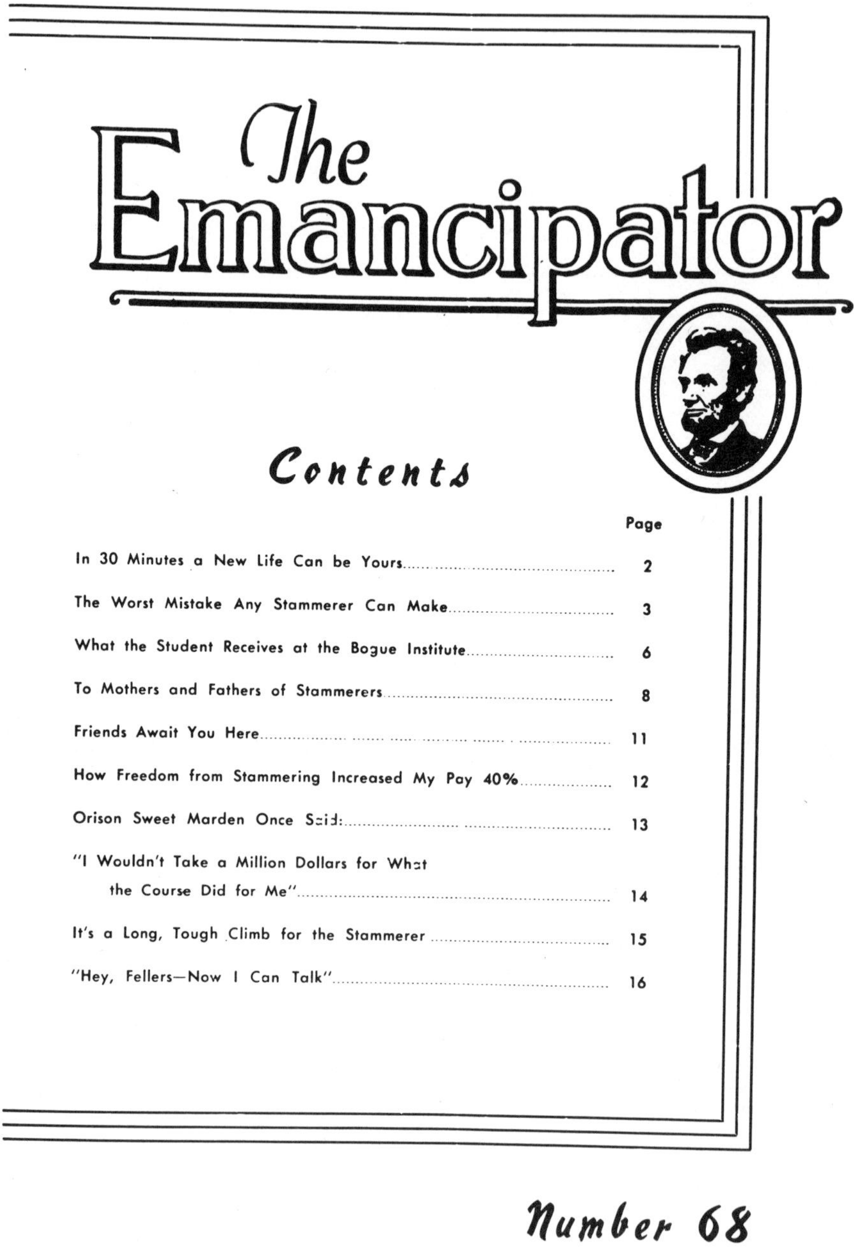

The Emancipator

Contents

Number 68

Figure 6:3 Description of "The Emancipator," a periodical published by the Bogue Institute. (From Stammering, Its Cause and Cure.)

THE EMANCIPATOR

Edited and Published by
Benjamin Nathaniel Bogue

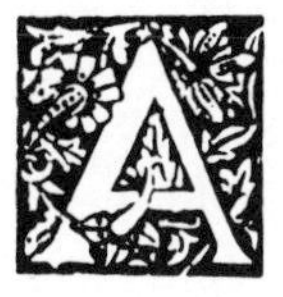
MAGAZINE devoted to the interests of perfect speech. The only magazine for stammerers published in the United States. The Emancipator teaches and believes in the philosophy of success, of achievement, of accomplishment. Ringing through the pages of The Emancipator is the clarion call to be what you wish to be, to do what you wish to do, and accomplish what you wish to accomplish.

The Emancipator has made dozens of people dissatisfied with the half-life of a stammerer. It has shown them the beauties and the advantages of the complete, successful, useful, overflowing, joyous life that can be theirs. The Emancipator has put ambition into the indifferent and listless, courage into the heart of the fearful, confidence into the hand of the timid and a positive will into the being of the negative personality.

The whole purpose of The Emancipator might be summed up in six words: *To better your condition in life.*

Subscription, $1.00 per year. **Sample copy, 10c**

Figure 6:4 Frontispiece of a copy of "The Emancipator."

"upwards of fifteen different methods" for the relief of his stuttering, among which he mentioned medical care, hypnotism, electrical treatments, training in breathing and vocal exercises, and elocution lessons. He traveled to a number of cities in this country and spent a good deal of money in the effort to resolve his problem. However, he continued to stutter until, after lengthy study and persistent efforts to improve his speech, he found "a method of control of the articulatory organs as well as of the brain centers controlling the organs of speech."

This system was formalized into the "Bogue Unit Method." The word "unit" simply referred to the fact that the system was organized into three units. The objective of the first unit was to build up physical efficiency, to assure that the person was in good health and the organs of his body were functioning properly. The second unit was to "restore the mental equilibrium" so that the mind would be able to properly control the organs of speech. The third unit " . . . synchronizes and harmonizes mental and physical actions and re-establishes normal coordination between the brain and the muscles of speech."

The foregoing represents the extent of Bogue's description of his method. The description is obviously quite vague, most likely by intention. We can offer the following analyses of the units.

Unit one seems quite straightforward; it sounds very much like that nonspecific recommendation found so often in our own literature, namely, "Keep the child in good health."

Units two and three appear to represent the two major features of the Bogue method as known from hearsay statements. Unit two—"restoring the mental equilibrium"—corresponds to what was reported to have been the initial phase of the treatment program. It consisted of a period of silence lasting at least several days. The student was required to observe strict silence, being permitted to communicate only by writing. Presumably the rationale for this was to erase or minimize the traces of the previous mental organization for speaking, thereby preparing the foundation for the new patterns.

Unit three is quite clearly the unit that incorporates the speech retraining effort. It is not difficult to see in "...synchronizes and harmonizes mental and physical actions . . ." the use of rhythm as Bogue is said to have used it: syllable-timed speech which was accompanied, at first, by some vigorous movement of the arm (such as swinging it) to emphasize the regular beat. The accompanying movement was gradually reduced to a very covert means of beating time (such as a slight unobtrusive tapping with a finger).

It is not known whether Bogue had any knowledge of the previous use of rhythm. In view of evidence that he was reasonably well read about stuttering it would seem quite unlikely that he was unaware that rhythm had been used before. Still, it remains possible that he did not have much knowledge of the matter—even some current writers have described the use of rhythm as a "new" method (e.g., Meyer and Mair, 1963; Van Dantzig, 1940).

It seems unfair to have accused Bogue of simply using rhythm in an artless and undiscriminating manner. Apparently other features were incorporated in the procedure; at least Bogue referred in several places to instruction in appropriate articulation and correct use of the voice. Moreover, he acknowledged that the development of his method was based on knowledge gained through his reading and in his experiences with the various teachers whose help he had sought. He gave particular credit to one who "had made speech defects almost a life study" and who "knew more about the true principles of speech and the underlying fundamentals of voice than all the rest put together."

Bogue's book contains sample letters of testimony which laud the effects of the treatment. These statements have to be taken at face value; it is unfortunate that we do not have others collected by an unbiased source. But there is no good reason not to believe that these testimonials were bona fide and unsolicited. It seems probable that many persons were helped by Bogue's method, if not cured. I am particularly persuaded of this by an admission made off-handedly by a fellow member of the profession a few years ago. This man, highly respected by those who know him for his research activities, once stuttered severely, and still stutters noticeably though minimally. His comment, made at the end of a short conversation in a hotel lobby during a convention was, "Say what you will about Benjamin Bogue, but that was the first time I had ever experienced fluency." He indicated that his experience at the Bogue Institute was an auspicious beginning to his personal success in dealing with his own stuttering.

The Lewis School

The Lewis School for Stammerers was established in 1894. In all major respects it was similar to the Bogue Institute[6]: it had a founder-proprietor; the school published a periodical (*The Phono-Meter*—not as clever a selection of title as the Bogue equivalent); it advertised actively, made expansive claims, and offered a money-back guarantee; and, the core technique of the method was the use of rhythm.

The founder-proprietor of the Lewis School was George Andrew Lewis, a man who Clark (1964) described as ". . . hardly notable for modesty and timidity." It would seem that he had particular talents as a promoter and public-relations man. At least by the year 1905 his return mail envelopes contained his picture and the words "Detroit, Mich.," plus a little note assuring the prospective respondent that nothing more than a stamp was required for the mail to reach him, since "Everybody knows me."

Probably this school's most lasting claim on history is that Charles S. Bluemel was once a student there. Bluemel, a stutterer from childhood, was born and raised in England. He first came to this country, at the age of 22, to attend the Lewis school. Later, having found during this first sojourn here that his asthma was improved in the climate of Colorado, he emigrated to the United States and lived here the rest of his life.

In his adolescence Bluemel had attended an English school for stutterers during a summer vacation. His stuttering had improved a good deal while receiving this instruction but relapsed after he returned to his boarding school in the fall. In 1906 he saw an advertisement of the Lewis school in an American magazine. He was impressed by the statement of guarantee, since in England, he said, one could expect a written guarantee to be fulfilled. So he went to Detroit, with great expectations that his stuttering would be cured.

However, Bluemel was very disappointed by the Lewis method; he felt that the means for achieving the goal were worse than the disorder itself. So, after three months of attendance, he left the Lewis school, disenchanted and discouraged. Somewhat later he returned to demand reimbursement of his tuition. It was refunded, although evidently not cheerfully.

Bluemel's experience with the Lewis school was an unhappy and unproductive one. Again, however, one must wonder if it appropriately represented the typical experience of students attending the school. It seems clear that Bluemel did not enter cooperatively into the treatment process. Clark (1964) relates:

> He preferred his stuttering to the pattern. It was at this time, in a reaction against such superficial treatment, that he first began to crystallize his own ideas on a nonorganic basis of stuttering. While at this school, he and other dissatisfied students experimented with Bluemel's idea (sic) of negative practice and several other methods, but none proved effective.[7]

As indicated earlier, there is essentially no existing evidence which bears favorably on the results or influence of the commercial schools. There is no evidence of this kind largely because it was never sought—and never sought because of the preclusion that there would be none to find. Within this context the story which follows stands out in dramatic relief.

This statement came to me quite by accident several years ago. A student in my introductory course on stuttering was somehow reminded that her father had at one time or another said something about having been a stutterer. She wrote to him inquiring about her recollection and received in reply the letter reproduced below. For our immediate purposes the letter has value as a sample of positive testimony for the methods of the commercial schools. Beyond this, however, it is a lovely story which reveals a man of character, warmth, honesty, sensitivity, and good humor—who also happens to stutter. The title of the letter is his own.

STARTS, STOPS AND STIGMAS OF A STUTTERER

This story of my life is made from a series of memory notes, and will be quite disconnected. It seems as I built new speaking habits my very bad memories have disappeared. I have to relive events that I don't want to bring back!

I always thought I stammered until you informed me there was no difference between stammering and stuttering. I still disagree unless you admit many, many kinds of stuttering. I always felt sorry for those poor individuals that repeated consonants. Mine was a much more subtle affliction. I picked out a word or a sentence that carried a memory of past difficulty in certain situations. I could see this word coming, I knew with a dread certainly that it would give me trouble and unless I could substitute another word, I did have trouble. And I did not repeat the beginning of that word. I came to a screeching halt. Set your diaphragm, tense every muscle in your arms and neck, clench your hands into tight fists, lean forward and try, just try to make a sound come out, not even a squeak. It didn't matter whether the word began with a vowel or a consonant. It was a memory chain of situations and words.

There were and still are situations and places where I talk very smoothly and easily, *so it appears to the listener*, and yet *I* am in a mental whirlpool. I know a word is coming up, I must substitute for it, but I can't find a substitute, God I'm going to get stuck on that word, but I make it, I'm talking OK, I got over that hurdle. A deep breath, try to relax, no one can tell you are in trouble, here comes another one I'd like to use but there is a synonym almost as good, got over that. Here comes another, keep talking smoothly, don't slow down or you'll be in trouble. Ha! Made it! Try to relax. Look your listener or audience in the eye. They are interested, they don't know but that you are a good speaker. Relax those hands and arms. Let them hang. God here comes another word. . . . How many times have I gone through that and no one knew but me.

There were many situations. Some I can recall were: Reading aloud, talking over the telephone, getting on my feet and answering a question in a class. (I could do much better seated.) Explain a problem to a class or group standing before them or at the blackboard, any foreign language (Latin and Spanish in High School). Telling a funny story, always get stuck on the punch line. Other silly ones but just as deadly to me. Like telling my parents about a show I had seen. Others will come to mind.

Right now I remember a word "tomato" that bothered me last summer when talking over the telephone to a customer. I mastered it by using METHOD which I will explain in detail later. Then there is a rhythm to this for me. A high point and a low point. Times when I forget that I ever had a speech difficulty and times when I am acutely aware of it.

I can remember, clearly, that up to school I enjoyed reciting pieces and poems that Dad taught me and had me give before groups of people. It didn't matter whether at home or in front of strangers or in the weekly "literary society" meetings that we attended in the one room school house. I can recall that I enjoyed and took a lot of pride in speaking. I've searched my memory many, many times, when did it start? Perhaps I rebelled against my parents, my teacher. I know it started about then.

Also about this time, came an event that I remember vividly. It was winter in ———, Idaho. Dad was a Forest Ranger and this was mountain country. The snow was about 5 feet deep, leaving only the tips of the fence posts peeking out in long straight lines across the level valley. It was the winter before school, so I must have been 5. School was from May to October. I enjoyed winters. People came with teams and sleds and played cards all night, and I was allowed to stay up late. Most of them stayed and had breakfast before leaving for home. Dances always lasted until dawn, and all the kids came and we danced, Dad played the fiddle and I could play the G chord on the piano and sometimes he asked me to chord for him. I thought I was smarter than most of the kids. I know I wondered if they had thoughts like I had. I resented adults talking down to me, because I knew that I knew a lot more than they thought I did. (I think many people, including teachers, sell short the 4 and 5 year olds.)

The snow was quite crusty this winter. Many coyotes had been seen and just a few days back Dad had shot at a big dark animal that he thought must have been a timber wolf. Everyone had talked about it and I was all ears. I was between the house and the outside toilet. It seemed a long ways, along the curved path, with the snow high over my head making it a narrow, deep, mysterious canyon. So I frequently traveled on the crust when it would hold me, as it barely would that day if I walked carefully. Then I saw it, a big animal, dark, and coming toward me, and not very far away. Timber Wolf! I started to run and broke through the crust to my knees. I tried to shout to mother, to scream, to say anything and I couldn't. I couldn't utter a sound. So I floundered there, utterly terrified, and that animal came up to me and was almost on top of me before I recognized it as my dog. My Dog. My big, black and tan, part bulldog. He licked my face and I sobbed big gasping sobs, thankful that I could get my breath. I finally got to the path and ran to the house to tell Mother and was scolded for acting like a baby and timber wolves never would come that close to the house anyway. I went out and climbed up on the snow to the roof of the wood shed and sat there for a long time looking for timber wolves and thinking it all over and really how silly I had been. I've never told anyone of this event and I'm sure Mother never remembered it. But I had dreams about it and nightmares when wolves were after me and I couldn't run and I couldn't shout for help. In a way this is the same feeling I get when I am unable to speak, and I've wondered about it. Was this such a shock that it left scars?

My first teacher boarded at our house and I rode to school with her on a horse, behind the saddle. A one room school with grades from one to eight, and kids from five to eighteen. There must have been about 20 altogether. I had looked forward to school because I had learned to recognize many words in a wonderful story about the little red hen. Dad had taught me to read by words not sounds. I remember vividly that first day. My teacher was no longer kind and considerate. She was stern, sharp, and "no back talk." She chalked my name on my desk top and I was to place beans over the letters. I could print my name easily and I recognized writing though I couldn't do it as easily as printing. And I had to use my right hand too and I thought it was all a lot of nonsense and I said so and got my hand slapped with a ruler. Do you know that hurts. That first day too, we started learning words on the blackboards by sounding the letters. Some of the words I knew and I felt much smarter than the rest of the kids and why sound them when I already knew them. I said as much and during recess when all the other kids were out playing I had to stay in and sound letters. I hated her from then on. She informed my parents that this left handed business was for the birds, I guess, because I was forced to learn to eat with my right hand. I had never realized until then that I was a southpaw. Was this a reason?? I have heard both pros and cons on this subject. I can't remember that I started having trouble then.

It was with another teacher, my second year, when we had to stand and read aloud to the class (the entire room in fact) that I dreaded to read aloud because the other kids in the class and the older boys too, laughed at me and mimicked me. Apparently I repeated consonants, I can't remember.

I don't remember having trouble reciting until my fifth grade in a two-classroom school. We had moved out of ——— that winter so we kids could go to school in the winter time. There were only certain words by then that I could see coming and I usually substituted other words until my teacher noticed and made me stop and say the word. That was when I first remember being unable to utter a sound without opening my mouth real wide, so wide that my jaws would hurt, and gasping and finally exploding with the word. The entire room enjoyed it and even the teacher LAUGHED AT ME AT TIMES. God, I'll never forget that school year.

Dad and mother had me read aloud to them that year at home. At times I could read with no difficulty. Other times I had to struggle. Mother had the same trouble with her speech, you know. Not really noticeable, but on some words she would stop and sort of gasp before she could go on. I could read by the hour to my younger sisters with no difficulty, but if I became aware that some older person was listening—BOOM.

On the phone, my first trouble that I remember, was when I was 12 years old. I was on a Forest Service Lookout that summer. Of course, just staying with the man in charge. It was the old crank phone and communications were sometimes real bad. We had to report in twice a day and I was asked to do it at times. I probably asked for the privilege. If connections were good, fine, but if I had to stop and repeat what I had just said, all of a sudden I was tense as a drum and gasping like a fish out of water, trying to say a simple sentence that I had said easily not 5 seconds before. I found I could cover the mouthpiece and swear fluently in cases like this, and usually be OK. Or sometimes a silly giggle would help when swearing was not fitting to the situation.

I can't recall that I was particularly shy in those days. I was liked at school. I was the champion wrestler of any kid my size. I read anything and everything I could get my hands on. Dad had taught me to ride and drive a team and throw a diamond hitch on a packsaddle. I had my own little rifle and could outshoot Dad. I got my first deer when I was 12. But when it came to talking there were situations I avoided at all costs, and my parents did not push me.

My Sophomore year in High School was in ———, Nev. We had two teachers for a student body of 26, I believe. For the first time in my life I found a teacher who understood my troubles. We talked a lot about it. I was learning to play the trombone and he told me I was trying to talk like trying to play the trombone by pushing on the mouthpiece. He made me try to relax on my feet. I actually took part in inter-class debates and found that by becoming intensely interested in my subject and knowing it real well, I could talk.

The next summer, I was 15, Mother and we kids moved to ———, Calif. I drove the car down, and took over as man of the house as Dad stayed in ———. There I took two months of speech correction with a little old lady in San Francisco, who had been recommended by the teacher in ———. There I learned all about relaxing from flat on my back to sitting to standing. We practiced until I could distinguish my heart beat in any part of my body. My ears, any of my fingers and toes. I learned correct breathing and to push my diaphragm as in singing. We practiced How now brown cow, etc. and etc. and etc. She was helping me. I knew it. I was gaining confidence. For the first time I knew that I didn't have to live with this speech difficulty all my life. I don't know how she did it, exactly. Just can't tell you. Unless it was relaxed breathing because it was nothing like the METHOD I later learned in Detroit, Mich.

From ———, Nev. we came to ———, Idaho and I enrolled as a Junior in the High School. I had more confidence in my speech than I had ever known before. I was active in student activities, was liked, and was elected Vice President of the Student Body. About 120 in those days.

I was trying to fly before I learned to walk! One morning when we were assembled to listen to the usual bible reading the Principal asked the Student Body Officers to come up front and give a brief talk. I was unprepared, I had to wait, standing there, for the President to give his talk. And I was next. My heart was pounding. I couldn't get a deep breath or relax. Adrenalin was pouring into me. When my turn came I stuck on the first words. After exploding with two or three words, I laughed and said very easily "I guess I have nothing to say." Everyone roared. They were laughing with me not at me but the damage had been done. I knew then, as I know now, that everyone that speaks has blank spots, that a speaker, no matter how experienced, is usually nervous at the start. But I never had the courage to try again, though I knew that was the thing to do. The Principal never asked me again.

All through school, from the first grade on up, I enjoyed and made every effort to get into plays. Sometimes in reading my lines I had speech difficulty but after they were memorized, *there was no more trouble.* Our drama teacher picked me for the lead in the Junior play. We really had turnouts, too, in those days for plays. Half the county, it seemed. Also I had one of the main parts in the Senior play. I dreaded it before I got started, but I did very well. I'm certain I wasn't as good as you are, but I thought I was and it gave me a lot of confidence in me. I didn't stutter in a play. Was it because I was living the part of a person who had no speech difficulty????

The summer after I graduated from high school we moved to ———, Idaho. There I worked for Grandad in the fruit orchards. Grandad spoke the King's English. He used words precisely with perfect grammar. I knew he had stuttered in his youth and had overcome it, he said, by concentrating on the precise language he used. I was miserable that summer because I wanted to go to college, but I didn't want to go until I could talk. I had lost the confidence gained in San Francisco and didn't know how to regain it. At Grandad's suggestion I went out alone and practiced speaking to imaginary audiences. I even tried pebbles in my mouth like one of the Roman what's-his-name orators. It didn't help much. Perhaps in general conversation but in memory-chain-trouble situations I was as bad as ever.

Then I met a Mr. Holbrook who was picking fruit for Grandad. He was a Chemistry and Physics teacher in a nearby high school. I discovered he had a speech impediment and I found a sympathetic listener to all my woes. He wanted to help me, so that Fall I enrolled as a post-graduate in the High School. Taking advanced Algebra which would help me in my intended career as a Chemical Engineer and helping Mr. Holbrook's Chem and Physics Lab. In the Lab with individual students, there was no trouble, but give me a problem to explain to the class or explain a problem on the blackboard, back came everything and I stuttered. Mr. Holbrook insisted that I keep trying. He said practice made perfect. It was good training. No one laughed or made fun of me. And there were times when I could talk easily and how wonderful I felt. But other times it was a struggle and with no reason for it, that I could see.

The following spring, at Mr. Holbrook's suggestion, I wrote to the Lewis Institute, Detroit, Mich. (for Stammering and Stuttering) and later enrolled in their Correspondence Course.

It was largely the same stuff I already knew. Proper breathing, relaxation exercises, reading aloud. There were other ways, they said, but I would have to come to Detroit. I practiced on the lessons that summer but I worked too because I knew I was going to Detroit. Dad and Mother helped and early in December I departed for Kansas City, Mo. as the man-in-charge of a car of apples and riding in style in the caboose of a freight train.

It was quite a trip. A bit of your time to hit the highlights. My car was diverted in Denver for Ft. Worth, Tex. There was no danger of freezing weather to the south, so I left my car of apples, grabbed my little suitcase and climbed on an empty boxcar heading East across Kansas in December. Boxcars, coalcars, oil tankers, locomotives, I tried them all before I reached Chicago. Cold, hungry, dirty and frequently hiding from railroad detectives, I met winos, hobos, prostitutes and homosexuals, tramps and pickpockets. They were usually friendly and willing to give a green kid advice in riding the rails. I learned too. One little girl, not over 15, but probably a professional, wanted to cuddle for warmth. Nothing more, it was too cold. She also wanted and took the four or five, one dollar bills I had in my overcoat pocket. In Chicago the mercury was close to zero and the wind blowing, so I parted with a few dollars and rode the Greyhound into Detroit.

The Institute was a huge 3-story house (home) on Woodward Avenue. It was home from the threshold. A huge negro mammy answered the bell. "Honey you're a sight for the chillun." She got me upstairs and into a hot bath with very few questions about who I was and what I was doing there. They knew I was enroute but no date of arrival had been set. My room was not pretentious, but carpeted and comfortable. I shared it with a young man seemingly little older than I, but who turned out to be our main instructor and who, wonders of wonders, was a second year University student in Chemistry. There were 16 men students in that combined dorm-school building, ranging in age from 17 to probably 50. They were all, without exception, friendly, sympathetic, quiet and serious. They were all there for a purpose. There were 8 or 10 women in my classes too. From pretty girls on up but they were housed in a different building, darn it.

That same day of arrival, as soon as I had bathed and got into clean clothes I was told that Mr. Lewis wanted to see me in his office. I dreaded the interview because I knew I'd have trouble. He was a huge, friendly, slow moving St. Bernard type. Before I could try to say a word he held his finger to his lips and said "Shush, you have just arrived into a new world, there will be no talking until you learn the language." He handed me a pencil and a small pad and told me that I was on strict silence for two weeks. That I couldn't hum, sing, talk or even whistle except in classroom. The interview was lengthy because all my answers were in writing. So I started on what they call METHOD and it proved to be, in my case anyway, what I needed, what I had been looking for.

In the classroom, the opening half hour was deep slow breathing with our arms hanging (we were sitting in chairs) our heads back, eyes closed and mouths hanging open. Our instructor checked individual ribs to make sure we *were* breathing properly. We were told to relax, relax, relax, deeper and deeper with each outgoing breath. It was hypnosis, pure and simple, but it worked. You did relax.

But relaxation, sitting and standing was an important part of METHOD.

To me, METHOD is nothing but a series of steps that one practiced until they become a habit. They were the proper steps in speaking that every person uses when speaking well. They put your attention on something that required concentration, making it impossible to think about having speech difficulty.

A new student was given a card on which was a large horizontal figure 8 like this

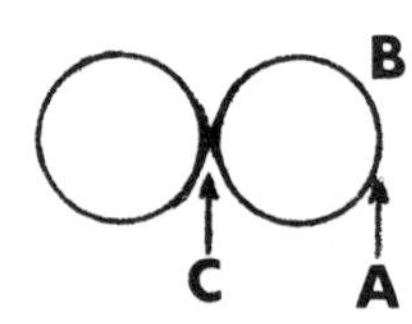

They were asked to visualize a ball resting at A. It must bring to mind these mental and physical steps. 1. I am poised, head up, chest out. 2. I am completely relaxed. 3. I am very deliberate and at ease.

The ball rises toward B. It is leading, I am following it. And as it rises I take a slow deep breath. The ball moves smoothly past B and as it starts down my breath starts coming out, I am exhaling easily through my forehead. As the ball passes C, I speak the first syllable, my voice tone arching from my forehead to the listener. Before a group of people it is directed to the ones in the back of the room. The second syllable is spoken when the ball has traveled around the left circle and come back to point C, the third syllable or word when the ball has completed the right circle and come back to C. And there it is. It is that simple. But it takes practice, practice and practice before it becomes easy and natural. Part of you. A habit.

The first and second day the new student is an observer only. He sees the advanced students use METHOD and speak and read easily and well. I wondered if I could ever be able to speak as easily as they did.

But I did in less than two months. Of course it was daily practice on speech and nothing else. Even now I can close my eyes and easily visualize the figure 8 outline. Or concentrate and see it plainly on the wall.

About the third or fourth day the student is asked to stand in front of the class, demonstrate the procedure of METHOD and sound only the vowels A, E,

I, O, and U. He can trace the movement of the ball on his card with his finger or on an imaginary 8 on the wall of the room. Next comes the reading of a short sentence, sounding only the vowel sounds. Then comes the consonants, and suddenly, one day you realize you are reading new material in front of the class as easily and naturally as if you had always done it.

During the silent period, you are given all kinds of assignments to do in town. All with a pad and pencil. You ask directions from a policeman, you buy an article in a store, you get a book from the library, etc. and etc. An advanced student goes with you the first time or two to make it easier for you. There are amusing situations. People usually think you are deaf and dumb, and they sometimes say some very silly things, thinking you can't hear them. You gain confidence, you feel superior, you get to enjoy these assignments.

All this time you are practicing METHOD. There are numerous class relaxation periods, and you get so proficient at relaxing that you can lose the feeling in your hand or arm if you want to. You listen to the advanced students give brief prepared talks, readings, or one minute talks on a subject the instructor gives them as they come to the front of the class. They are all good speakers. You are sure that some of them never had a speech difficulty. It is all done in a fun atmosphere, and there are times when the instructor gets the entire class going with almost uncontrolled laughter. You listen to outside speakers give brief talks. They are usually from the local Toastmasters Club and you take notes and criticize both the faults of a poor speaker and the mannerisms and little tricks a good speaker uses to hold his audience.

Breathing becomes almost a Yoga ritual. You practice inhaling and exhaling as you walk down the street. There is a series of movements that you practice to music. Deliberately and slowly moving the hands and arms like a Balinese dancer.

Other assignments come when you end the silent period. You go out and ask questions of people, but this time you wave your finger in front of you as you talk following the figure 8. An advanced student is along and he does the same thing as though he were a beginner. You are nervous but you discover people's thoughts can't hurt you. And usually they are a little afraid of you. Policemen do a double take but they are always courteous and answer your question.

You gradually speed up as you become more proficient. You no longer use your finger but follow the ball on an imaginary 8 with the center between the eyes of the person you are speaking to. You have practiced the steps of METHOD until it is now easy to talk relaxed and sure of yourself.

Now comes all the problems and situations that have bothered you all your life. You write them down and dig them out one by one. There is an intercom phone that you practice on. You tell funny stories. You can and do get help in any situation that gave you trouble. But by now it isn't difficult. And now you are helping the new students, you are an advanced student and they think you are pulling their leg when you tell them that you used to have a speech difficulty.

So in three months I changed my life. I came home so changed that people remarked about it. I got home late at night after my parents were in bed. I was telling them some of the highlights of the trip, and Mother started crying out of pure happiness I guess because that had always been one of my trouble spots, talking to them in the bedroom after coming home from a show. It just never occurred to me that I might have trouble.

I hope you can get something out of all this. I have backslid. There are also bad times now. That rhythm again. But the monkey is no longer on my back. I have never gotten over being nervous and having my heart pound before I get up to speak to a group of people, but I have deliberately pushed myself into situations like that. That was the main reason I took advanced R.O.T.C. and became an Officer. Why I accepted the Presidency of the State Floral Assoc. Why I talk to the Garden Clubs and teach advanced Military Tactics at Boise and Ft. Lewis. Why I like to sell fertilizer to people in my present job.

Perhaps my troubles are why I like to hear the personal problems of people and try to help them. I see the little boy and little girl in people and their inherent need to confide in someone. Perhaps they sense this because many people frequently tell me surprising things!

These were all *my* problems. I'm sure that every person that has a speech difficulty has his own unique problems. But I believe there is a general background or pattern common to all who stutter.

With love,
Dad

P.S. This isn't very much in spelling or grammar but perhaps it will give you a talking point with your teacher. I don't care in the least if you let them read it. Until again,
Love, Dad

For ease of reference we will identify the author of the letter as Mr. A. In most respects his letter speaks eloquently for itself; however, there are certain matters which merit recapitulation.

We might note first that he derived considerable benefit from his initial efforts with relaxation, but that relaxation alone was inadequate. At the same time, relaxation was important adjunctively in the method to which he credits his success.

From the description he gives of what was done at the Lewis school it is obvious that the approach employed was considerably more complex and planned than criticism has suggested. That is, it clearly was not just a simple and crude use of rhythm. In fact, some of the features of the treatment are typically found in "respectable" therapies—such as: relaxation, breath control, prescription of various pertinent assignments, exposure to real-life situations, supportive activity by the therapist, attention to aspects of good normal speech. Further, he clearly speaks of procedures which, in the idiom currently in favor, would be called "shaping" and "systematic desensitization." We should bear in mind that new names do not mean new techniques.

Note in particular Mr. A's references to the amount of practice involved and the clear indication that he was persistent in his efforts and willing to apply himself. Practice, persistence, and application are elements that figured prominently in the findings relative to recovery from stuttering reviewed in the preceding chapter.

Certain other material in the previous chapter is also recalled by Mr. A's reference to his maternal grandfather. The grandfather is said to have overcome his stuttering "by concentrating on the precise language he used," evidently another case of self-recovery achieved through working at careful speaking.

Mr. A reveals several bits of information about himself which deserve notice. He is a recovered stutterer, and has been for some time; much of the time he is unaware of ever having had a speech problem. Yet he still has a residual tendency to stutter, a tendency which recurs sporadically and without discernible cause—as his actual stuttering had. Reports of waxing and waning of stuttering occur repeatedly in case histories of stutterers. He mentions a history of stuttering in at least one person in each of the two generations preceding him. And, it is of interest that he is left-handed.

But we are interested most immediately in the evidence that the method of a commercial school was effective. The description Mr. A gives of other students in his class leads one to suspect that a sizable number of them achieved results similar to his.

We have very limited means for estimating the number of individuals who passed through the commercial schools. Mr. A mentioned about 25 students in residence during the three-month period he was there, and Clark (1964) refers to a class portrait in which Lewis posed with 156 students. If one were to make even a conservative estimate from these values, extrapolate it in reference to the enrollment that would be represented by a period of only ten years, and consider just the two schools discussed in this chapter, one can envision a very substantial number of individuals. Certainly if the majority of a population of such size turned out to be failures one could expect that there would be an impressive account of them somewhere.

Unfortunately, there is evidently no record anywhere of the extent of successes and failures of the commercial schools. Lacking that information we have lost much valuable knowledge regarding important influences in the amelioration of stuttering. There are many possible reasons for the successes and failures, but there is probably little point in conjecturing about them here. It is entirely conceivable that a certain number of the students thought the method had "erased" their stuttering, or expected it to continue to work for them in an essentially automatic way. In contrast, those who experienced success may have been less literal in their acceptance of the method.

Certainly Mr. A is a good example of one who did not expect a magical end to his stuttering. He followed instructions, worked hard at the assignments, and assumed responsibility for continuing to employ the method long after leaving the school. And he is still not "cured" in any absolute sense of the word. Yet he is certainly a success.

EPILOGUE

An adequate story of the commercial schools and their era is yet to be pieced together. Perhaps no one will ever have appropriate or sufficient motivation to attempt it. Quite possibly the story's primary value would be its historical interest. However, I am persuaded that there would be a good deal more that would be of interest and value to us, from both a negative and a positive standpoint.

Be that as it may, there is at least one matter of relevance to stuttering therapy that has been clearly identified in what little we know about the commercial schools—namely, there is some very potent effect on stuttering embodied in the matter of rhythm and it can be useful in the treatment of the disorder. We cannot afford to ignore this effect or to repudiate it.

We will consider the matter of rhythm more fully in the next chapter.

Notes

1. The original name of the association was American Academy of Speech Correction (see Paden, 1970, for early history of the association).
2. This man appeared in Seattle while I was at the University of Washington. He advertised in a local paper and gave two free public lectures, at which time locally obtained "assistants" handed out his literature. He then spent five days giving consultations, for a fee.
3. First published in 1919, the book had gone through six printings at the date noted in this reference.
4. A neat Madison Avenue type of touch. See example in Figure 6:3.
5. There is no need to review here the points on which Bogue's information was correct or incorrect in comparison to present day knowledge. Some of his errors, for instance his statements regarding the role of imitation and fright and the probability of outgrowing stuttering, were common for his day. In fact, some of them have been repeated in more recent times and in more respected sources.

6. Since the Lewis School was established first, there is a possibility that the Bogue Institute was modeled after it, but to my knowledge there is no evidence bearing on this conjecture.

7. Perhaps the refund of Bluemel's tuition was not made cheerfully because he had not complied with the conditions of the guarantee. The guarantee of cure was made " . . . provided the pupil will carry out and obey my instructions." (See Clark, 1964.)

A similar provision was part of the Bogue guarantee. This does not seem to be either misleading or unreasonable.

References

Bogue, B. N. *Stammering: Its Cause and Cure*, Hammond, Chicago, 1927.

Clark, Ruth M. Our enterprising predecessors and Charles Sydney Bluemel. *Asha*, **6**, 108–114, 1964.

Goldiamond, I. Operant analysis in the control of stuttering. *Program of 42nd Annual Convention, Am. Sp. Hearing Assn.*, 54, 1966 (abstr.).

———The treatment of stuttering: A case management symposium. *Program of 47th Annual Convention, Am. Sp. Hearing Assn.*, 37, 1971 (abstr.).

Klingbeil, G. M. The historical background of the modern speech clinic. *J. Speech Dis.*, **4**, 115–132, 1939.

Meyer, V. and J. M. Mair. A new technique to control stammering: A preliminary report. *Behav. Res. Ther.*, **1**, 251–254, 1963.

Paden, Elaine P. *A History of the American Speech and Hearing Association 1925–1958*, American Speech and Hearing Assn., Washington, 1970.

Van Dantzig, M. Syllable-tapping, a new method for the help of stammerers. *J. Speech Dis.*, **5**, 127–131, 1940.

7

RHYTHM: PAST AND PRESENT

The use of rhythm in the treatment of stuttering did not originate—or end—with the commercial schools. Our recorded history of the matter identifies a number of names associated with its use over a long period of time, and these accounts are probably not exhaustive. Perhaps it has been known for centuries and our very early records are simply incomplete. There is at least a suggestion of therapy through rhythm in one account of the means by which Demosthenes was helped to overcome his stuttering.[1] Reportedly he was advised to "declaim loudly while walking uphill" (cf. Klingbeil, 1939). The inference here is that this activity would readily induce synchrony of the pace of speaking with the rhythm of walking.

Whatever the situation may have been with Demosthenes, we do know that the beneficial effect of rhythm has been recognized for at least 150 years.

EARLY TIMES

There is adequate record of the use of rhythm in stuttering therapy from the beginning of the 19th century. The name most often associated with the use of rhythm in this early period is Colombat de l'Isere. Often references to him are accompanied by an air of ridicule for having promoted the use of rhythm in stuttering therapy. Although he might be spared the opprobrium that is accorded the commercial schools, there is often the clear implication that his treatment of stuttering was superficial and uneducated. One even finds an implication of ignorant gullibility directed at the action of the French Academy of the day for awarding Colombat the Monthyon prize for his achievements in working with stuttering.

The memory of Colombat and his contributions to the field of stuttering are maligned by the typically brief references to him which mention only his time-beating method. Colombat was seriously and sincerely committed to the study of stuttering and other speech disorders, as his writings reveal (Colombat, 1830, 1834, 1840). He employed techniques other than time-beating, and his use of rhythm was based upon a rationale that was reasonable for his time. He believed, with others, that stuttering was caused by a lack of harmony between nervous activity and the musculature of the organs that must function together to produce speech. He therefore devised a series of "orthophonic exercises" which involved all of the musculature of the speech system. The object of the exercises was to restore the necessary physiologic harmony. The most effective agent in the implementation of these exercises was rhythm, and to assist in this implementation he developed the "muthonome," a metronomic device pictured in Figure 7:1 and described by Colombat as follows:

> Muthonome, or *orthophonic lyre* for producing and regulating the rhythm. AAAAA, strings of the lyre or copper bars on which is indicated by the figures the number of oscillations per minute made by the pendulum, CC. B, bell on which a little spring-loaded hammer indicates the first time or the *beat time* of the measure. D, key for winding the instrument. E, bolt on which the measures of 1,2,3,4, & 6 time are marked with numbers. One pulls or pushes it a little either way according to the rhythm one wants to follow in the orthophonic exercises. F, a little slide in the shape of an owl by means of which one speeds up or slows down the oscillations of the pendulum CC.

Perhaps Colombat has come to be the main historical figure associated with the use of rhythm because of the recognition he received. However, he was not the first to use time-beating, even in his era. Before him it had been used by Serre d'Alais and Dupuytren (circa 1820), both Frenchmen, and earlier still (circa 1800) by Thelwall, an Englishman. A statement by Thelwall about his method should be of interest. In a letter written in 1801 he gave this description:

> From one simple and original principle I trace the fundamental and physical

distinctions of heavy and light syllables and from the unavaoidable alterations of these, I demonstrate the formation of those simple cadences of common and triple measure out of which arise all the beauties of rhythmus and all the facilities of fluent and harmonious utterance. (From Bluemel, 1913, Vol. 2, p. 81.)

The use of rhythm in treating stuttering evidently reached its zenith with Colombat and waned thereafter. One can only guess at the actual reasons. There was evident dissatisfaction with the fact that the early impressive improvement was often misleading in respect to eventual effect; but there were other salient influences too, such as the dramatic advent of surgical treatment, and the use of other "methods." Nonetheless, rhythm was included as part of a therapy program by many other

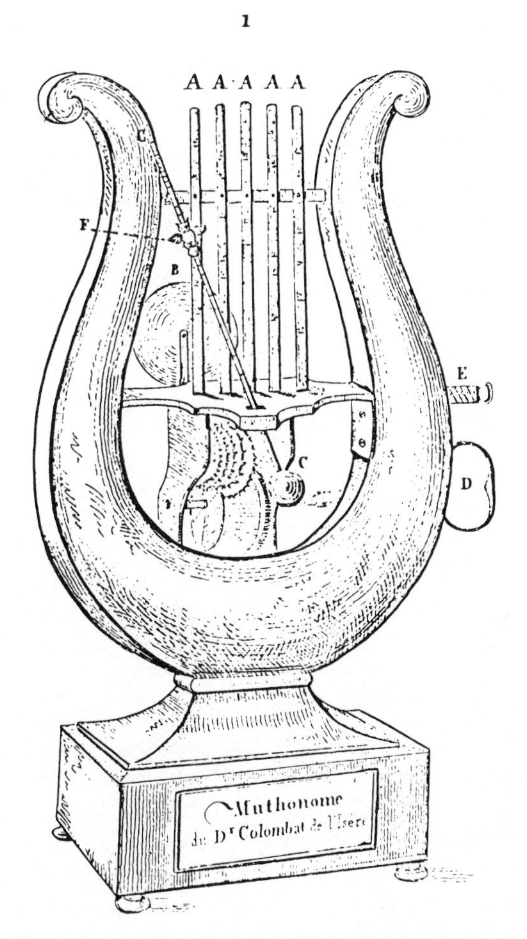

Figure 7:1 Muthonome, developed by Colombat (see text for description).

practitioners during the remainder of the 19th century; for instance, Cull and Shuldham in England; Violette and Rouma in France; Blume, Lehwess, Wyneken, Kussmaul, and Gunther in Germany; Graves in Ireland; and Hammond in the United States (cf. Potter, 1882 and Bluemel, 1913).

The efforts of these early workers should not be dismissed lightly, as it seems they have been, on the presumption of a sophisticated perspective from a more recent vantage point in history. Actually, a presumption of present-day sophistication in the treatment of stuttering is highly questionable in view of several considerations, such as: the many approaches in current use; the generally poor recovery rate; the very doubtful value of some approaches in active current use; the persisting disagreements about therapy techniques; the continuing search for some new method; and the myopia that sees revelation in new names applied to old procedures.

The profession's comparative view of past and present has been rather astigmatic and its position arbitrary. Certainly it should be recognized that the outright rejection of the use of rhythm has been particularly inappropriate in view of the fact that currently, more than 100 years after Colombat, we still do not know very much about the influence of rhythm and how it affects stuttering.

MODERN TIMES

A Brief Interlude

Attention to the matter of rhythm was scant in the early years of the profession's growth. When evidence of it did appear briefly in the late 1930s the interest was along experimental lines, and only some of it was very incisive.

The most analytic of these few investigations was the one published earliest. Robbins (1935) reported the culmination of some research that had extended over 14 years. This work had been undertaken originally in reference to earlier evidence that in stuttering " . . . there is a marked disturbance of rhythm in verbal expression." Robbins studied the temporal dimensions of several speech features of both stutterers and nonstutterers: the comparative lengths of accented and unaccented vowels, intersyllabic pause time, and the ratio of vocalization to expiration.

He found certain very impressive differences between stutterers and nonstutterers on these several dimensions.

It is noteworthy that these findings evidently generated no interest within the profession; Robbins' work did not stimulate further investigation. Apparently the profession was not ready for curiosity about rhythm. Probably this was due in large measure to the fact that there was at that time very limited attention to the kind of speech-language variables that occupy our interest today. But there is little doubt that the atmosphere was also substantially influenced by the aura of reaction to the commercial schools and their predecessors in the use of rhythm. For instance, Robbins himself noted that various forms of rhythmic speech had been used therapeutically with stuttering "since 1775," but he contended that most forms of rhythmic speech violated one or more of the "principles of rhythm" in normal speech. He concluded, therefore, that such artificial rhythms should not be used in the therapy of stuttering.

Within a few years two other studies addressed to the effect of rhythm appeared in the literature. They were items in a series entitled "Studies in the Psychology of Stuttering" carried out under the direction of Wendell Johnson. The title clearly announced the conceptual orientation (and the interpretive scope) of the investigations.

In the first study Johnson and Rosen (1937) compared the effects on stuttering of 12 kinds of imposed pattern. Three of these conditions embodied a regularly recurring rhythm: metronome, arm-swing, and sing-song. The other conditions were: singing; whispering; speaking slowly, rapidly, loudly, softly, in a high pitch, and in chorus. Fluency was enhanced quite regularly in all of these conditions except speaking rapidly. The rhythm conditions, however, had the most pronounced effect.

Shortly thereafter Barber (1940) studied the effectiveness of different patterns of rhythm and different modes of rhythmic stimulation. Essentially, she used several variations of two basic patterns, one involving syllable timing and the other word timing. The modes of stimulation were visual, auditory, and tactual. She found stuttering to be significantly reduced in all conditions, though some were much more effective than others. The least effective condition was the one calling for speaking with emphasis on every third word—a difficult pattern to follow.

The rationale and objectives of these two studies is not clear, other than to have made the obvious comparisons reported. The authors made no reference to the source of their interest in speech patterning or the influence of rhythm. Further, their conclusions simply reiterated the presumption made at the outset, namely, that the salutary effect on stuttering was due to "distraction."

Actually, several important findings were revealed by these studies.

First, any kind of pattern (including such an odd one as every third word) resulted in a significant reduction in stuttering. Second, patterns with an apparent regularity produce a dramatic effect. Third, the matter of pattern regularity may be somewhat misleading, since it did not matter if the pattern was related to syllables or to words. Fourth, the effect can evidently be induced through any sense modality.

The only article in our professional literature of this era which dealt specifically with the use of rhythm in therapy was written by Van Dantzig (1940), a Dutchman, who described a "new" method for the treatment of stuttering which he called "syllable-tapping." This method consists of speaking in syllables to the accompaniment of "noiseless (sequential) taps of the fingers of one hand." Van Dantzig recommended that the patient be encouraged to use his preferred hand, and the sequence of the tapping was to begin with the little finger and continue toward the thumb. He emphasized that one should not make the sequential movements in the opposite direction, but gave no rationale for this recommendation.

The method proceeded in three stages. The first stage was devoted to extensive practice in deliberate and emphatic execution of the finger movements in time with syllable utterance. The second stage was characterized by minimizing the finger movements and executing them with the fingers obscured from view. In the third stage the patient learned to perform "impulse movements," that is, to think or imagine the movements instead of actually moving the fingers. Van Dantzig said that when the patient reached the level of proficiency represented in stage three "he can be considered completely cured." He added, however, that some stutterers are unable to reach this stage.

Van Dantzig acknowledged that his method presented " . . . a certain analogy with an old expedient recommended for the help of stammerers, namely beatime time with one's hand." This was his only reference to precedents. He noted that speech therapists had considered time-beating with the hand to be a mere trick and to have no value, and he seemed to agree with this assessment. He contended that his method was superior, first because of its refinement of motor movement, but more importantly because of its "*methodical application*" and "*final sublimation to ideo-motoric impulses.*" He claimed it to be the most suitable method "for regulating the speech rhythm and for keeping a legato[2] manner of speaking at the same time."

Van Dantzig indicated that he had described the method in the hope that he might induce some American speech therapists to try it and correspond with him about their experiences with it. Apparently he did not arouse much interest.

The Recent Resurgence of Interest in Rhythm

Approximately a quarter of a century after the brief attention to rhythm reflected in the foregoing publications, the matter of rhythm suddenly reappeared in the relevant literature. Beginning in 1963, articles appeared sporadically for a few years and then with increasing frequency until by 1972 there were some 25 actual publications, and several more unpublished manuscripts, dealing with rhythm and stuttering. The matter has attracted the attention of the press several times during this period (*London Sunday Times*, 1966; *Medical World News*, 1967; *Newsweek*, 1968).

There are several very interesting facets to this resurgence of attention to rhythm; we will mention them in increasing order of "interest." First, the contributions have come mainly from outside the United States. Second, within the United States interest has been quite localized and expressed largely by persons other than speech pathologists. Third, the major focus has been on the therapeutic use of rhythm. Fourth, one rarely finds reference to the previous use of rhythm in therapy. Fifth, the "prime mover" of this renewed interest in rhythm was the development of a device—the electronic metronome.

A better instrument.—The electronic metronome, made possible by the capability of modern technology to miniaturize circuitry, is a very small, lightweight, self-contained, battery-operated device so designed that it can be worn in the fashion of a behind-the-ear hearing aid. The instrument has manually set volume and rate controls.

The prototype of the miniaturized metronome was the featured item of the first publication in this new era of attention to rhythm (Meyer and Mair, 1963). The article included a description, schematic diagram, and pictures of the device. It consisted of two behind-the-ear hearing aid cases, each containing half of an "astatic multivibrator." The two aids were connected by a fine-wire cable of sufficient length to cross the back of the head when the aids were in place, one behind each ear.

Subsequent publications (Brady, 1968; Horan, 1968; Wohl, 1968) have described other models of electronic metronome. They are basically the same kind of instrument but vary in size and convenience. The most successful model[3], described by Brady (1968), was developed in the United States as an improvement of the Meyer and Mair prototype. It is a single self-contained behind-the-ear instrument that has readily accessible and easily adjusted rate and volume controls. Figures 7:2 and 7:3 show the unit against a standard rule and in place as worn.

The "Pacemaster" was developed through the cooperative efforts of three men in Philadelphia who had an interest in the use of rhythm as a therapy technique for stuttering. E. Robert Libby's interest in the instrument was personal; he is a stutterer who had experience with a metronome for many years. Irwin Rothman, an osteopathic psychiatrist, and John Brady, a psychiatrist, had a professional interest in the use of rhythm, having employed a standard desk model in therapy for several years.

Because Mr. Libby's experience with a metronome provides another

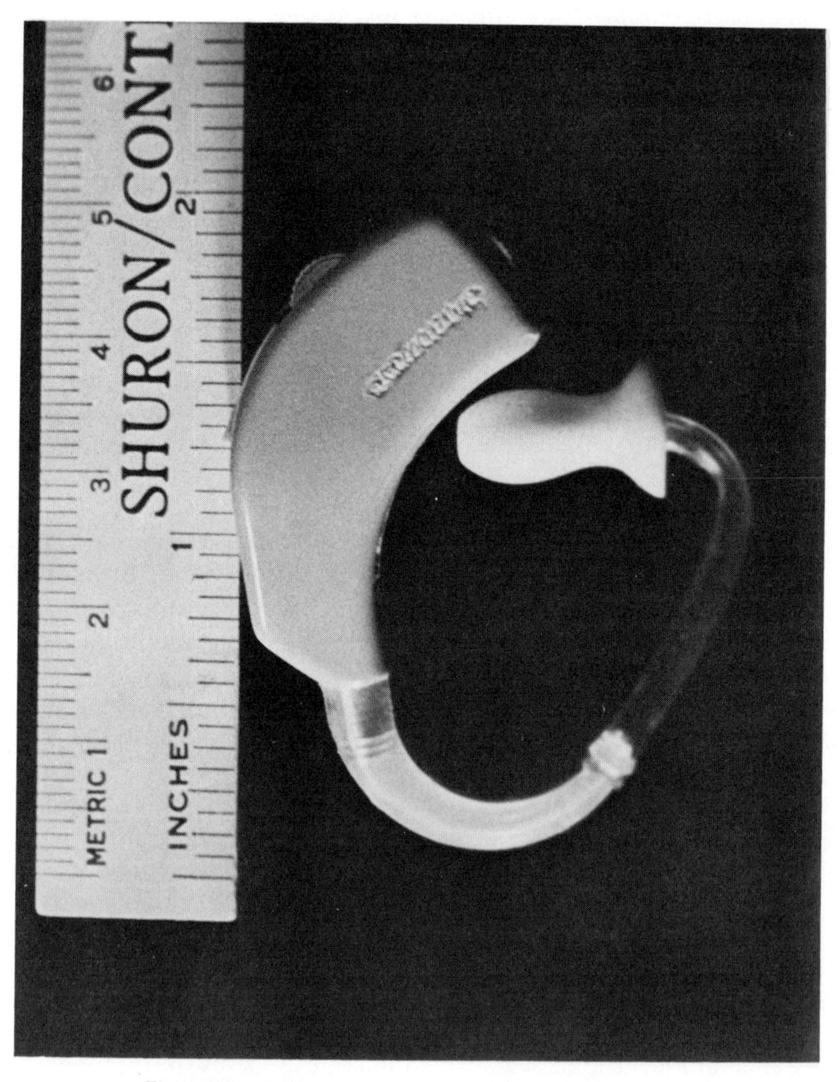

Figure 7:2 The "Pacemaster," miniaturized electronic metronome.

dimension of information about the use of rhythm, which otherwise would remain obscure, we will devote some space to briefly chronicle his story.[4]

Mr. Libby's earliest recollection of stuttering was at age 6. He stuttered rather badly throughout his childhood and adolescence and could not recall that his stuttering changed very much during this time. He received therapy through the schools while in the elementary grades and

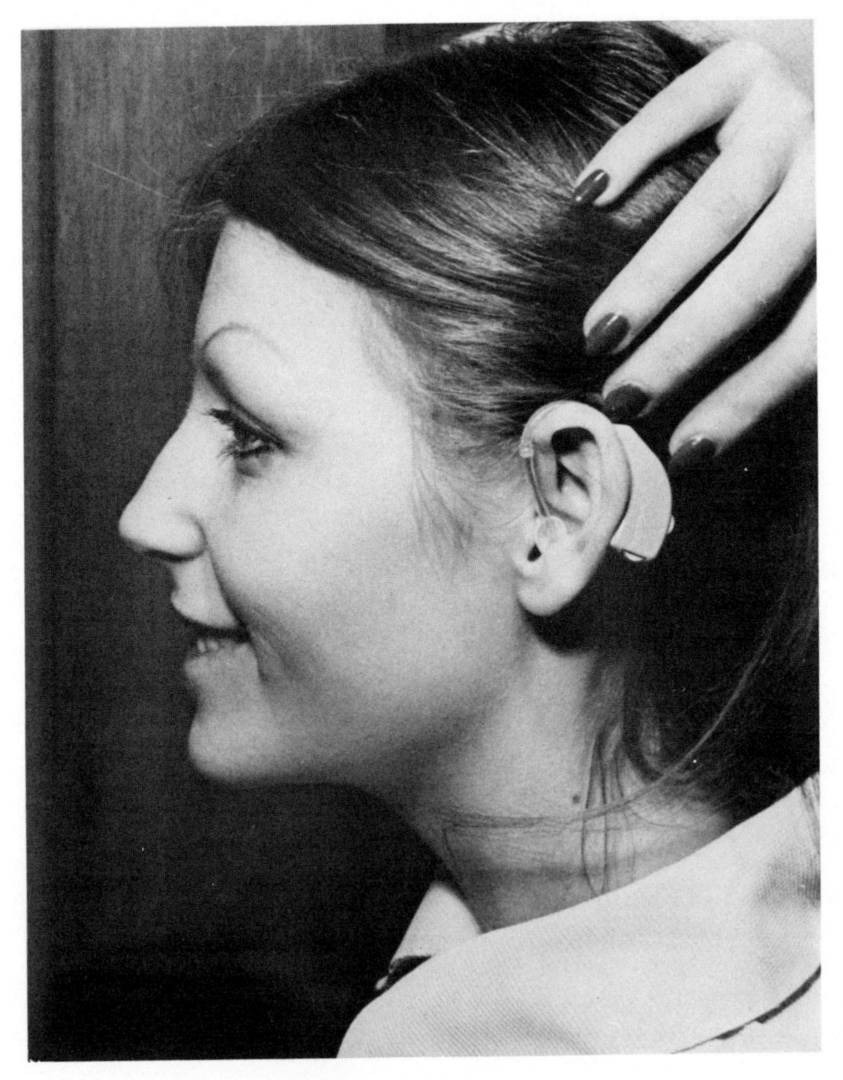

Figure 7:3 The "Pacemaster" in place as worn by a patient.

during his junior high school years but remembered it as more frustrating than helpful. He struggled on through high school and college, again without much evident change in his stuttering. However, he found he was having great difficulty communicating when he began to practice his profession as an optometrist, and felt he should try to obtain some help with his stuttering.

Upon the advice of his physician he obtained psychiatric treatment and persisted with it for two years. He said that he learned a great deal about his anxieties and personal problems, but his stuttering did not improve. Psychiatric treatment was another disappointment.

Following this he sought the help of a well-known speech therapist in the Philadelphia area who, after examination, advised him that his problem was irremediable and that his best alternative was to make his personal adjustment to it. He was very distressed and discouraged by this professional opinion.

Shortly thereafter he noticed a small ad in the newspaper that invited anyone who stuttered to join a nonprofit club for stutterers. It was called the "Kingsley Club," after Canon Kingsley, the well-known 19th century English author and lecturer who was also a stutterer. The Kingsley Club was originated and led by an attorney, William Smith, who practiced law actively in spite of his own stutter. The organization of the club was very informal; it was essentially a vehicle to provide interested adult stutterers the opportunity to continue to do something about their stuttering. The membership of the club was usually not large; over the years its size ranged between 25 and 50 persons. Most of the members had had previous experience with several methods of therapy that had not been successful.

Club meetings were held one evening a week with the primary objective being the experience of better speech. To this end their activities centered around the use of a standard desk metronome. Each member had his chance to speak to the ohers while using the instrument. Everyone was more fluent with the use of this aid; many of them spoke with no stuttering at all. Whenever a new member joined the club the conversational content for the first few weeks seemed to center around personal problems related to their stuttering, but after this initial period, which seemed to exhaust the topic, they simply talked about what they had done that day. Basically, their interest was in the experience of more fluent speech. The group support they felt focused around this shared, yet personal, achievement. Mr. Libby said that he always felt euphoric after leaving the group. Unfortunately, the euphoria—and the more fluent speech—were short-lived.

The club did have a social aspect which, however, subserved the interest in better speech. Every three months they met for dinner—and giving speeches. With Martinis added to metronome the club members were even more fluent—speeches ran "interminably," and the meetings lasted far into the night.

Because the weekly meetings, though supportive, had little consistent effect on his daily speech, Mr. Libby began to practice with a metronome at home after work. Over a period of many years of steady practice with the instrument his speech gradually improved and he became less and less dependent upon regular practice with the metronome. However, he has continued to "refresh" his greatly improved fluency with occasional practice, especially when there is, for some reason, a brief period of increase in his stuttering. Today his speech is fluent most of the time, and the stutterings that occur are mild and intermittent. Understandably, he is enthusiastic about the use of a metronome in stuttering therapy.

Variations on the basic theme of a miniaturized metronome have been reported. Azrin et al. (1968) described a device for delivering rhythmic tactual pulses. This instrument was developed primarily for use in experimentation and was quite cumbersome. It required a battery pack using standard size batteries and long wires running from the pack to the pulsor, which was attached to the wrist. Donovan (1971) reported the construction of a combination portable metronome and masking tone generator. The instrument is said to be of convenient size and weight. It will deliver either a rhythmic pulse, a continuous masking tone, or an intermittent, regularly recurring masking tone. The supposed advantage of this instrument is that it includes the masking provision, which is otherwise available only in a separate instrument. We will make note of masking devices in the next chapter.

Present-day efforts with rhythm.—Now, 130 years after Colombat developed a version of the metronome specifically for use in stuttering therapy, we have a new version of the instrument—one which is more refined, compact, convenient, and easily regulated. But the advance is largely one of mechanical technology. The basic principle and the manner of implementation remain unchanged. This might explain in part why there is so little reference to prior work with rhythm. Those who know nothing of the history of stuttering therapy cannot, of course, be expected to be knowledgeable about the previous use of rhythm. Those who are cognizant of the prior experience with rhythm in stuttering therapy could well have little motivation to review the record. As we noted earlier, the written record would neither support nor generate great enthusiasm. (At the same time, we also pointed out that the unwritten record, if recoverable, might yield a substantially different picture.)

The apparently unimpressive record of rhythm therapy in previous application to stuttering does not automatically discredit it as a useful technique, as its detractors wish to contend. Nonetheless, a renewed interest in rhythm should proceed with all due recognition of its past. In this way we are less likely to repeat previous mistakes and more likely to build in a constructive manner. It seems quite clear that, so far, the new use of rhythm has failed to take account of what has gone before. To this extent, at least, it is suspect as a professional undertaking.

A related reservation about the new rhythm era is that much of the current writing is infused with the jargon of the day. Rhythm therapy is now "behavior therapy," changes that occur are "conditioned," fluency is "shaped." At best the terms are innocuous, in that they refer to nothing that was not known or done before. At the same time, their use reflects either ignorance of, or indifference to, what is known about rhythm and stuttering. Furthermore, what the terms suggest is misleading, at least in the sense of implying a knowledge and understanding that really does not exist. That is, we do not know that stuttering is some learned function or disturbance in learning (see Chapter 2), which is what this orientation implies.

There is no reason to think that the current use of rhythm in stuttering therapy involves any particular advance in respect to a *method* of therapy. Obviously the inducing instrument has changed certain practicalities of usage—mainly because it is portable—but the essential method remains the same as before. This should be clearly evident once we have reviewed the reports of recent work that seems to herald the beginning of a new rhythm era. Much of this material provides grounds for encouragement and a certain degree of optimism, but it should be appraised judiciously.

Rhythm therapy with the device.—Meyer and Mair (1963) were the first to report the use of the electronic metronome in stuttering therapy. They indicated that their work was initiated "from the observation that metronome beats eliminate stuttering." They reported the use of their instrument with 10 subjects between the ages of 15 and 43, all but one of whom had had previous therapy which included routine speech therapy, shadowing, hypnosis, and psychotherapy.

All of their patients spoke fluently with the metronome; the most satisfactory rates were found to be between 75 and 95 beats per minute. There seemed to be an optimal rate for each patient, which was determined subjectively in terms of the ease and fluency of his speech.

After each patient's optimal rate was established, he was fitted with an aid and instructed to wear the device in all situations and to speak with the rhythm. Progression toward speaking fluently without use of the aid was undertaken gradually in a sort of trial-and-error fashion. The patient was instructed to test periodically his ability to speak with the device turned off, in the anticipation that these periods would gradually lengthen. Any occurrence of difficulty was to be met by reverting to use of the apparatus. As periods of fluency increased without use of the device the patient was to try removing it entirely. If he encountered difficulty after this point, he was to first try slowing down his speech, using a rhythmic pattern in doing so. If this was not sufficient to reinstate fluency, he was to return again to the use of the instrument. Patients were advised to explain the purpose of the device to strangers before engaging in long conversations with them.

The authors reviewed the progress of five patients some time after the initial training period, which had varied from one to ten weeks. Four of these individuals were improving, without the use of the instrument. The fifth had had difficulty but he had also lost interest in improving his speech due to a major change in occupation.

Somewhat later Meyer and Comley (1969)[5] reported on their experience with 48 stutterers, ranging in age from 11 to 58.

The objective of these investigators was to teach the patients "rhythmic speech"; those who failed to develop this skill were taught "syllabic speech." The authors did not specify the difference; however, "syllabic speech" almost certainly refers to speaking in time to a metronome beat at the rate of one syllable per beat. "Rhythmic speech," in comparison, most likely means speech that is conditioned and supported by the cadence of a metronome but is not "locked in" to syllable-by-syllable timing.

In the beginning period of the treatment a standard desk metronome was used with all patients and an optimal "beat" was established for each person. After this initial period, some patients were fitted with the small electronic metronome while others continued treatment with unaided rhythmic speech. Each patient was seen once weekly for about 12 weeks. The treatment sessions were spent mainly in attempting to help the patients with their own specific difficulties; the treatment often utilized relaxation and sometimes simulated social situations.

Seventeen patients failed to master "rhythmic speech"; the authors did not report what subsequently became of these individuals.

Those who had responded to training in rhythmic speech were seen for reevaluation 24 weeks after the termination of treatment. All of them were reported to have remained significantly improved. In fact, six were said to have achieved complete fluency. Three of these patients were ones who had worn the miniature metronome in the period of treatment following the basic training with the desk metronome; the other three had received unaided rhythmic speech therapy during that period.

Wohl (1968) reported the improvement attained by 139 patients, ages 15 to 68, during a one-year pilot study of the use of the portable metronome. Nineteen of the patients were treated through a clinic therapy program which included the use of rhythm as a means to "establish correct timing" within a broader objective of "making good the deficiencies in language learning and memory." The procedure began with having the patient listen to several beats in order to appreciate the timing. He then moved into saying a list of words in time to a "comparatively slow beat." Gradually the patient worked up to saying word combinations of increasing length and complexity of composition.

One hundred and twenty of the patients were reported to have been "self-treated." The author did not indicate that anything more was involved in this self-therapy beyond the personal use of the electronic metronome. The results, presented in Table 7:1, reveal a very favorable outcome for both groups.

In a later publication Wohl (1970) described an elaborate training program which involved structured help in the use of the portable metronome, desensitization, and attitude reeducation. She indicated, however, that something less than 10 percent of the cases needed this program, even for purposes of using the instrument in public. Also, attention to personal reactions to the problem was unnecessary.

Brady (1968, 1971) has given the most extensive description of a therapy program involving the use of the electronic metronome. His description spells out what is only suggested or alluded to briefly in some other reports.

The first stage involves the use of a desk metronome set at a very slow rate (around 80 beats per minute, though possibly much lower for a severe stutterer); the patient speaks by pacing one word to a beat. In the second stage, usually beginning with the second session, the approxima-

Table 7:1 Success rate in use of the electronic metronome by 139 patients (From Wohl, 1968.)

	Therapy	*Self-treated*
Acquired fluency	4	10
Great improvement	15	62
Some improvement	0	47
No improvement	0	1

tion to more usual rate and cadence begins. The rate of the metronome beat is gradually increased, the pacing of speech to the beats is less regularized (i.e., one beat might pace two or three syllables, or a pause, etc.), and longer units of speech are paced to the beats. This phase is completed when the patient can speak with the metronome at a rate of 100 to 160 words per minute with minimal stuttering. At stage three the miniature metronome is substituted for the desk metronome. The patient makes use of the aid in situations of increasing "difficulty level" in his daily life. In phase four, the final stage of actual treatment, the patient gradually abandons the use of the metronome, following the difficulty-graded procedure of the previous stage.

The move to speaking without the metronome "proceeds in a cautious, trial-and-error manner," i.e., if the patient runs into difficulty, he immediately reverts to a temporary use of the metronome. This principle—reversion to an earlier stage—actually runs throughout the entire treatment process. That is, if at any point in treatment the patient shows signs of relapse, he is instructed to revert to a slower rate and a more definite pacing. Brady emphasizes the importance of this principle of reversion to an earlier stage and says that it "sometimes requires much coaching by the therapist."

The principle also extends into the period beyond the formal therapy process. Brady recognizes that the tendency to stutter often waxes and wanes, and that patients may be beset by unexplained episodes of stuttering tendency long after therapy has been "successful." In such instances the patient is urged to return to the use of his device in order to minimize the temporary recurrence of actual or incipient stuttering.

Brady wove into the rationale of his procedures the theoretical bases of "anticipatory tension" and "conditioned anxiety." Originally this called for the inclusion of certain "behavior therapy" procedures of the Wolpian "reciprocal inhibition" type. Particularly since Brady continued to maintain his theoretical position, it is of considerable interest to find his later acknowledgement that, "Now we find it is not necessary to do so [i.e., include the Wolpian procedures] in most cases." The same experience and conclusion were reported by Wohl (1970). On the other hand, Brady reported an apparent need for *adjunctive* counseling and supportive psychotherapy in many cases. However, these are implemented only after the patient has shown substantial improvement with his stuttering.

Brady reported the results obtained with 23 severe chronic stutterers between the ages of 12 and 53. All had previously had some form of therapy, which included speech therapy, psychotherapy, and behavior therapy. Actual treatment time per patient in the rhythm therapy varied from five one-hour sessions for several patients to 31 sessions with one patient. The average length of treatment was 12 sessions and extended over a period of several months.

Reevaluation of the patients' speech was made between six and 44 months after treatment, the average follow-up period being 14 months. Two patients did not show any significant improvement while speaking without the metronome.[6] The remaining 21 showed substantial improvement in their unaided speech, as reflected in an average reduction in stuttering of 67 percent. Eleven of these patients no longer used the metronome at all, and eight more were using it only some of the time. All of them felt that carry-over to unaided fluent speech increased proportionately with continued use of the device.

Comparison of pre- and post-treatment interview data and the results of two measures of personal adjustment provided evidence of favorable changes in the patients' general adjustment at the time of follow-up. Similar findings are reported by Andrews and Harris (1964) and Brandon and Harris (1967).

Rhythm therapy without an instrument.—Some efforts have been made to implement rhythm in a manner like that of the metronome but without the use of mechanical devices or timing movements of some part of the body (e.g., Van Dantzig's "syllable-tapping").

Andrews and Harris (1964) reported their experience with a training program utilizing "syllable-timed" speech, which consists of speaking syllable by syllable, stressing each syllable evenly, and saying the syllables in time to a regular thythm.

Andrews and Harris worked with 35 patients, ages 11 to 45, in a 10-day intensive therapy program, followed by an extended less formalized period, which then led into eventual follow-up at three-month intervals. The patients were separated into two adult groups, one adolescent group (ages 16-19), and one children's group (five boys age 11).

The basic initial work within each group was individual. They began with easy things to say, progressing from simple sentences to short prose passages according to a prescribed routine. Each patient first said each simple item in unison with the therapist, then in repetition of him, and then by himself—all in syllable-timed pattern. These items were practiced repeatedly until all patients could say them error-free.

The next step was to employ syllable-timed speech in spontaneous expression. This was begun in a very structured and formal manner by such means as playing formalized word games. The subsequent objective was the use of syllable-timed speech in the ordinary verbal interaction of group discussion.

At the end of the first two-hour session all patients except the 11-year-olds were speaking at 80 syllables per minute with no stuttering. The 11-year-olds were able to perform adequately when speaking in unison but they did not progress so rapidly in the use of syllable-timed speech. With them the teaching of syllable-timed speech had to begin with a general discussion about syllables. They took considerably longer to use syllable-timed speech in ordinary conversation and did not do well with it consistently until the fourth or fifth day.

The authors pointed out that syllable-timed speech is not difficult to execute but that if stutterers are to become proficient they must practice. Their patients were required to practice—100 hours—mostly in the first 10 days of the organized therapy program. Each day began with practice in reading and speaking in slow syllable-timed speech; the discussion period was not started until everyone had completed this initial work satisfactorily. Syllable-timed speech was constantly required in the discussion periods as well.

Gradually the rate of fluent syllable-timed speech increased until "normal speeds" of 100 to 150 syllables per minute[7] were attained. As the rate of speech increased there was a gradual return of normal stress contrast; this evidently occurred quite naturally, since the patients were unaware of the change. This return of normal stress contrast was permitted to happen as long as no stuttering recurred.

Most of the first few days were spent in the clinic, but thereafter an increasing number of excursions were arranged. Patient reaction to use of syllable-timed speech in the community varied. Some patients, excited about the fluency thus made possible, were eager to use it; others were reluctant to speak in this manner because it sounded artificial. Support of the group was felt to be valuable in these circumstances, not only in providing encouragement for those more hesitant but also in exerting some restraint on those who were overly enthusiastic. Eventually the patients spent less time in the group and more on individual assignments calculated to test their skill in speaking.

The groups were not planned or conducted as psychotherapeutic groups, but group members "became aware of the individual needs and anxieties and endeavored collectively to deal with them." In one adult group this aspect of group function was intentionally encouraged; in the other it received little attention.

Following the intensive treatment period, the separate adult and adolescent groups all met together as one large group at least 10 times in the next 10 weeks. These meetings were hour-long sessions in which they discussed individual experiences and problems with speaking that had occurred in the interim between meetings. These weekly sessions were devoted mainly to discussing effective use of syllable-timed speech. With the dissolution of the more cohesive small groups, there was an end to the spontaneous discussion of attitudes and anxieties. Andrews and Harris felt that, for this reason, it had been a mistake to combine the three groups in this period. However, this would seem a mistake only if one assumed that the discussion of attitudes and anxieties was somehow important to improvement in fluency. Actually, their results revealed that both of the original adult groups achieved comparable levels of success, even though in one group considerable time was spent "working through the problems and anxieties concerned with stuttering" and in the other this aspect was ignored.

During these weekly meetings the patients were all encouraged to use formal, slow, syllable-timed speech, and metronomes were used to insure that this was done. They were given continued advice about syllable-timed speech, particularly regarding the likelihood that their natural tendency would be to revert to syllable-contrast speech. They were advised that if stuttering recurred as they began to return to normal speech, they should immediately revert to syllable-timed speech and persist in using it for the rest of that day. Use of formal syllable-timed reading was recommended in case the recurrence of stuttering "reached significant levels."

All patients except one[8] experienced a marked reduction in stuttering (to the "mild" level or better) by the end of the treatment period. They were then reevaluated at three-month intervals, which extended from six to twelve months after treatment. Most of the cases showed some amount of relapse at the first three-month review; however, there was no further relapse among those followed for nine and twelve months.

The authors indicated that the degree of improvement seemed to be linked to initial severity of the stutter, in that the method was proportionately more effective with severe stutterers. They also commented that those who did best were the patients who were "reasonably free from anxiety and other neurotic symptoms," although it is not clear how this was determined.

Actually, age was the variable most impressively associated with change. The group of 11-year-olds made the greatest amount of initial improvement, showed the least amount of relapse, and had maintained this level of improvement when last seen nine months after treatment. This record is of particular interest in view of the fact that they had the most difficulty learning syllable-timed speech, and that in their group no particular attention was directed to matters of attitude or possible anxieties.

Several years later Brandon and Harris (1967) reported the results of a therapy program using syllable-timed speech with 28 stutterers, presumably all adults. Treatment was initiated by a simplified explanation of the approach and then demonstration with simple sentences. These were first repeated by each patient in unison with the therapist and then alone. Further progression followed a carefully graded scale of difficulty in reading and speaking practice using syllable-timed speech. The rate of speaking in the early stages was considered to be very important; 70 syllables per minute seemed to be the most effective.

In the initial two-week training period patients were seen three times daily. Each day started with an intensive period of reading practice using syllable-timed speech. General conversation within these sessions was increasingly encouraged as long as the regular rhythm was maintained. Gradually the speaking situations were extended into the community, especially during the second week. After this initial two-week period, the patients were seen two times a week for three months, then once a week for another three months.

A four-level scale was developed to assess each patient's speech before treatment and in follow-up. Each level on the scale was a composite of the percentage of words stuttered, word per minute rate, type of stutter, and associated symptoms. Personality measures and assessment through psychiatric interview were also employed pretreatment and at follow-up.

At the time of reevaluation a year and a half after termination of treatment 18 cases showed 60 percent or greater improvement on the scale described above. Ten cases showed less improvement than this; six showed very little change. In consideration of the severe criticisms leveled at the commercial schools for the supposed adverse effects of the use of rhythm in treating stuttering, Brandon and Harris made a particular point of noting that the method had not had the effect of exacerbating stuttering in any of these individuals. Furthermore, personality assessments indicated no adverse personal reactions, even in the six cases whose speech was virtually unchanged.

The patients who showed little change in their speech did not differ much either in age or intelligence from those who had improved substantially. However, the personality assessments indicated, interestingly, that those who showed the least improvement tended to be sociable, outgoing, rather egocentric, and *free from anxiety*. The latter finding is contradictory to the statement regarding improvement and anxiety made by Andrews and Harris. However, it is consistent with evidence from other areas of investigation of human function that motivation is an important contributor to change.

EXPERIMENTAL STUDY OF RHYTHM

Some of the recent work with rhythm has been concerned with an assessment of the explanations given for its beneficial effect. Actually, most of this work has been addressed to assessing the adequacy of two of the explanations that have been offered. One of these explanations—that the effect of rhythm is due to distraction—has been expressed much more often and accepted much more widely than any other conjecture. The other, less frequently voiced, explanation is that rhythm achieves its effect because it induces the stutterer to slow down. It has also been claimed that rhythm minimizes stuttering through a form of "masking" effect, or because it induces regularity in speaking. There is some experimental evidence bearing on these interpretations as well.

Rhythm as Distraction

It was mentioned previously that a logical appraisal of distraction alone will reveal it to be a fallacious explanation of the effect of rhythm. Again, we will defer that appraisal to an even more appropriate context (see p. 187), since "distraction" has been offered as the explanation of effects other than rhythm. However, it is appropriate at this point to call the reader's attention to the fact that the explanation of rhythm as a distraction is essentially groundless. One never hears, for instance, *how* it distracts or *why* it should be distracting. For the time being, let us consider some experimental evidence that contradicts the "distraction" account.

Several investigations have assessed the effect on stuttering of conditions other than rhythm which could logically be expected to act as distractions. This section reviews investigations of the influence on stuttering of random noise, irregular rhythms, and "subsidiary tasks."

Noise.—Beech and Dubbane (1962) compared stutterers' fluency in normal circumstances with that observed while they talked under conditions of random, loud, ambient noise. The noise condition did not improve the level of fluency.

Irregular rhythm.—Meyer and Mair (1963) commented on their observations with two patients that irregular but predictable rhythms were less effective than regular rhythms, and that irregular and unpredictable rhythms had no influence on fluency.

The report by Meyer and Mair is consistent with the earlier findings of Barber (1940), who investigated the influence of twelve different rhythmic conditions. Eleven of these conditions involved saying either a word or a syllable in time to some regular rhythm. Some of these rhythms were externally imposed; others were self-generated and accompanied by some simple and routinized body movement. The twelfth condition called for accenting every third word. All conditions had a markedly beneficial effect on fluency, but the latter condition was clearly inferior to the others.

Fransella and Beech (1965) compared the fluency of eighteen stutterers reading aloud under normal circumstances to their level of fluency when reading in time to a rhythmic metronome and to an arrhythmic metronome. Each subject was instructed, for reading with the rhythmic beat, to say each word or syllable in time with the beats, whichever pattern he found to be easier. With the arrhythmic instrument the subject was instructed to listen carefully to the beats to see if he was able to discern any recurrent pattern which he could reproduce in his speech. The authors found the condition using the rhythmic metronome to be significantly superior to the other conditions. Speaking in time to the arrhythmic metronome was only slightly better than speaking with no metronome at all. (Evidently both metronomes had the same overall average rate. The authors did not identify the range of aperiodic rate of their arrhythmic metronome, a matter which is of some importance.)

Azrin *et al.* (1968) compared the effects of a rhythmic and arrhythmic tactual pulse in reducing stuttering during reading. The rhythmic device delivered a pulse at 90 beats per minute. The arrhythmic instrument generated a pulse rate which, on the whole, averaged 90 beats per minute but delivered them at irregular intervals varying from 0.3 to 1.3 seconds. Subjects were instructed to speak one word per pulse unless the word was too long, in which case they could divide the word syllabically between pulses. The rhythmic pulse resulted in approximately a 90 percent reduction in stuttering for each stutterer. In contrast, the arrhythmic pulse had no discernible effect on the stuttering of any of the subjects.

Brady (1969) also compared the effects of an arrhythmic and rhythmic metronome on stutterers' speech. In both metronome conditions subjects were asked to speak extemporaneously, one syllable per beat, in time to the metronome. The rate for the rhythmic metronome was regular at 120 beats per minute. The overall average rate of the arrhythmic metronome was the same but the intervals between beats varied randomly between 0.3 and 0.7 seconds. Brady found that both of the metronome conditions produced significant improvements in fluency. However, the rhythmic condition was significantly more effective than the arrhythmic. He noted that speaking with the arrhythmic metronome was "a difficult confusing task" and that although the patient's speech was quite fluent it did not have the smooth cadence that comes with speaking to a rhythmic metronome.

The Brady report is the only one that makes reference to the *quality* of the subjects' speech under the influence of the arrhythmic metronome. Even his description is very brief, indicating only that the cadence was not as smooth as that found when talking in time to a rhythmic metronome. The implication here is that there was a cadence of some sort in the speech of his subjects when they were attempting to speak to the pattern of the arrhythmic metronome. This possibility seems the more likely when it is recalled that the range of aperiodicity of this metronome was not marked. The range was less than half a second (0.3 sec to 0.7 sec) and this difference would be attenuated perceptually by the occurrence of the beats at an average rate of 120 per second. This relatively narrow range of irregularity might have permitted support of some more-or-less regular cadence, even though evidently not as regular as with a standard metronome.

Such factors might well reconcile the difference between Brady's findings and those of Azrin *et al.* (1968) and Fransella and Beech (1965), both of whom found that the speech of their subjects was no better with the arrhythmic metronome than with no metronome at all. Fransella and Beech did not report the range of aperiodic intervals covered by their device. However, the range of the instrument employed by Azrin *et al.* was from 0.3 to 1.3 seconds, at an average rate of 90 beats per minute. Thus, the actual range of random irregularity was over twice as great as that employed by Brady and, further, the slower rate would have had the effect of perceptually exaggerating the irregularity. It seems unlikely that this sequence would support any kind of speaking pattern. Although the results of these three investigations do not reveal consistently that the effect of an arrhythmic instrument is no better than no instrument at all, they all clearly agree that a regular beat is significantly superior to an irregular beat in reducing stuttering.

The finding that reduced stuttering was associated with an arrhythmic beat in one of these studies is a matter deserving further study in the effort to discover how rhythm functions to ameliorate stuttering. For the moment, however, we are most interested in the fact that in all the studies a rhythmic beat was found to be significantly superior.

The comparisons of rhythmic and arrhythmic pulses have proceeded on the grounds that the two conditions could be assumed to be equally distracting. This would seem to be a very defensible assumption. In fact, there is good reason to contend that attempting to follow an arrhythmic beat should be much *more* distracting than following a regular one. This would follow not only from introspection and subjective analysis; it is clearly indicated in Brady's description of it as a "difficult confusing task."

This common finding that speaking to a more-or-less regular rhythm is superior to attempting to speak to an irregular rhythm is sufficient evidence to contradict the claim that rhythm represents a distraction. However, there is other contradictory evidence.

Subsidiary task.—Fransella (1967) compared the influence of a rhythmic metronome with the effect produced by a number-writing task. In this task subjects, while reading aloud, were required to listen for and write numbers presented by tape recording. The numbers had been recorded at irregular intervals which ranged from one to four seconds. It was assumed that this task was clearly a distraction, since it obviously required the subjects to direct their attention to some other activity.

Again the results were clear-cut: there was a significant reduction of stuttering with the metronome whereas fluency during the number-writing task was no different than under ordinary conditions.

Brady (1969) subsequently replicated Fransella's work with the number-writing task. He also found that this condition did not have any noticeable influence on stuttering but, again, that a rhythmic metronome had its characteristic effect.

The findings of a study by Greenberg (1970) bear directly on the matter of distraction although this was not the objective of the study. Greenberg studied the effect of a standard metronome on the fluency of 20 stuttering children while they talked about toys. The metronome was set at a rate of 98 beats per minute. Ten of the children were instructed to pace their speech to the beat of the metronome. The other ten subjects were not given any instructions but simply spoke while the metronome "provided a rhythmic auditory background noise" which was not in the clear attentional focus of the subjects.

The fluency of both groups was significantly better with the metronome than without it. Those subjects instructed to pace their speech to the beat of the metronome showed somewhat more improvement in fluency, but it was not significantly different from those who did not receive these instructions. Here we have a situation in which stutterers' fluency was markedly improved, evidently through the influence of a metronome beat of which they were hardly aware. "Distraction" is a very improbable explanation of these findings.

Greenberg did not analyze differences in the pattern of her subjects' speech between the ordinary and the metronome conditions. However, she did remark that when listening to the recordings obtained it was "very often easy to tell when the subject has 'fallen into a rhythm' with the metronome." This strongly suggests that the metronome unobtrusively influenced the pattern of the subjects' speech in much the same way that a definite, perceptible rhythm induces many forms of rhythmic activity. We are all familiar with the tendency to "keep time" to the music of a band, an inclination which expresses itself quite naturally. In fact, infants at least as young as ten months evidence the effect quite readily. Work songs and sea chanteys have developed from this principle and are a natural expression of it.

The phenomenon has been referred to as a "synchronization effect" by Azrin *et al.* (1968), who demonstrated it experimentally on very simple motor and vocal acts. "Synchronization" is an attractive description of the phenomenon but it does not tell us very much. It does not suggest any explanation of the nature of the phenomenon—its possible dimensions or bases. Certainly it provides no indication of what might underlie the beneficial influence of rhythm on stuttering.

Nonetheless, in the case of Greenberg's subjects we can see the operation of the general principle of synchronization and note that the reduction in stuttering associated with it presents another contradiction to the explanation that rhythm has its effect on stuttering through distraction. That is, since improved fluency was evidently associated with a rhythm induced through the synchronization effect, and since synchronization occurred without involving an awareness of it or attention to it, any improvement due to rhythm could hardly be explained in terms of distraction.

Rhythm and Slowing Down

A second explanation of the rhythm effect is that it induces the stutterer to decrease his speech rate. This seems a plausible explanation in view of the observation that—at least among normal speakers and mild stutterers—more time is needed to speak to rhythm than when speaking in ordinary cadence. The evidence bearing on this matter is not as extensive as that relating to the "distraction" account, but what is available seems to be rather definitive.

Some of the findings reported by Barber (1940) are relevant to the issue. She found that stuttering was significantly reduced at both a slow rate of 92 beats per minute and at a fast rate of 184 beats per minute, with no substantial difference between the two rates.

Fransella and Beech (1965) had their stutterers read at their usual rate and at a slow rate (not specified, but evidently an average rate of 75 beats per minute) in time to the beat of a rhythmic metronome, an arrhythmic metronome, and with no metronome. They found that the effect of rhythm was independent of rate. It should be noted, however, that there was also less stuttering in all three conditions with the slower rate.

Brady (1969) approached the problem somewhat differently, in that he kept rate constant in a metronome and a no-metronome condition. He first obtained a speech sample from each of the subjects reading at his usual rate under normal conditions. From these samples he determined the subject's speech rate in words per minute. He then had the subject read in time to a metronome set at his individual rate. He found that all subjects stuttered significantly less when speaking in time to the metronome.

The evidence provided by these studies indicates quite consistently that rhythm has a beneficial effect on stuttering independent of a decrease in rate, although slowing down also was found to be salutary.

Other Accounts of Rhythm

Two other explanations of the rhythm effect have been offered. One explanation, that the effect is due to "masking," has been made in reference to the influence of a metronome. According to this view, the ticking of the beats operates in some way to damp the stutterer's auditory feedback function, and this effect is considered to be the real agent responsible for the reduction in stuttering.

The masking explanation is clearly not tenable for two reasons. Most importantly, rhythm is effective through other sensory channels; it has been demonstrated that tactual pulses (Barber, 1940; Meyer and Mair, 1963; Azrin *et al.*, 1968) and visual flashes (Barber, 1940; Meyer and Mair, 1963; Brady, 1969) are as effective as audible beats. Since the effect is not limited to the auditory sense, it cannot very well be a function of auditory masking.

A second contradiction of the masking explanation derives from the findings regarding the ineffectiveness of an arrhythmic metronome. Auditory masking should be produced as well by certain arrhythmic patterns as by rhythmic ones.

The other explanation of the rhythm effect is that the improvement in fluency is occasioned by the induced regularity in speech. This explanation would seem to follow logically from the repeated evidence of the potency of a regular rhythm. However, regularity of the inducing beat does not necessarily mean that the accompanying speech will evidence the same regularity. Also, fluency can be maintained without attaining the degree of regularity expressed by a device. Figure 7:4 shows Graphic Level Recorder tracings of the same seven-syllable phrase[9] spoken by six stutterers who were instructed to speak in the manner of one syllable per beat, self-induced. Each major deflection represents a syllable. The sample from subject 1 was spoken at a rate of 182 syllables per minute; the sample from subject 6 is at 120 syllables per minute. Note the amount of temporal variation between the midpoints of the syllable pulses (the variation would have been greater had the reference lines been set at the intensity peaks). Also, this variation tends to increase as the syllabic rate decreases.

Perhaps the amount of temporal variation reflected here is not of much consequence. Assuming for the moment that it is not, then the explanation of regularity in speech assumes some cogency—but only when considering the special case of speaking in a pattern of one syllable per beat. For patterns other than this—including the pattern of one *word* per beat—the correspondence of speech units and rhythm beats is not

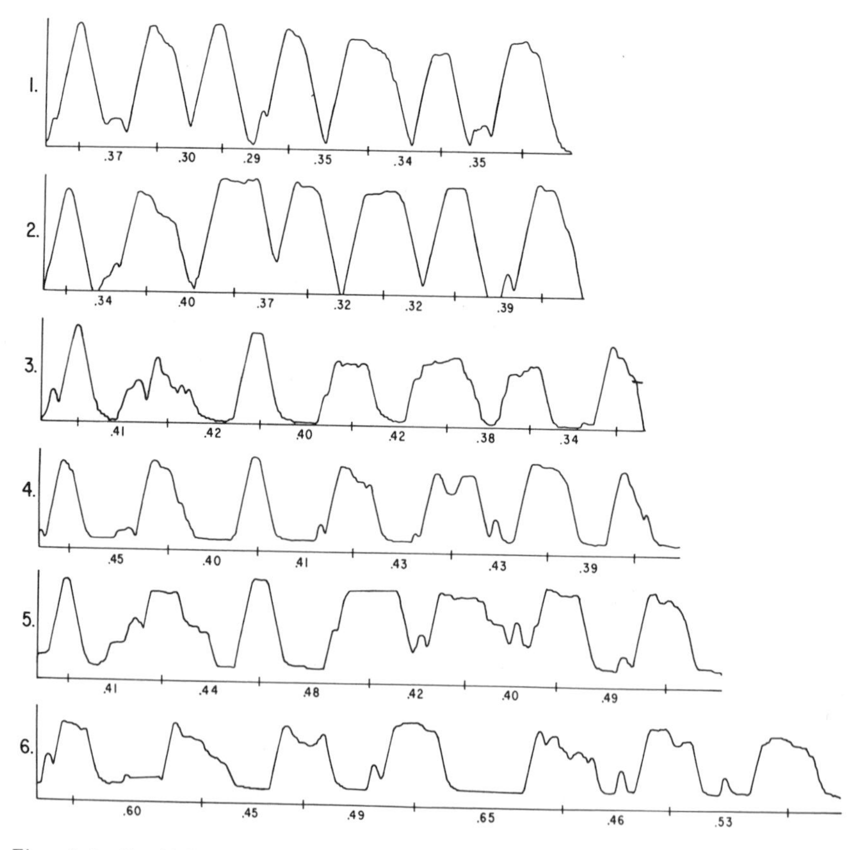

Figure 7:4 Graphic Level Recorder tracings of the phrase "put some butter on a plate" as spoken by six stutterers at a rate of one syllable per beat, performed without a regulating aid.

consistent. There is then much less regularity in the accompanying speech, and the lack of regularity becomes more pronounced as one moves away from syllable-timed speech. This is shown clearly in Figure 7:5, which contains two relevant tracings from Jones and Azrin (1969).

In view of the above it seems doubtful that the salutary effect of rhythm is due entirely to an induced regularity in speech. Undoubtedly the regularity of the inducing pattern is important, but it must function more as a guide, or support, in the execution of a modified speech pattern. Experimental support for this conjecture is supplied in the finding that an arrhythmic pulse, if not markedly irregular, may occasion a significant reduction in stuttering (Brady, 1969). There is also other relevant experimental data, which we will consider in the next chapter.

SUMMARY AND DISCUSSION

There is overwhelming evidence that stuttering is dramatically reduced whenever a stutterer speaks in a more-or-less regular rhythm. The potency of rhythm in the reduction of stuttering is revealed in several ways.

Rhythm is effective regardless of the means by which it induces a speech pattern. In the case of instrumental induction and support, it makes no difference whether the cue for the "beat" is auditory, tactual, or visual—the end result is the same. Induction without the use of an instrument is also effective, and a pattern can be achieved through the agency of some actual body movement, either gross (e.g., arm-swing) or fine (e.g., finger taps); or by attending to some internally conceived pattern ("ideomotor impulses," or visualizing a ball touring a horizontal figure eight); or by consciously intending to follow a pattern while speaking (syllable-timing).

Relevant experimental data show no difference in effectiveness between the rhythm of instrumental aids and the self-generated rhythms associated with some body movement. To date no attempt has been made to compare the effectiveness of these "induction source" methods to a technique in which the patient simply attempts to speak rhythmically without some external supportive rhythm (e.g., syllable-timed speech). It would be of considerable interest and value to know if such comparison would also reveal no difference.

In practice it has been common to find the use of some form of "induction source." This practice may have developed for several reasons but very likely the principal basis was the intentional implementation of the

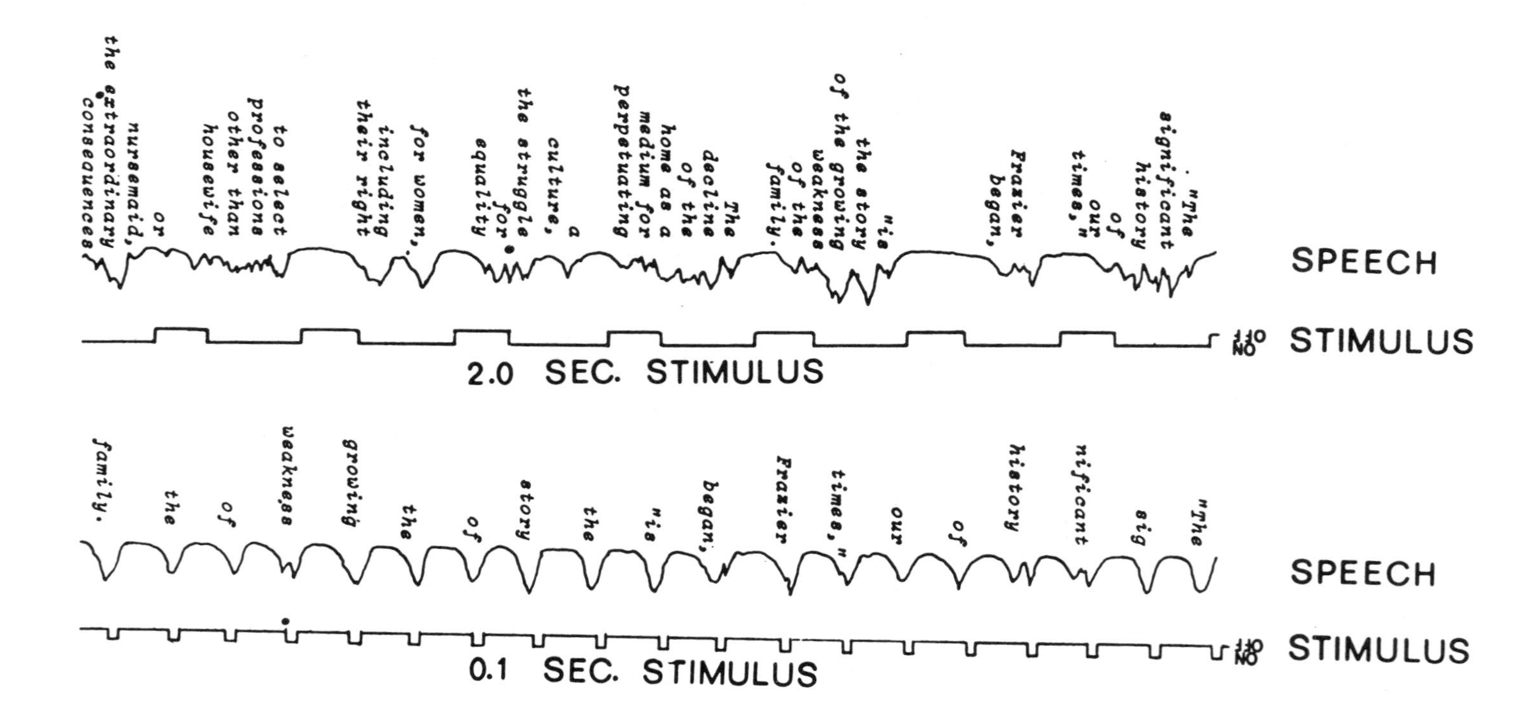

Figure 7:5 *Tracings demonstrate that beneficial effect of a rhythmic beat is not adequately explained as an induction of regularity in speech. (From Jones and Azrin, 1969.)*

synchronization effect. That is, putting to work the knowledge that a patterning of activity is set up almost compellingly through the presence of a definite beat.

Another indication of the potency of rhythm is that the effect is *immediate* and *continuous* as well as pronounced. The clear-cut reduction in stuttering is achieved as soon as the stutterer begins to speak in this manner, and the effect is thereafter neither intermittent nor relative. When the stutterer speaks to a rhythm, he either does not stutter at all or he stutters very infrequently.

A third feature of great significance in respect to the power of rhythm—and of special interest in regard to the immediacy of its effect—is that in most cases the "accessory" features of the stuttering pattern are eradicated along with the speech features. The apparent exceptions are some very severe stutterers whose accessory features may not disappear immediately; but even in these cases the nonspeech aspects of their stuttering fade fairly quickly. From the standpoint of therapy this means great savings in time and effort that are otherwise devoted to the consideration, appraisal, analysis, and attempts at reduction of this apparent superstructure.

One might consider that a corollary of the foregoing point is the evidence of improvement in personal adjustment following successful use of rhythm therapy, *without* concurrent use of other therapy forms.

A fourth feature of substantial significance is that with the improvement in speech achieved through the use of rhythm there is less need for "attitude" therapy or preoccupation with "anxiety," which represents another saving in time and effort. In addition to their practical value these features offer a substantial contribution to our understanding of the nature of stuttering, in that they provide another dimension of evidence that fear and anxiety are not as paramount in stuttering as has been claimed.

A fifth testimony to the power of rhythm is the substantial evidence, accumulated from various sources and times, which indicates that the effect of rhythm is practically universal. It is an exceedingly rare stutterer who does not show at least substantial reduction in stuttering when speaking under the influence of rhythm. This suggests very strongly that whatever is embodied in the effect of rhythm has applicability to all stuttering. This would mean that as far as therapy is concerned, the questions of different etiologies of stuttering or different kinds of stuttering become relatively academic—at least for the foreseeable future.

There is one subsidiary feature which merits consideration within the purview of the "universality" of the effect of rhythm. Some work has suggested evidence of individual preferences for particular rhythm rates. This finding would not be entirely unexpected in view of the reality of individual differences in all kinds of human function. However, it is of special significance for our purposes that, regardless of possible individual differences in rate preference, it is obvious from the findings of all the work reviewed that individuals respond favorably to rates set arbitrarily without any consideration for individual preference. Moreover, they respond well to a variety of set speeds within a fairly wide range of rates. In other words, the matter of individual preferences for some particular rate seems to be immaterial, at least for practical purposes.

At the beginning of this section we indicated that significant improvement in fluency is occasioned by speaking in a "more-or-less regular rhythm." It is appropriate to describe the effect in this way because there is abundant evidence that under the circumstances of rhythm induction the patterns of (fluent) speaking vary considerably.

When speaking of the regularity involved in the use of rhythm it is necessary to distinguish between the regularity of the pulse of the inducing source and the regularity of the speech that results. Instruments used in the rhythm therapy of stuttering always have had a regular beat. Regularity of pulse has been standard probably because a regular rhythm seems more "natural" and also because tradition and simplicity of construction have provided instruments which generate a regular beat. Clearly a regular rhythm is probably easier to follow and does produce an excellent effect, but we have seen that it is not necessary for the inducing rhythm to be regular in order to substantially reduce stuttering occurrence. Both the odd rhythm included in Barber's study (every third word) and Brady's randomly arrhythmic metronome occasioned significant reductions in stuttering. These influences were not as pronounced as those effected with the use of more regular rhythms, but the important point is that, even so, stuttering was substantially reduced.

We do not know what limits of "regularity" of the inducing rhythm must be observed in order to achieve maximization of the rhythm effect, but perhaps identifying these limits is unimportant. We do know that a regular rhythm is simplest to produce, easiest to follow, and evidently has the most marked effect. These are important considerations in respect to decisions regarding the use of an inducing source. However, they are misleading considerations if one infers that they identify what is responsible for the effect produced. It does seem that regularity in the inducing source is desirable; but it is also clear that strict regularity in *speaking* is not the automatic result, nor is it necessary in order for the effect of rhythm to be realized. In fact, there is evidence of considerable latitude in the resulting speech patterns which will still support fluency.

Even when the inducing source is an instrument that generates a regular pulse the pattern of speech accompanying the beat is not routinely the same as the pattern developed by the instrument itself. It is more likely to be so in the case of speaking in time to the instrument at a rate of one *syllable* per beat. Often, however, it is not; for instance, even speaking in the pattern of one *word* per beat is not the same, yet evidently a rhythm of one word per beat is just as beneficial as speaking one syllable per beat. Recall that in some of the work reviewed in this chapter, subjects were given their choice of speaking to a pulse by syllable *or* word, and the reduction in stuttering resulted regardless of their choice. Similarly, other subjects were advised to speak in a certain pattern (say, one word per beat) but to adjust this pattern *as necessary* to accommodate words of varying length. Again, there was marked reduction in stuttering. Further, in many cases the rhythm effect is maintained even when whole clauses or phrases are "keyed" to a pulse, with the clauses and phrases varying in length.

It can be said, then, that in the case of speech which accompanies the pulse of an instrument the "regularity" of the speech pattern is not the regularity of the instrument pulse, except possibly in the case of syllable correspondence. In the case of self-generated rhythm the "regularity" of even the syllable-per-beat pattern varies more than might appear to casual observation.

In contrast to all the positive features of the effect of rhythm there exists one very major reservation: the effect seems "bound," that is, it shows a clear tendency to be limited to the time the inducing rhythm is operative. While this does not detract in any way from the essential potency of the rhythm effect, it does pose certain real problems for its practical use. Hopefully these problems will be more easily circumvented when the nature of the rhythm effect is better understood. However, even at this time a good deal of the work done strongly suggests that there are ways of capitalizing the effect of rhythm and utilizing it to support a progression toward unaided fluent speech.

Very interestingly, the two means of capitalizing rhythm are two processes we have encountered before as playing significant roles in recovery from stuttering: *slowing down* and *practice*.

The reader should recall that in all the references to the therapeutic use of rhythm one invariably finds that treatment begins with a slow rate—usually less than 95 syllables per minute[10]—and continues at a slow rate for some time. Typically the rate is gradually increased, but if difficulty is encountered at any stage there is always the provision for return to a slower rate. At any stage there is also the continual recourse to slow-rate exercises, both as a part of clinic function or self-administered. Thus, while slowing down is not the *reason* for the beneficial effect of rhythm, in practice it is certainly a concurrent process of evident importance.

Once again practice shows up as an important variable in effecting a change in stuttering. Whatever may be the real agent through which the potency of rhythm is implemented, it is clear that the stutterer must work persistently at incorporating its benefits.

The principal agent of the rhythm effect remains unknown. There is ample evidence that the effect is not due to distraction or masking, and that it is not due simply to reduced rate. The most obvious feature about rhythm—regularity—also does not in itself provide an adequate explanation of the effect. As the preceding discussion indicates, the inducing rhythm occasions changes of some sort in the way the individual speaks. The nature of these changes is yet to be determined. In the following chapter we will consider what these changes might be, looking to an understanding of the principles embodied in the effect of rhythm which also might have significant corollaries in other fluency-inducing conditions.

Notes

1. A certain amount of argument centers around the identity of Demosthenes' speech problem. It is most often said to have been stuttering, but some writers claim that, instead, it was an articulation or a voice problem. Lately Bien (1969) has added the speculation of hypernasality due to cleft palate, but the bases for his guess are quite flimsy. Actually, certain of the quotations he gives are much more suggestive of stuttering. So are many other original quotations and references.

2. "Legato" is a musical term meaning "in a smooth, even style, with no noticeable interruption between the notes." (see Webster's *New World Dictionary of the American Language*, 1966 Ed.) We will encounter this term again.

3. Called the "Pacemaster" it is available from Associated Auditory Instruments, 6796 Market Street, Upper Darby, Pennsylvania, 19082.

4. Personal correspondence.

5. This report was actually made in 1966 at the Monterey conference. The proceedings of the conference were not published until 1969.

6. The percentage of stuttering for most patients while wearing the metronome was near zero.

7. This is actually rather slow for "normal speech." Various sources (Cotton, 1936; Johnson, 1961; Kelly and Steer, 1949; Ptacek and Sander, 1966) indicate that the normal rate of speech is a little above 200 syllables per minute.

8. This man was able to learn the technique initially but then began to have trouble; in spite of continued effort he did not make any progress. It is of interest that he was one of that adult group in which particular attention was paid to the emotional aspects of stuttering.

9. The phrase was embedded in a much longer speech sample.

10. Actually a very slow rate; anything under 100 syllables per minute is very slow, considering that the average rate of spontaneous speech is slightly over 200 syllables per minute.

References

Andrews, G. and Mary Harris. *The Syndrome of Stuttering*, Lavenham, Suffolk, Eng., 1964.

Azrin, N., R. J. Jones, and Barbara Flye. A snychronization effect and its application to stuttering by a portable apparatus. *J. Appl. Behav. Analysis*, **1**, 283–295, 1968.

Barber, Virginia. Studies in the psychology of stuttering: XVI Rhythm as a distraction in stuttering. *J. Speech Dis.*, **5**, 29–42, 1940.

Beech, H. R. and J. Dubbane. Unpublished study, Institute of Psychiatry, London, 1962. (Cited in Beech, H. R. and Fay Fransella, Explanations of the "rhythm effect" in stuttering, pp. 141–151 in Gray, B. B. and G. England, (eds.), *Stuttering and the Conditioning Therapies*, The Monterey Institute for Speech and Hearing, Monterey, Calif., 1969.

Berman, P. A. and J. P. Brady. Miniaturized metronomes in the treatment of stuttering: A survey of clinicians' experience. *J. Behav. Ther. and Exper. Psychiat.*, **4**, 117–119, 1973.

Bien, S. M. Was a pebble in Demosthene's mouth a primitive obturator? *Ann. Dentistry*, **28**, 10–18, 1969.

Bluemel, C. S. *Stammering and Cognate Defects of Speech*, Vol. 2, G. E. Stechert, New York, 1913.

Brady, J. P. A behavioral approach to the treatment of stuttering. *Amer. J. Psychiat.*, **125**, 843–848, 1968.

———Metronome conditioned speech retaining for stuttering. *Behav. Ther.*, **2**, 129–150, 1971.

———Studies of the metronome effect on stuttering. *Behav. Res. Ther.*, **7**, 197–204, 1969.

Brandon, S. and Mary Harris. Stammering: An experimental treatment program using syllable-timed speech. *Brit. J. Dis. Commun.*, **2**, 64–68, 1967.

Colombat de l' Isere, *Du Begaiement et tous les autres vices de la parole*. Mansut Fils, Paris, 1830.

———*Traite de tous les vices de la parole et en particulier du Begaiement*. Bechet et Labe, Paris, 1840.

———*Traite medico-chirugical des maladies des organes de la voix*. Mansut Fils, Paris, 1834.

Cotton, J. Syllabic rate: a new concept in the study of speech rate variation. *Sp. Monogr.*, **3**, 112–117, 1936.

Donovan, G. E. A new device for the treatment of stuttering. *Brit. J. Dis. Commun.*, **6**, 86–88, 1971.

Fransella, Fay. Rhythm as a distraction in the modification of stuttering. *Behav. Res. Ther.*, **5**, 253–255, 1967.

———and H. R. Beech. An experimental analysis of the effect of rhythm on the speech of stutterers. *Behav. Res. Ther.*, **3**, 195–201, 1965.

Greenberg, Janet B. The effect of the metronome on the speech of young stutterers. *Behav. Ther.*, **1**, 240–244, 1970.

Horan, M. C. An improved device for inducing rhythmic speech in stutterers. *Australian Psychol.*, **3**, 19–25, 1968.

Johnson, W. Measurements of oral reading and speaking rate and disfluency of adult male and female stutterers and nonstutterers. *J. Speech Hearing Dis., Monogr. Suppl.* **7**, 1–20, 1961.

———and L. Rosen. Studies in the psychology of stuttering: VIII Effects of certain changes in speech pattern upon frequency of stuttering. *J. Speech Dis.*, **2**, 105–109, 1937.

Jones, R. J. and N. H. Azrin. Behavioral engineering: Stuttering as a function of stimulus duration during speech synchronization. *J. Appl. Behav. Analysis*, **2**, 223–229, 1969.

Kelly, J. C. and M. D. Steer. Revised concept of rate. *J. Speech Hearing Dis.*, **14**, 222–226, 1949.

London Sunday Times, Dec. 11, 1966. Vest-pocket device aids stammerer.

Medical World News, March 17, 1967. Metronome helpts to beat stammering.

Meyer, V. and J. Comley. A preliminary report of the treatment of stammer by the use of rhythmic stimulation. In Gray, B.B. and G. England (eds.), *Stuttering and the Conditioning Therapies*, Monterey Institute for Speech and Hearing, Monterey, Calif., 1969, pp. 153–158.

Meyer, V. and J. M. Mair. A new technique to control stammering: A preliminary report. *Behav. Res. Ther.*, **1**, 251–254, 1963.

Newsweek, July 8, 1968. A real rhythm method.

Potter, S.O.L. *Speech and Its Defects*, P. Blakiston, Son and Co., Philadelphia, 1882.

Ptacek, P. H. and E. K. Sander. Age recognition from voice. *J. Speech Hearing Res.*, **9**, 273–277, 1966.

Robbins, S. D. The role of rhythm in the correction of stammering. *Quart. J. Speech*, **21**, 331–342, 1935.

Van Dantzig, M. Syllable-tapping, a new method for the help of stammerers. *J. Speech Dis.*, **5**, 127–131, 1940.

Wohl, Maud. The electronic metronome—an evaluative study. *Brit. J. Dis. Commun.*, **3**, 89–98, 1968.

———The treatment of non-fluent utterance: A behavioral approach. *Brit. J. Dis. Commun.*, **5**, 66–76, 1970.

8

CONDITIONS THAT AMELIORATE STUTTERING

It is appropriate once again to mention that at least in the past 30 years too much attention has been directed to purported differences, and not enough to similarities and relevant commonalities, in the speech of stutterers. This criticism has special relevance to stuttering therapy, since a set of observations exists, in what might be called an area of "fluency induction," which strongly suggest a fruitful direction in which to explore the matter of commonalities.

A number of conditions, other than speaking under the influence of rhythm, are known to have an ameliorative effect on stuttering. These conditions are: singing, choral speaking, shadowing, severe hearing loss, auditory masking, and delayed auditory feedback. We will consider each of these categories separately, as well as a group of miscellaneous external conditions that have a less pronounced, but still notable, effect.

Most of these conditions have been said to produce their effect because they create a "distraction."[1] Distraction has been used frequently to explain the beneficial effect of many conditions, yet it is an explanation that must be questioned. As mentioned earlier, distraction is never elaborated; that is, no adequate account is ever made of *how* a condition is distracting or *why* it should be distracting.

It seems very likely that the distraction explanation had its origin in the claim made by some stutterers that they do not stutter when they do not think about their stuttering. This sort of testimony has a kind of homespun appeal, and it is particularly credible if one is already persuaded that stuttering is a psychological problem caused or conditioned by fear and reaction. From this has come a kind of professional folklore "rule"—if a stutterer does not think about his stuttering, he will not stutter.

However, if one considers such testimony circumspectly it has very little plausibility. Speaking generally for the moment, we should question: How can someone report what he does *not* do when he is *not* thinking about it (i.e., is not aware of it)? Brief reflection should assure the reader that this is quite impossible. At best, one can only make a vague, retrospective, and inaccurate judgment about matters of this kind. Yet invariably it is just this sort of circumstance on which the stutterer's testimony is based. For instance, he will recall an episode and report that at some particular time in that episode he suddenly "realized" that he had not been stuttering. He had not been stuttering, he will explain, because he had not been thinking about it. Sometimes the report is elaborated: he had not stuttered until the moment he realized he had not stuttered, but *then* he really *did* stutter.

How can one accept such testimony at face value? Not only is the basic situation hardly credible, but one's doubts should be raised by the fact that the same stutterer, often in the same conversation, will relate that sometimes he does not stutter in a situation where he felt sure he would, that is, when he was thinking about it!

One's credulity should be further tested by such evidence as that presented in Chapter 3 (page 25) that stutterers are not very accurate observers of their own stuttering even when they are alerted to make a judgment about it.

There is no intention here to disavow the claim made by some stutterers that their stuttering tends to become worse when they have to speak under circumstances where they are particularly nervous, embarrassed, or worried about how well they will speak. But these must be considered to be special circumstances which permit only the inference that stuttering may be exacerbated by certain events. Of course there may be some relationship between the occurrence of stuttering and thinking about it, but the relationship is very irregular and relative; it is certainly not a relationship of the order that subtends a "rule."

We can look to even more compelling reasons for considering distraction an ingenuous and superficial explanation in stuttering. The essential meaning of distraction is "to draw (the mind, etc.) away in another direction; divert."[2] The word is used appropriately in circumstances such as the following. If a mother wishes to avoid a tearful episode when taking from a young child something he likes but should not have, she offers him a *distraction*, often in the form of another attractive object. Libraries maintain quiet because noise presents a *distraction* to reading concentration. A motorist misses a freeway exit because of the *distraction* of a view further ahead. The essential point is that the person is now preoccupied with the distraction and *is no longer thinking about* that from which he was distracted.

We should note that a distraction may be momentary or long-term. A long-term distraction has to be very persisting and powerful in order to maintain its effect. The "distractions" claimed for stuttering would have to be of the latter type.

Now, how can distraction be what occurs in the case of conditions that induce an amelioration of stuttering? Supposedly the stutterer is distracted from "his stuttering" or from his "expectancy to stutter" (Johnson, 1937). Actually it makes no difference. Either account means that when a stutterer speaks to rhythm, sings, reads in chorus, etc., *he is no longer thinking about his stuttering*. How can this be? Why should a stutterer, who supposedly is constantly preoccupied with his stuttering, suddenly no longer think about it simply because he speaks under one of the conditions being considered here? He is still required to speak and still has to give some attention to what he is saying—and therefore to the fact that he is saying it. If his concern about fluency (his preoccupation with stuttering, his expectancy to stutter, etc.) is bound up with the act of speaking, as is contended, then how can he possibly not think about his stuttering or suddenly no longer expect it? To come at it from another direction, one should ask: To what is his mind supposedly diverted? Why should it be diverted there, and how can it be kept there so long?

There is one answer that will suffice to answer all of these questions: namely, that the distraction explanation of stuttering reduction is logically impossible.

While a logical analysis is sufficient to discredit distraction, we should not fail to mention that this explanation has always been completely conjectural. There is nowhere any evidence of its supposed operation that would endure even casual scrutiny. If one asks stutterers themselves why they do not stutter under these conditions, they will say they do not know—unless, of course, they have been taught to say it is due to distraction. In such cases, questioning them about how the distraction supposedly operates will quickly reveal that they do not know.

At this point one might well expect to encounter "suggestion" as the explanation of next recourse. Here several rejoinders are pertinent. First, "suggestion" represents a departure from the distraction explanation; it is not a buttress for it, as is sometimes implied. Second, if suggestion is to be considered as a possible explanation, one must account for what underlies the suggestion. The effect of the ameliorating conditions can be produced with entirely naive stutterers, those who have no idea whatsoever of what they are likely to experience. In such instances there has been no suggestion. Third, if suggestion is ever in any way a meaningful account, then why do we not find that almost any condition will have an ameliorative effect through suggestion? For instance, why should we not find that a stutterer will stutter less when it is suggested to him that he will be more fluent if he holds a large red handkerchief at waist level while he speaks; or that he will not stutter if he speaks while balancing a pencil on his head; or many other conditions one might fancy?

Neither distraction nor suggestion are reasonable explanations for the induced amelioration of stuttering. The reason for devoting time to a critical appraisal of these explanations is not only because they are so inappropriate and incorrect, but because they have for so long stood in the way of progress in both therapy and theory of stuttering. From the standpoint of therapy, the identification of some effect as a distraction has been tantamount to dismissing it as trivial and of no consequence to therapeutic effort. In respect to theory, the explanation of distraction has conveyed the false implication that the effect is well understood, and thereby accounted for and not deserving of further investigation. Progress in both domains has been stultified by this superficial and hollow explanation that does not even merit designation as an hypothesis.

We must generate realistic hypotheses if we expect to arrive at an understanding of the nature of stuttering and of the requirements for its effective treatment. To generate realistic hypotheses we must begin with realistic facts—that is, with data that are neither personalized nor preferred—and then proceed to develop reasonable accounts based firmly on these data. Some of the most neglected data in the field of stuttering are those having to do with these ameliorating conditions. It is past time to look at them carefully and objectively.

It must be emphasized that only *certain* conditions have this temporary ameliorative effect on stuttering. This in itself is an important fact, suggesting that the agents responsible for the change may be few in number. Possibly each of the several conditions known to induce fluency in stutterers has an effect unique to iself, or it may be that several effects, in different combinations, find expression in some conditions and not in others. Again, it may be that one, or several, effects are common to all of these conditions. Whatever is found to be the case, the answer will be of considerable significance at least to stuttering therapy.

The ideal solution would be to find that in all of these conditions there is a common feature, or core of features, that represent recurring principles underlying the salutary effect on stuttering. Identification of a common agent, or cluster of agents, operative in these several conditions would be of great importance for two reasons: (a) the simplicity and economy of explanation, and (b) the broad base of application and implementation. Identification of certain core principles would provide a foundation of therapy method which should serve as a sound frame of reference for the efficient implementation of existing techniques and the development of new ones.

The objective of this chapter is to analyze each of the known fluency-inducing conditions for features that either are, or represent, the possible common agent(s).

The several conditions listed at the beginning of this chapter have been viewed and dealt with in the literature as though they belong in two different categories: those which involve auditory function and those which do not. Probably certain historical influences contribute to this view. For instance, the effect of conditions like rhythm and singing have been recognized and discussed for a very long time and these conditions have been associated with each other for a number of years. In contrast, awareness of the influence of auditory-based conditions has developed only in quite recent times. Nonetheless, the principal reason for believing that these conditions represent two different categories is simply because several of them involve audition and the rest do not.

Because of this obvious, albeit surface, difference it has been assumed that conditions assignable to one or the other of these two categories function in basically different manners in fluency induction. While the analysis to be developed in this chapter will illuminate features common to all of these conditions, we will adhere to this twofold classification primarily for purposes of organization in discussion.

CHANGE IN MANNER OF VERBAL EXPRESSION

Singing

Undoubtedly singing is the most widely known of the conditions having a salutary influence on stuttering. It is frequently reported in the professional literature, and casual sources as well, that stutterers are fluent when they sing (see, for example, Fletcher, 1928; Johnson and

Rosen, 1937; Reid, 1946; Bloodstein, 1950). Most likely the salutary effect of singing is best known because almost everyone has occasion to sing at one time or another, whereas the other ameliorative conditions are not as likely to be as commonly experienced or as clearly observed.

Speaking of this matter recalls a remarkable initial interview I once had with a 10-year-old stutterer. One question that I include routinely in examination is to ask the patient for some statement regarding his view of the reason for his stuttering. This youngster reflected a bit and then said, "Well, I don't really know. My doctor says it's because I get nervous. . . . But I don't stutter when I sing, and I'm really nervous when I sing." He meant singing solo. "Nervousness"—meaning uneasiness, apprehension, embarrassment, etc.—about singing solo is a feeling shared by probably most lay people, normal speakers and stutterers alike.

This 10-year-old's statement reflects a simple observation and a trenchant reflection. It is unfortunate that the field of stuttering has not seen more of such straightforward yet provocative analysis. The statement has a double-edged significance. On the one hand, it exposes another flaw in the contention that stuttering is due to "fear" or "anxiety" or the like. Here there is "fear" focused on, and operative during, a very speechlike, oral, personal performance, yet there is no stuttering. On the other hand, the statement calls attention to the dramatic reduction of stuttering in a condition which, though very speechlike, is in certain ways quite different from speech. This is a matter that deserves much more investigation than it has received.

Apparently it cannot be said that every stutterer can attain fluency through singing. A few contradictory cases have been reported. Robinson (1964, p. 10) claims to have recordings of two stutterers who evidence "considerable stuttering" while singing. However, he does not describe what this stuttering (while singing) is like, nor does he relate this to the severity and character of the stuttering when speaking.

A colleague once sent me a recording of an individual who supposedly stutters while singing. Actually, there is no stuttering "while singing"; the man is simply talking, with abortive attempts at singing. He does not develop any song. From the brief speech samples included on the tape it is evident that he is a very severe tonic stutterer.

The influence of singing has been interpreted as a special instance of the effect of rhythm, since song is known to have rhythm. However, it is doubtful that the effect of singing is to be explained in this way. A meter of some kind does underlie song, but frequently the beat is not clearly evident and often the words of the song do not have a close correspondence to the melody, which expresses the meter. Also, most songs do not have a simple redundant pattern, even though there is an underlying "beat." The tune of a song varies, and many times a syllable may extend beyond one beat of the "time" (meter) or, in contrast, a beat may contain more than one syllable. However—and this would seem to be the crucial matter—syllabic units do correspond to the musical notes. That is, in song syllables are expressed as tones of the song; the significance of this point should become evident from the succeeding discussion.

Clearly there are differences between the acts of speaking and singing. Unfortunately these differences have not been explored very extensively. The relevant publications have developed the topic in reference to the training of professional singers, with the objective being the improvement of singing technique. For the most part the analysis and discussion in these sources have been rather general and descriptive, illustrative by example rather than presenting actual comparison of samples. Further, the few actual comparisons made have employed samples obtained from trained singers. For instance, in a study by Vennard and Irwin (1966), the only study known to the author in which a direct comparison was made of spoken and sung versions of a complete sentence, the subject who provided the two samples was a professional singer. Also, his delivery of the spoken version of the sentence was done ". . . in a voice such as might be used for a Scripture reading in a service of worship." Similarly, studies by DeLattre (1958) and Sundberg (1970), both of which made comparisons of spoken and sung vowels, used a trained singer as the source of the samples.

Our interest in speaking-singing comparison is concerned with the difference between conversational speech and casual singing as produced by untrained voices. The studies mentioned above do not literally meet these conditions; nonetheless, most of the findings are clearly relevant and appropriate. There is a substantial consistency within all of this material, with the content of the more general references receiving specific corroboration from the more detailed studies. The latter, while fairly limited in number, yield results that are very much to the point.

Several features of singing serve to distinguish it from speaking. Significantly, they are quite closely interrelated. The most basic distinctive feature is that singing is predominantly phonation, i.e., singing is primarily vocalized sound. A second feature is that singing requires more time than speaking; it takes considerably longer to sing something than to speak it. In terms of the units of speech (syllables, phonemes) this clearly means a slowing down of rate. This slower rate is expressed through the extended duration of the speech units, especially the vocalized phonemes. A third major difference is that singing involves more volume (loudness, amplitude).

These three features find expression in all vocalized sounds, but predominantly in vowels. This is tantamount to saying that the principal differences between speaking and singing involve what happens with vowel production. A graphic display of the first two features is contained in Figure 8:1, which presents a comparison of the spoken and sung versions of a 15-syllable (49-phoneme) utterance. Note that the sung version takes slightly over three times as long as the spoken version. All phonemes are lengthened in the sung version but the predominant difference is on the vowels.[3] This increased duration of voiced phonemes, particularly vowels, represents a kind of "steady state" condition that

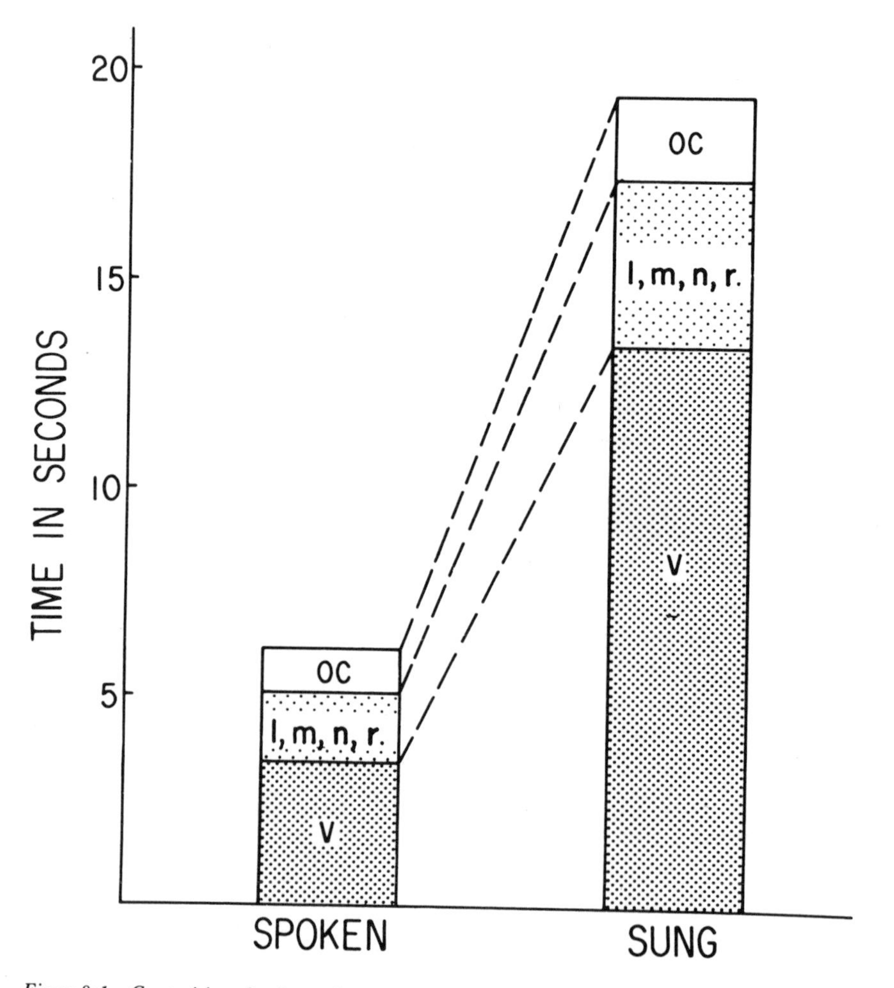

Figure 8:1 Composition of spoken and sung versions of the same utterance. V vowels; l, m, n, r = /l/, /m/, /n/, and /r/; oc = other consonants. (Data for figure from Vennard and Irwin, 1966.)

characterizes song and is known as "line" or "legato" (Vennard and Irwin, 1966).

There is a natural, commonplace tendency to emphasize vowels—and concurrently minimize consonants—when singing. In fact, this natural occurrence commands a considerable amount of attention among teachers of singing in their concern for the intelligibility of what is being sung. Appelman (1967), in a statement representative of writers in the field, cautions against this common tendency to minimize consonants; yet at the same time he says that " . . . . great care must be taken so that the formation of the consonant does not interfere with the proper resonation of each phoneme in a manner that would destroy the vocal line." The importance of the vowels is further emphasized in his statement that, "The maintenance of a legato line depends upon a rapid movement from one vowel position through the consonant to the following vowel in such a manner that neither vowel is affected by the consonantal articulation." (p. 238.)

There are some other notable features of singing which either are expressions of, or closely related to, the ones identified above. In certain ways singing can be said to be simpler than speaking: the syllabics are less complex, and variations in pitch, intensity and timing are not as great as in speaking. Contrasts, particularly stress contrasts, are less marked in singing. Because tone is generally louder in singing, there is need for more breath support (and hence more participation of the respiratory musculature), and breathing is more regulated. Singing produces a richer series of harmonics; resonator adjustments are more open, and sound energy is distributed more narrowly and in greater concentration.

Still other features are not quite so apparent: for example, changes in pitch and timing in singing are expressions of a ratio scale. Eventually it may be determined that such features contribute significantly to the effect of inducing and supporting fluency. However, we can easily find in the features already identified sufficient basis for a meaningful explanation of why stuttering does not occur in singing. This claim is not made simply on grounds of the prominence of these features, nor the fact that they relate closely to a broad spectrum of differences between speaking and singing, but also because, as we shall see, they embody principles that recur in the several conditions known to have an ameliorative effect on stuttering.

To objectify our present reference to these features, we should call attention especially to the predominating feature of increased phonation. In doing so we intend to make note of the attendant decrease in rate and, as well, the subordination of consonant articulation. Finally, we would point to the indications of general simplification, particularly the modulated contrasts in expression.

Before going on to a consideration of other conditions widely known to have a salutary influence on stuttering, it is appropriate to call attention to some findings that are particularly relevant to the matter of the effect of singing on stuttering. This material is especially germane because it contradicts an explanation sometimes made for the effect of singing, and at the same time provides additional support for the potency of the features identified above.

From time to time the salutary influence of singing has been attributed to the matter of familiarity; i.e., it is said that the stutterer becomes fluent when singing because he knows the words of the song he is singing. Actually, this explanation is credible only in respect to the tune (melody) of the song. The tune is the most easily learned and best-remembered part of a song; in contrast, most people cannot be relied upon to produce all of the words of even those songs with which they should be familiar. (Doubts about this claim can be tested easily by asking a random sample of one's acquaintances to sing "America" alone.) The melody of a song is the part that is the primary focus of a person's efforts when he attempts to sing a song.

But familiarity with either the words or the tune is relatively immaterial in regard to the effect of singing on stuttering. It does not really matter whether the stutterer does or does not remember all the words, nor is it important that he sing the tune accurately (the correct melody) or "in tune" (on key). What *is* important is that he make the kind of vocal adjustments that are characteristic of singing.

These considerations have led the author to deduce that if these features are primarily responsible for the salutary effect of singing, then one should find that stuttering is also dramatically reduced by chanting, an activity that is similar to singing on these dimensions. In addition, spontaneous chanting has no "tune," no rhythmic beat, no set pattern, and no familiar lyrics. Also, individuals are reluctant to perform solo chanting, perhaps even more than solo singing, because they feel conspicuous and embarrassed when doing it. Nonetheless, among those stutterers who I have persuaded to chant while reading something or while relating something spontaneously generated, none has stuttered while doing so.

Choral Speaking

It has been noted repeatedly that the frequency of stuttering is markedly reduced when the stutterer speaks in the immediate presence of others who are speaking at the same time. Originally this effect was observed casually in circumstances like recitative or responsive reading, such as in church; or in unison statements, such as saying the Pledge of Allegiance or other group-spoken oaths. The observation has been confirmed experimentally many times (Barber, 1939; Bloodstein, 1950; Eisenson and Wells, 1942; Johnson and Rosen, 1937; Pattie and Knight, 1944).

The experimental evidence accumulated so far has involved reading aloud rather than spontaneous speech. Of course this is a reasonable duplication of the circumstances in which casual observation has noted the marked increase in fluency. However, there are some data which indirectly suggest that spontaneous speech would be influenced in the same manner and degree. We will refer to these data shortly.

The bulk of the investigation to be considered in this section has involved actual choral, or "unison," reading, where all the participants (subjects and "chorus") read aloud the same material. However, interest in the effect of choral speaking has led to the extension of investigation into other conditions which, though similar and related, are not really choral reading. In some of this work the "chorus" has read material different from that read by the subject. In still other work the conditions employed have departed even further from choral reading in its absolute sense. For instance, subjects have been required to speak to the accompaniment of spoken nonsense syllables, continuous phonation of a vowel, recordings of gibberish, and of normal speech played backward. Such departures represent efforts to better understand the phenomenon of choral reading, and their findings have told us a great deal.

Johnson and Rosen (1937) included two choral reading situations among the twelve conditions[4] they investigated: one in which a stutterer served as the "chorus," and the other in which a normal speaker served this function. These conditions were among the most effective, being comparable to singing, arm swing, metronome, and a sing-song pattern. In all of these conditions stuttering was practically eliminated in their 18 subjects.

Johnson and Rosen viewed chorus reading as one form of "imposed rhythm" and interpreted its effect as due to distraction. Their explanation was that the choral accompaniment diverted the stutterer from making too critical an evaluation of his speech. They assumed that stuttering is caused by critical self-evaluation of speech and that choral reading, like singing and speaking to rhythm, is somehow distracting.

Barber (1939) also assumed that choral reading acted as a distraction. In fact her work was undertaken " . . . to investigate the effect of distraction and perhaps to contribute to the understanding of the fundamental nature of this phenomenon." The several conditions she employed were devised to assess: whether it was necessary for the subject and "chorus" to read the same material; whether meaningfulness of the choral material was important, or if just noise would do as well; or if the effect were simply due to the presence of another person engaged in a similar activity.

She used 13 different conditions, some with only slight variations, in which the accompaniment, when "live," was performed sometimes by stutterers and sometimes by normal speakers. The different accompanying activities included: reading the same material, different material, or nonsense syllables; phonating "ah"; and, making an unpatterned metallic noise.

Her findings showed that some of these conditions were more effective than others. The most dramatic improvement occurred in the several conditions of true choral reading, that is, where all participants read the same material. The least effective conditions were those in which a single reader read nonsense syllables. Barber's appraisal of her findings emphasized this difference, which she thought was due to the amount of "support" the stutterer could feel from the accompanying activity. Her explanation was that in such circumstances, where his performance is not easily differentiated, the stutterer does not evaluate his own speech so critically and therefore speaks better.

The superior effect of true choral reading is a matter of interest deserving further investigation. However, Barber's emphasis on this superiority as the basis for her interpretation ignored the fact that *all* the conditions she employed resulted in a significant reduction[5] in stuttering.

Bloodstein (1950) obtained interview testimony from 50 stutterers regarding the extent to which their fluency was improved when reading with other persons. All of them reported either that they stuttered very little or not at all when they read aloud with someone who was reading the same material. Seventeen of his informants could also report the experience of reading material different from that read by the accompanying speaker(s). Thirteen said that in this situation too they stuttered "hardly, or not at all"; one said he stuttered considerably less under such circumstances.

In this article Bloodstein identified unison reading as a "change in speech pattern," and the reading of different material as "strong or unusual stimulation." In a subsequent publication (Bloodstein, 1951) he incorporated the two effects into an interpretation which explained them both as due to lessened anxiety, similar to the explanations made by Johnson and Rosen, and Barber.

Eisenson and Wells (1942) attempted to assess whether stutterers' improved fluency in choral reading is due to "reduced communicative responsibility." It may be recognized that "communicative responsibility" has certain similarities to the type of interpretation offered by the foregoing authors, in that it also implies that the stutterer ordinarily feels an emotional burden when communicating and that this is the reason he stutters.

These authors had their subjects perform in two conditions, in each of which the subject read the same material as that read by a normal-speaking accompanist. In the first condition the subject was told that the reading was a rehearsal and that no one else was listening to him. In the second condition he was told that his performance was to be a test of his reading ability in "a radio situation," and that his voice would be transmitted to students in another room who would be tested later on the content of his reading. Just prior to the second reading he was given an "all ready" signal and the reading began when they were supposedly "on the air."

The authors gave no data regarding whether subjects' fluency in the first (rehearsal) condition represented an improvement over their usual fluency. In view of the findings of other studies it seems safe to assume that these subjects stuttered markedly less in this first condition than in their ordinary speech. However, the authors reported only the change in fluency between the first and second conditions of the study, and stated that as a group the subjects showed a decrease in the quality of their speech performance. However, this conclusion was heavily biased by the deviant performance of just one subject. Actually, only eight of the 19 subjects performed less well in the second condition; the rest showed either no change or slight improvement. Furthermore, the authors included "errors" other than stutterings. If their computations were to be limited only to "blocks" and "repetitions" (sic), the change for all (except one) of the subjects was minimal; the average increase in stuttering would amount to 0.2 instance. In fact it is quite remarkable that in spite of the obvious communicative pressure put on these subjects for the second condition, only one showed any notable reaction.

The notion of "communicative responsibility" may have somewhat more plausibility than the "critical evaluation" notion, yet the experimental evidence is not very persuasive. Certainly the data from the foregoing study make it impossible to agree with the authors' expressed belief that reduced communicative responsibility is the essence of the choral reading effect.

There is other compelling evidence that communicative responsibility is not an adequate explanation for the ameliorative influence of choral reading. Pattie and Knight (1944) employed a situation which provided a more appropriate test of communicative responsibility. Each subject first read alone to an audience (a control condition which was repeated as the last condition of the study). Then in one experimental condition the subject read to the audience while someone read beside him. In the other experimental condition he read alone to the audience with the voice of the other speaker transmitted to him from another room by telephone. The latter circumstance was found to be essentially as effective as when the accompanying reader was physically present with the subject, in spite of the fact that the transmitted speech was "less loud and less intelligible."

These same conditions were repeated with the accompanying speaker reading different material than that read by the subject. Reading different material was found to be less effective than reading the same material, but still a substantial decrease in stuttering resulted. Again, the effect was the same whether the accompanying speaker was physically present or speaking from the next room.

Pattie and Knight mentioned that this salutary effect might result through "reinforcing the nervous patterns which are preliminary to the act of speech." They thought that true choral reading (same material) might be superior because it acted as a pacesetter,[6] in essence imposing a rhythm similar to that of a metronome.

Pattie and Knight's findings clearly contradict explanations centering around the stutterer's self-reactions, whether such accounts are phrased in terms of reducing the stutterer's burden of communication or minimizing the prominence of his speech. However, their inference that the effect was like that of rhythm, based on the assumption of a metronome-like regularity in the reading of the accompanist, is not tenable. Choral reading does not express or induce the regularity that is apparent in speaking to rhythm.

The general idea of pacesetting, at least in respect to unison reading, would seem to have some plausibility. Still, it is difficult to see how the accompanist can be considered to set the pace or to lead. When choral reading is unrehearsed and no preplanned scheme is involved, the unison reading is undertaken—and proceeds—jointly; there is no "leader." The two (or more) voices rarely coincide exactly, and who is "in the lead" may change often (Wingate, 1973).

Cherry, Sayres, and Marland (1956a) reported that, in their experience with "a very wide sample"[7] of stutterers, choral reading was always successful, with no negative results. They also reported that conditions similar to unison reading were of comparable effectiveness in inducing fluency. They found that the stutterer would continue to read without stuttering even though the accompanying speaker suddenly shifted to reading different material. The same results were observed if the accompanist suddenly shifted to speaking "gibberish"—essentially speechlike utterance containing no true words though conforming to the phonetic structure of the language.

Note that in this approach of shifting to dissimilar material the accompanying speaker and the subject begin by reading the same material. Thus, the subject is started out with true unison reading and the shift is made after he has gotten "under way"—when he has reached a "steady state" in the terms of Cherry *et al.* It may be that this difference in technique accounts for the fact that these authors found conditions employing dissimilar expression to be as effective as unison reading, whereas other sources have found such conditions to be less effective. This suggests that if the most effective procedure is used to get the stutterer going, maintenance of his fluency can be achieved more easily. Results from another condition they employed suggest that it is not necessary to start with unison reading in order to obtain the level of effect typically reported for unison reading. They had their subjects speak while listening through earphones to a recording of speech played backwards. This condition was said to yield results similar to the other conditions, including unison reading. These findings clearly seem to qualify earlier evidence of a superiority of unison reading. The differences need to be reconciled.

Cherry, Sayres, and Marland believed that the influence on stuttering of these several forms of concurrent speech was evidence that stuttering is some sort of *basic* perceptual[8] problem. They pointed out that in all the conditions they (and others) have employed using concert speaking, the sounds contained in the accompanying utterances have conformed to the phonetic structure of the language. They suggested that this implied some sort of perceptual correction which damped or minimized those "components of the speech stimulus (that) take control in the perceptual habits which appear to give rise to stuttering." This suggestion is highly conjectural, particularly as applied to the influence of concert reading. Actually, the authors seem to have developed the notion first in relation to their work with "shadowing," where it is somewhat more credible, and then added to this the implications from their findings in work with masking. We will consider these matters shortly.

It should be mentioned that in a number of these conditions, particularly those other than unison reading, it is possible that some influence might be expressed through auditory masking. None of the studies have mentioned the loudness level of the sound accompanying the stutterer's reading, and this could be of some importance. Apparently all investigators have assumed that the sound intensity was at normal conversational level, which would be about 60–65 dB, SPL. As we will see shortly, two studies of auditory masking have included loudness levels in this range and both indicate some effect on stuttering. However, it must be conceded that masking noise effect at this level is not comparable to the effect produced by concert speaking. Additionally, Pattie and Knight did report a substantial effect of both same and dissimilar material in their telephone condition, in which the sound was reported to be noticeably below normal conversational level. We may safely conclude that auditory masking does not contribute substantially to an explanation of the effect of concert speaking.

Lee (1951) once suggested that the beneficial effect of concert reading might be due to the correct feedback supplied by the other speaker(s). However, this interpretation is contradicted by the recurring evidence that the effect is generated even when the accompaniment is different meaningful material or when it is one or another form of verbal nonsense.

Such findings also provide additional reason to doubt that "pacesetting" offers a very adequate explanation of concert reading, at least if pacesetting is understood to mean the regulation of a temporal pattern. Among the several different conditions in which the accompaniment has used dissimilar material, the supposed pacing pattern would have to have varied considerably. Yet evidently in all of these conditions the subjects continued to produce the standard pattern of English—the pattern they naturally produce as native speakers of the language. There may be some change in manner of speaking but it is doubtful that there would be much alteration in pattern, at least not the amount of change sufficient to approximate the pattern of the nonunison accompaniments.

The findings in a study by Wingate (1973) point out a factor that might be significant in the choral speaking effect, at least in the circumstance of unison reading, which is typically the most effective. Significantly, each speaker spoke more slowly during unison reading, with an average decrease of 20 percent below his solo reading rate. Evidently in choral speaking each speaker makes the effort not to "outrun" his companion, with the result that each of them speaks considerably more slowly than his ordinary rate. This occurred with such uniformity that it seems reasonable to assume that this is a regular occurrence in choral speaking. We might infer, then, that in the studies reviewed here subjects' speech rate was slower in the choral speaking conditions.

However, while reduced rate is evidently to be expected where two (or more) speakers are in physical proximity to each other, it is not certain that such would be the case in circumstances where the subjects were physically separated. For instance, in the telephone conditions employed by Pattie and Knight the subject and the accompanist were in different rooms; therefore, the accompanist was not reciprocally influenced by the speaking of the subject. Of course, it is possible that the accompanist might have slowed down as an unwitting act of consideration for the subject.[9] Such matters deserve further investigation.

The findings of this study of choral and solo reading also yielded information relevant to the matter of "pacing" in choral speaking. It was noted that the speakers of each pair were not regularly "in step" with each other. Their patterns of utterance showed a fluctuating overlap, which varied from nearly exact concordance to divergences of as much as three syllables. Also, while one speaker—usually the one having the voice with the greater volume or the lower pitch—generally held the lead, his lead was intermittent. Each of the voices would advance or trail, almost in alternating fashion. This phenomenon is portrayed graphically in Figure 8:2, which presents Graphic Level Recorder tracings of a representative example segment from a recording of two subjects reading the same passage together.

The effect of choral speaking on the speech rate of individual participants was the most impressive finding of the study. Perhaps the reported superiority of unison reading is substantially due to this factor. However, it may be that conditions such as backward speech, dissimilar reading material, or gibberish also influence a decrease in rate; these matters have not been investigated. Still, chorus speaking is clearly attended by a reduction in individual speaking rate. Once again the matter of slowing down reappears as a potentially substantive element in conditions that induce improved fluency in stutterers.

Other features of choral reading, closely interrelated with reduced rate, seem likely to be even more fundamental influences in inducing the improvement in stutterers' fluency.

Almost everyone should be familiar with the "droning" sound of unison reading when done by groups of people. This quality is not just an epiphenomenon of massed voices; it reflects adjustments in manner of speaking that are made by all individuals in the group. The same quality characterizes the choral reading of just two individuals; and, further, if the voice of each speaker of the pair can be isolated, it will also be found to have this "intoning" quality.

The significance of this phenomenon is that the intoning reflects a modification of both phonatory and articulatory aspects of oral expression. The predominant change is in phonation, expressed on the one hand through increased duration—primarily of vowels—and on the other by modulation of stress contrasts and some increase in volume. Also,

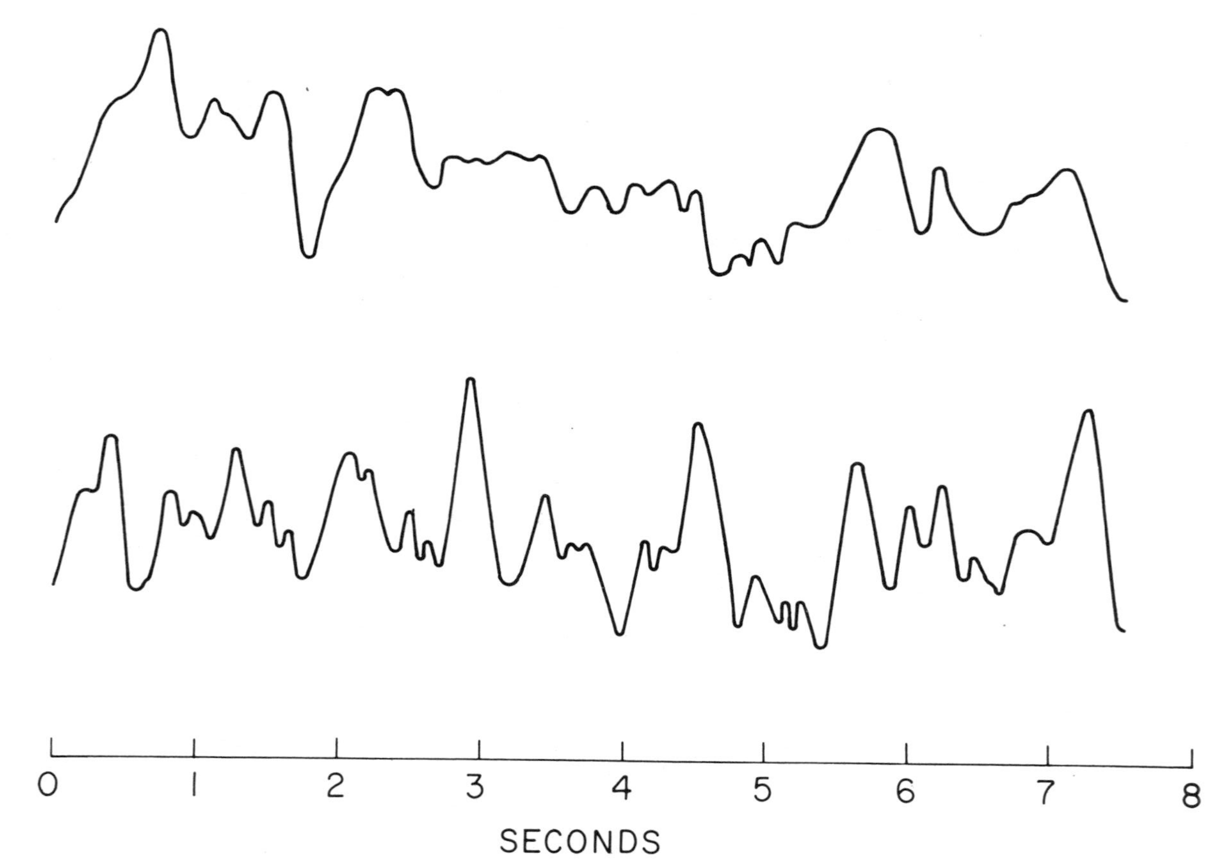

Figure 8:2 Amplitude tracings (Graphic Level Recorder) of the voices of two male speakers reading the same material in chorus. The sample is a three phrase sentence: "From within the small ship the passengers felt the movement of the heavy swells, though now the ship

consonant articulatory gestures are essentially subordinated, relative to their status in ordinary speaking.

Thus, the significant differentiating features identified in the section on singing are seen to recur in a careful appraisal of the changes in manner of speaking that are occasioned by choral speaking.

Shadowing

Shadowing is a procedure in which a speaker immediately copies (orally) what another speaker is saying. It is not a process of repeating phrases or brief sentences from memory, but of reproducing continuous connected speech as it is heard and while the "lead" speaker continues to talk. The "shadower" is following, within fractions of a second, what the lead speaker says. He thus has, at best, only a vague idea of what words he will speak until immediately before he must reproduce them.

The ability to shadow speech was first noted by Cherry, a British telecommunications engineer, in the course of some of his experimentation on human detection and recognition of speech signals (Cherry, 1953). Initially he found that his subjects, all normal speakers, could shadow what they were hearing over earphones, but it was soon determined that they could also do so in free-field listening. To Cherry these findings were evidence of the strength of "ingrained speech habits" of producing well-learned speech sounds and sequences. Throughout his writing, he dealt with the phenomenon of shadowing within a general framework of feedback concepts, and he emphasized the importance of auditory perception in the process.

Cherry's work with normal-speaking subjects was extended to use with stutterers by Pauline Marland, who evidently gave the phenomenon of "shadowing" its very apt name (cf. Marland, 1957). The decision to try the procedure with stutterers evidently was based on three assumptions. First, that auditory perception is significantly involved in stuttering. This assumption was founded essentially on the phenomenon of delayed auditory feedback, which, interestingly, was the serendipitous finding of another communications engineer, Bernard Lee (Lee, 1950b). Second, that in shadowing the subject's auditory perception is transferred to a large extent from his own voice to that of the lead speaker. Third, that through this procedure stutterers could automatically be trained into new "habits" of auditory perception—and therefore into performing the motor acts which these "habits" presumably regulate.

Cherry, Marland, and Sayers described the use of shadowing with stutterers in several publications (Cherry, Sayers, and Marland, 1955,

1956a, 1956b; Marland, 1957) and regularly reported good results with both children and adults.[10] The total number of cases on which their findings were based is indeterminate, since they did not routinely report this information. It seems that a generous estimate would be in the neighborhood of about 70 subjects altogether.

Evidently shadowing is not as universally effective with stutterers as are singing and choral speaking. In the Cherry *et al.* publication (1956a) reporting the largest sample studied—51 adult stutterers—four were unable to shadow sufficiently well to complete the task of shadowing a 120-word passage. Another eight subjects had a fair amount of difficulty and stuttered sufficiently to cause them to miss from 6 to 20 words of the passage. However, particularly in view of the fact that these eight subjects stuttered a good deal under normal conditions they were considered to have performed adequately in the shadowing task. The remaining 39 cases experienced relatively few stutterings while shadowing, such that no one missed more than five of the words in the passage.

If we may presume to use this subject sample as a reference, one could estimate that in about 92 percent of cases shadowing is moderately to highly effective in reducing stuttering. A more casual estimate relative to findings indicated in other reports would corroborate this estimate as a sort of minimum figure.

It seems that neither Cherry, Sayers, nor Marland published any further reports on shadowing subsequent to their brief series of articles in the late 1950's. However, reports of the therapeutic use of shadowing have appeared sporadically from other sources (Walton and Black, 1958; Maclaren, 1960; Walton and Mather, 1963; Kelham and McHale, 1966; Kondas, 1967). On the whole, the data reported in these publications leave us with some uncertainty about the value of shadowing as a therapy technique. Quite regularly other methods were incorporated in the procedures described, and it is therefore not at all clear to what extent shadowing was responsible for, or contributed materially to, the improvements reported. Also, the quality of the evidence varies a great deal. The Maclaren source provides simply a narrative review of a few cases. The reports by Walton and his collaborators each refer to just one case. Only two of the publications (Kelham and McHale, 1966; Kondas, 1967) report actual studies of a research character. Unfortunately, the methodological confounding in these studies too makes it difficult to be comfortable about the success they claim or the indication that the improvement was primarily due to shadowing. Also, neither study took into account the factor of spontaneous remission, which, as we have seen (Chapter 5), is most likely to be an important variable when considering children. At the same time, one cannot fail to be impressed with the claim of over 70 percent improvement made in both studies, particularly in Kondas' record of stability of improvement in children, maintained three years after treatment.

It seems very likely that the shadowing technique has benefited a fair number of stutterers, but we have no reasonable basis for making any estimate of the frequency with which benefit might have occurred. We have even less of an idea how the technique might have had its salutary effect. Authors reporting the therapeutic use of shadowing typically have made an early reference to the explanation of its effect originally advanced by Cherry *et al.*—namely, that the effect is due to a "transfer of (the shadower's) auditory perception." Evidently the authors assumed that Cherry's conjecture was accurate and that this "transfer" automatically takes place. Therefore they pay little attention to details of the procedure used. There is no specification of how the shadowing is implemented, and thus we have little idea of what the subject actually may have been led into doing. Kelham and McHale mention that in their use of the technique " . . . patients had to concentrate on imitating the rhythm of the therapist's speech." Kondas' description of the "cured" speech status mentioned that "some slowness of speech may eventually appear."

None of the reports on shadowing have provided much description of procedure, particularly certain details likely to be of considerable significance to the understanding of the shadowing phenomenon and its influence on stuttering. There has been little systematic description of the subjects' speech while shadowing. Such matters as speech rate and variations therein, the frequency and type of errors made, qualitative aspects of the subjects' speech, etc., are very relevant to the understanding of how shadowing operates.

Occasional references to such matters reflect the extent of their importance. Cherry, Sayers, and Marland (1956a) indicated that the lead speaker's speech rate varied between 50 to 100 words per minute. This is equivalent to a range of 75 to 150 syllables per minute, quite a slow rate when one considers that the average rate of speech is slightly over 200 syllables per minute. A slow rate is also clearly implied in the report of Cherry, Sayers, and Marland (1955) and Marland (1957). It is not known that this slow rate was intentional; it seems quite probable that in shadowing, as in choral speaking, the lead speaker may quite subconsciously adjust his rate to assure more likely success by the subject.[11] One must immediately suspect that a slow rate has characterized all the reported use of shadowing. If we accept this as a likely probability, we find once more that "slowing down" is at least a prominent part of another condition that has a salutary effect on stuttering.

There are other modifications of speech induced by shadowing which probably contribute substantially to the reduction in stuttering, but that have received little attention or interest. Cherry made a passing reference to such changes in both the original article (Cherry, 1953) and later in his book (Cherry, 1957). Speaking of the shadowing speaker's reproduction of the message, he noted, in the first publication, that "very little emotional content or stressing of the words occurs at all," and later described this speech as occurring "in irregular, detached phrases and . . . in a singularly emotionless voice as though intoning." (p. 279.)

To put the matter in other terms, shadow speech is not a very faithful copy of ordinary speech, primarily because it lacks normal prosody. This "intoning" character of shadow speech is without doubt its most distinctive feature and is readily observable if one makes a point of attending to the subject's manner of speaking.

Another prominent characteristic of shadow speech is that it is rather mumbled, i.e., poorly articulated. This characteristic, typically not mentioned in reports on shadowing, was investigated experimentally by Sergeant (1961), whose study of "concurrent repetition" stemmed from quite different interests. Sergeant measured the intelligibility of shadow speech as a function of certain variations in the intensity and rate with which subjects spoke 10-word sequences consisting of words from PB-50 lists. Averaged results from 24 subjects indicated that if rate of presentation were less than 115 words per minute (172 syllables per minute) and intensity greater than 33dB above SRT an intelligibility score of 50 percent could be expected. Intelligibility scores improved with further decrease in rate and increase in intensity, but even at the slow rate of 102 syllables per minute and an intensity level of 60 dB, intelligibility did not exceed 68 percent. Sergeant found that intelligibility did show some increase through twice-daily practice over an eight-day period, yet most of the subjects participating in the practice program did not increase their intelligibility above 80 percent. These findings provide experimental evidence of a feature of shadow speech that is never mentioned in the sources dealing with its use in stuttering, yet which is also readily observable if one attends to the subject's manner of speaking.

It is indeed curious that Cherry's explanation of shadowing has been so uncritically accepted. On the surface his account might seem to make a kind of sense in that the "shadower" is obviously listening to what the lead speaker says. But beyond this very obvious and superficial connection there is very little logic to the explanation. It does not accommodate certain observations made by Cherry himself, viz., that a shadower will substitute his culture-specific equivalents for the slightly different words used by a lead speaker. As examples, Cherry (1957, p. 129) reported that an American shadower will say "railroad," "airplane," "ash can," or "gotten" in place of the "railway," "aeroplane," "ashbin," and "got" used by his British "leader." Further, a shadower sometimes omits or adds a word, or uses a word that is quite different from its counterpart in the leader's speech; that is, the words are quite different on the dimensions of perception and production, though usually having a semantic equivalence (e.g., "on" for "over"; "car" for "auto"). Such evidence clearly contradicts the idea that the shadower's speech is "controlled" by a transfer of his auditory perception.

Comparisons of the speech of leader and shadower have never been made. If this were done, one would certainly find a set of differences, which would include more than the features just mentioned. For instance, it would also be found that while the shadower's speech has an intoning quality the leader's does not.

Matters of this kind have evidently received no consideration. The phenomenon of shadowing has been locked in to a well-entrenched conception about how it operates. As with rhythm and choral speaking, there is a favored, but inaccurate, explanation for how fluency is produced. In the case of shadowing the favored explanation most certainly originated in the excitement attending the burgeoning awareness of feedback concepts, and it evidently has maintained its unchallenged status through the persistence of a poorly reasoned enthusiasm for such views.

If one looks at shadowing without preconception but simply in terms of analyzing the observable changes in speech that evidently are induced by it, one finds features that characterize the effects of other conditions that have a salutary effect on stuttering. We have already identified these features in the foregoing discussion. They are: (1) reduced rate, (2) emphasis on phonation, with reduction of stress contrasts, and (3) subordination of consonant articulatory gestures. These are the same features identified in our analyses of singing and choral speaking.

Another Look at Rhythm

In Chapter 7 our discussion of rhythm arrived at several conclusions about the rhythm effect. First, although a decrease in rate is a natural consequence of speaking to rhythm, and is in fact exaggerated when rhythm is intentionally used therapeutically, the evidence seemed to indicate quite clearly that the effect of rhythm is not due solely to a decrease in rate. Second, although regularity is the most obvious feature of rhythm, especially simple rhythm, regularity *per se* probably contributes only in the sense that it simplifies the guiding function of rhythm. It was suggested that this guiding function provides the vehicle through which the central element of rhythm in speaking can have its effect. We can now consider the particulars of this function and its operation.

By a "guiding function" we mean that the beats of a rhythm, whether regular or irregular, provide a series of foci for organization of the speaker's verbal expression. The aspect of regularity in rhythm is of secondary significance; a regular rhythm is superior to an irregular one simply because it is easier to organize anything in reference to a regular system than to an irregular one. The important matter is how speech is linked to the foci provided in the beats of a rhythm.

The speaker links syllables to these foci—essentially, certain kinds of syllables, and according to a particular pattern. These "certain kinds of syllables" are the stressed syllables, especially those syllables which in English receive primary stress (meaning primary phrasal stress—to assure a distinction to word stress).

This principle of linkage of rhythm beats to syllables carrying primary stress may not be readily apparent in the casual observation of speaking to rhythm. For instance, in the simplest pattern of speaking at one syllable per beat one will find that normally unstressed syllables will also concur with beats (see illustration below). On the other hand when someone simply speaks to the accompaniment of a rhythmic pulse, certain beats will be associated with pauses as well as with both stressed and unstressed syllables.

For purposes of clarification the relationships being described here can be diagrammed as in the following examples, in which the same sentence is said in three different patterns of syllable-beat concurrence. The spots below each line represent the recurring beats of a regular rhythm. In the first line the rhythm is one syllable per beat. Lines **2** and **3** are intended to represent two levels of increased rate of rhythm, although such patterns might be expressed without an increase in rate. Note that in both **2** and **3** certain beats are associated with pauses. Note also that the syllables that would receive major stress in ordinary speaking (identified by small arrows) remain the same in all three patterns. If one were to listen to a speaker expressing these three patterns, one would be able to hear a special prominence given to these ordinarily stressed syllables, even in the pattern of one syllable per beat, where one would expect to find the greatest uniformity of stress.

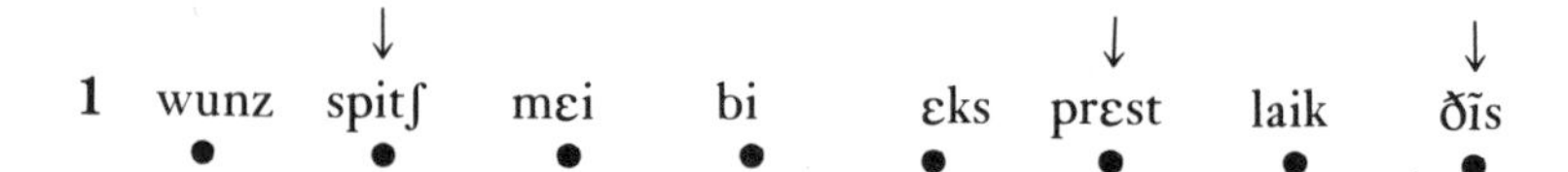

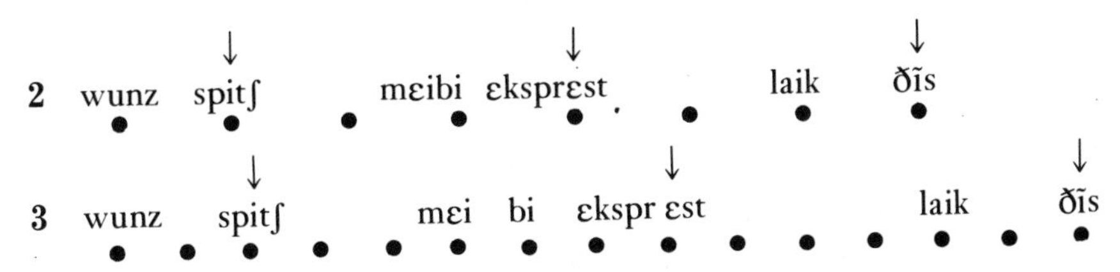

So, through the guiding function of rhythm the speaker is led to align syllables with beats. Moreover, he does this in a particular way: he aligns normally stressed syllables with certain beats of the rhythm. These particular alignments are the foci of organization for speaking to rhythm; they constitute the basic structure of the pattern. When an individual speaks in time to rhythm, his basic pattern is to move from one such focus to another. The syllable-beat relationships in the intervals between these foci depend upon the nature, usually the rate, of the rhythm. Most often there are other syllable-beat concurrences, but beats will also concur with pauses as the speaker "marks time" in order to have a normally stressed syllable match with a beat of the rhythm.[12] (The reader should be reminded that regularity in speaking, when talking to rhythm, is a possibility only in the limiting case of speaking one syllable per beat.)

Significantly, the execution of any rhythm pattern is implemented by placing emphasis on syllable nuclei. This fact, which would seem to be clearly evident to careful direct observation, has been substantiated experimentally. Boomsliter and Hastings (1971) investigated the locus of occurrence of syllable peaks in the speech of normal subjects speaking in time to a metronome. They found that what they referred to as the "instant" of the syllable is almost exclusively within its vowel section.

This action of placing emphasis on syllable nuclei is the means by which the guiding function of rhythm sets in motion and supports the central element of the rhythm effect—emphasis on phonation. Syllable nuclei are predominantly vowels, which are the major phonatory component of speech. Expressive emphasis of these components produces primarily an increase in their duration and some increase in volume. It is undoubtedly significant to the overall effect on stuttering that ordinarily this emphasis also involves other vowels in addition to those of the normally stressed syllables. This is especially true of the simpler rhythms, and the simpler rhythms have the most dramatic effect on stuttering.

When a person speaks in time to rhythm, there is an accompanying reduction in stress contrasts. Also, with more emphasis now placed on vowels, there is a corresponding relative subordination of consonant articulation. The whole effect of rhythm is enhanced, of course, with slow rates. As noted in Chapter 7, use of rhythm in the therapy of stuttering always begins with a very slow rate. It should be remembered that this slow rate is expressed essentially in extended duration of voiced elements.

The effect of rhythm, then, can be understood to be occasioned by the same factors as in singing and the other major salutary effects: increase in phonation, slower rate, and moderation of contrasts and consonant articulation.

Miscellaneous Conditions

Discussion in the previous sections of this chapter has proceeded with the recognition that the conditions being assessed were highly effective (i.e., inducing minimal or no stuttering) with almost all (i.e., 90 percent or more) stutterers. In the present section we will take note of certain other conditions reported to have a beneficial influence on stuttering.

The relevant information is presented in a report by Bloodstein (1949) based on his search through a wide variety of sources in which some mention had been made of circumstances that purportedly had occasioned improvement in a stutterer's fluency. Some of these reports were based on experience with a number of cases; others were essentially anecdotal reports referring to single cases. Bloodstein collected and compiled descriptions of 115 different circumstances of this nature. Then, through interview and questionnaire, he obtained statements from stutterers regarding their personal experiences with the various circumstances. The respondents were asked whether, when speaking under each condition, they stuttered (1) the same as usual, (2) definitely less, (3) hardly any, or (4) not at all.

Because these are questionnaire data based on rather small samples, certain reservations arise in respect to how to deal with them and what may properly be inferred from them. With the appropriate cautions in mind let us undertake an appraisal of this additional material.

Table 8:1 contains a list of those conditions for which a substantial majority (85 percent or more)[13] of the stutterers questioned indicated a marked improvement in fluency. It should be noted that the number of subjects (first column) varies for each condition included. In some cases the number is quite small; in no instance were there more than 50 respondents per item. The entries in the second column are the percentage of subjects who reported that their stuttering was at least "definitely less" (i.e., response categories 2, 3, and 4). Actually, most of these values represent replies of "hardly any" or "not at all" and reflect the salutary effect of these conditions on the majority of these respondents.

The entries in the columns at the right of the table are coded by letters that signify the present author's interpretations of the effect of these conditions. The "d" signifies duplication of conditions already considered in previous sections of this chapter. These conditions constitute a third of the items in the list. The code letter "p" is an abbreviation for phonation. It seems clear that these conditions induce a speaker to change his manner of speaking in a way that emphasizes, or principally involves, modifications in the phonatory aspects of speech production. Almost all of these conditions can be reasonably understood to involve some definite change in phonation. For instance, imitation of a dialect or another person's man-

Table 8:1 Conditions reported to result in substantial reduction of stuttering (From Bloodstein, 1949.)

			Agent			
N	*Percent*	*Condition*	*d*	*p*	*lp*	*r*
50	100.0	Chorus reading, same material	x			
50	100.0	Speaking to an animal			x	
46	100.0	Singing	x			
37	100.0	Speaking to an infant			x	
28	100.0	Simultaneous speaking and writing*				
47	97.7	Swearing		x	x	
45	97.8	Speaking with no one else present				x
26	96.2	Speaking to a rhythmic swing of the arm	x			
49	95.9	Reading aloud with no one else present				x
42	95.2	Imitating a regional dialect		x		
40	95.0	When feeling calm and relaxed				x
36	94.4	Imitating another person's manner of speaking		x		
17	94.1	Speaking in time to walking	x			
17	94.1	Speaking to a rhythmic twist of the wrist	x			
33	93.9	Imitating a foreign dialect		x		
24	91.7	Speaking to rhythmic foot tapping	x			
48	91.7	Making an inconsequential remark			x	x
31	90.3	When putting on a jocular manner		x		
18	88.9	Speaking through closed teeth		x		
33	87.9	Speaking in a sing-song manner	x			
30	86.7	Speaking on a lower pitch		x		
35	85.8	When you have handed the listener a written slip with the information you wish to convey				x
34	85.3	When assuming a bold front and speaking in a confident and boisterous manner		x		
27	85.2	Speaking to your girl (or boy) friend				x
47	85.1	Speaking while engaged in a sport	x			

*See text.

ner of speaking clearly involves mimicry of resonance characteristics and a unique intonation of prosodic pattern. Similarly, speaking in a confident and boisterous manner, or when genuinely amused or jocular, or swearing, share the common feature of increase in vocalization.

It seems most likely that the effect of "simultaneous speaking and writing" is achieved through the agency of slowing down and a concurrent exaggeration of prosodic elements. It should be mentioned here that 84 percent of 47 subjects reported at least substantial benefit from "speaking more slowly than usual."

The code "lp" refers to "low propositionality," indicating that there is some reason to claim that speech under these conditions is of reduced propositional value. Many authors contend that the beneficial effect of conditions such as these is due to the stutterer being more at ease and less concerned about himself, what he says and how he says it. However, there is another interpretation for these observations, consistent with the principles developed here. One should consider the kinds of things a person is likely to say in speaking to an animal, an infant, or when swearing, etc. Such utterances are most likely to be simple, brief, overlearned, and routinized. As such they are also likely to be spoken with a distinctive and familiar speech "melody," which is the focal core of the expression.

For the conditions coded "r" it seemed that the only apparent explanation would be in terms of relaxation. Here we should first recall that stutterers' testimony about their stuttering when alone is rather questionable, even though there also is little doubt that many stutterers do stutter less when they are relaxed. However, it must be recognized that a relaxed state does not have some magical direct effect on fluency: the effect is wrought indirectly, through changes in the individual's physiologic state and the resulting modifications in the speech acts. Most likely all systems involved in speech production are importantly influenced by such changes; however, the voice has most often been recognized to be especially sensitive to emotional states. In effect, then, while relaxation is the superficially evident circumstance of change, the agent of change can once again be traced to modifications of the speech process, particularly the phonatory aspect.

Thus, the effect on stuttering of these less widely known circumstances can also be accounted for in terms of the principles isolated in the major conditions having a salutary effect. The nature of the relevant changes in these conditions might not be so clearly apparent here as in the material covered in the preceding sections, but this is due essentially to the fact that we have little pertinent data with which to procede beyond rational inference.

CHANGES IN AUDITORY PERCEPTION

The remaining conditions to be discussed in this chapter—hearing loss, auditory masking, and delayed auditory feedback—involve some change in auditory perception. However, it is by no means certain that a change in auditory perception provides the appropriate dimension for explaining the effect of these conditions on stuttering. In fact, it is the purpose of this part of the chapter to illuminate and evaluate such an explanation and its origins, as well as to develop an analysis that penetrates beyond this level of explanation.

Before going on to an analysis of these conditions it seems appropriate to call attention to certain matters that have special relevance to the attempts made so far to explain these ameliorative influences on stuttering. Of the three conditions included in this section, it would hardly be sensible for anyone to suggest that the influence of hearing loss is due to "distraction". But it is of considerable interest that distraction also has not been offered as the explanation for the effect auditory masking or delayed auditory feedback. Actually, if one considers the grounds on which distraction has been offered as the explanation for other fluency-inducing conditions, it could be just as suitably invoked to account for masking and delay.

In the case of auditory masking and delay there is a very obvious alternative that also makes a certain kind of sense. As anyone knows, audition is clearly involved in learning to speak and it plays some role in maintaining speech function; therefore, if speech is disturbed, the disturbance might be due to some problem in audition. As we shall see, explanations of stuttering which have focused on a hypothesized auditory dysfunction have been widely attractive and well accepted. We shall also see, however, that such explanations have some very substantial limitations, and that there are other more credible explanations for the fluency-inducing effect of these conditions.

Some interest in a cause-effect relationship between stuttering and hearing has existed for a long time. This interest can be described as having passed through three eras, which were determined more by the professional intellectual climate of the times than by limitations of knowledge and technical capability.

The earliest era extended from at least the beginning of this century to the middle of the 1940s. During that time information about the relationship between stuttering and hearing was limited to observations made of individuals with marked hearing deficit—the deaf and severely hard-of-hearing. One finds little evidence in that era of an inclination to explore the relationship experimentally, even though the technical capabilities of the time would have made this possible.

The second era was marked by the appearance of an experimental approach to the problem embodied in the use of auditory masking technique to simulate artificially the conditions of diminished audition found in the hearing handicapped. The third era, which began a few years later, was primarily a technical extension of the second era, occasioned by the accidental discovery of a more exotic means of altering auditory perception—namely, delayed auditory feedback.

Several years intervened between the time the phenomenon of delayed auditory feedback was initially reported and the time it was implemented in the study of stuttering. However, since that time it has accrued a great deal of favor within the profession, primarily because it is thought to provide a model for the explanation of stuttering. Many errors of analysis and deduction have been made in the pursuit of substantiating this model. We will encounter them as we proceed toward our primary objective, the analysis of the beneficial effect on stuttering that is generated by alterations in auditory function.

Hearing Deficit and Stuttering

Apparently Bluemel (1913) was the first person in this country to make a point of the evidence that auditory function seemed to be involved in stuttering in some way. Bluemel's ideas of the nature of stuttering changed over the years, but at that time he believed stuttering to be a form of transient auditory amnesia. According to this notion, instances of stuttering occurred when the verbal image required for that particular moment was faint. In support of this general conjecture Bluemel pointed to the observations made by others which indicated a connection between auditory dysfunction and stuttering. For instance, he referred to a statement by Gutzmann (1912) to the effect that it was "well known" that the congenitally deaf never stutter. He also quoted testimony from Gallaudet himself that in 50 years of work with the deaf he had visited many schools in this country and in Europe and had met thousands of deaf people but could not recall ever having known a congenitally deaf person who stuttered. Bluemel surmised that the deaf person, lacking auditory function, would not have auditory imagery. He would, therefore, not be susceptible to disturbances in auditory imagery that could affect his "mental and oral speech." Consequently, the deaf person would be invulnerable to stuttering.

A number of years elapsed before investigations were undertaken which were to contribute more objective data to these casual reports. While the findings that emerged contradicted the sweeping claim that stuttering does not occur among the deaf, they did document quite consistently that the incidence of stuttering among the deaf and hard of hearing is considerably lower than among people with normal hearing.

In 1937 Voelker and Voelker published a case study of a congenitally deaf boy who stuttered and who evidenced certain so-called "secondary manifestations" as well. This case at least provided clear evidence that stuttering does occur among the deaf, and it was all the more impressive evidence because the youngster was known to have been deaf since birth. Other, more broadly based data was soon to come.

The following year Backus (1938) reported the results of a questionnaire survey sent to 206 schools for the deaf that taught oral means of communication. The teachers in these schools were asked to report any totally or partially deaf persons who stuttered at that time or who had ever shown signs of stuttering. Only 55 stutterers were identified in a total population of 13,691 children attending these schools, a ratio of 0.4 percent. This value is substantially lower than the figure of 0.7 to 1.0 percent usually reported for the general population. Backus indicated that the ratio could not be determined more precisely for several reasons inherent in the manner of data collection; however, it seems improbable that a more exacting form of inquiry would have revealed a ratio approaching that reported for the general population. Support for this surmise is provided in Backus' report that teachers in 70 percent of the participating institutions had stated, as had Gallaudet, that they had never heard of deaf persons who stuttered.

Actually, only six of these 55 stuttering children could be said to be deaf. The format of the investigation did not provide extensive information regarding the extent, nature, or duration of the hearing loss, nor the nature and extent of stuttering in individual cases. Thus the data did not permit analysis of the extent to which stuttering may have been related to amount, type, or character of hearing loss.

Since these findings did reveal a substantially lower occurrence of stuttering among persons with severe hearing handicap, they provided evidence for the existence of some kind of relationship between stuttering and auditory function. At the same time, however, the nature of that relationship is qualified by the finding that some individuals with a severe hearing impairment do stutter. This evidence is itself sufficient to indicate that no *basic* relationship exists between stuttering and auditory function. This fact has been overlooked repeatedly in recently popular efforts to formulate an explanation based on such a basic relationship.

A year later Harms and Malone (1939) presented material they had collected in an attempt "to determine if hearing acuity is an etiological factor in stuttering." They undertook to approach the problem from two directions: investigation of the extent of stuttering among the deaf and appraisal of the extent to which hearing loss occurs in stutterers.

Their information regarding the former question was obtained in essentially a replication of the Backus study. By means of a questionnaire, they obtained data regarding the occurrence of stuttering among pupils in 209 "oral" schools for the deaf and hard of hearing. They received reports of only 42 cases of stuttering in a total original population of 14,458 children. These figures yield a ratio of 0.29 percent, somewhat less than in the Backus study. Actually, only 8 of these 42 children were totally deaf; the remainder had varying amounts of residual hearing, although in none was the level of hearing better than 22 percent. As in the Backus study, the authors did not obtain the information necessary to assess a possible correlation between level of hearing acuity and extent of stuttering.

The authors obtained data regarding the question of hearing acuity in stutterers from routine audiometric examination of 62 stutterers seen consecutively in their speech clinic. These individuals had not been referred for hearing evaluation, and evidently they also had not considered that they might have a hearing loss. The audiometric examination indicated that all of them did have a slight loss, ranging from 10 to 22 percent. The nature of the losses, the etiology, and length of time in existence were not determined.

In reference to the data they had gathered, Harms and Malone concluded that since stuttering "is negligible" among the deaf but does occur in association with reduced but usable hearing, loss of hearing acuity in the period of speech formation is a cause of stuttering. The reasoning involved in arriving at this conclusion is itself unclear, especially since it is contradictory to several aspects of the data they reported. Additionally, it omitted from consideration the many hard of hearing individuals who do not stutter, and also the many stutterers who have no hearing handicap.[14] In sum, the meaningful contribution of this report is its corroboration of the findings reported by Backus.

Several explanations have been offered to account for the infrequent occurrence of stuttering among the deaf. In recent times these early findings have been incorporated, largely by implication, within the feedback interpretation of stuttering. We have already suggested that there are major limitations to this interpretation, but we will defer further comment for a later special section. For the moment we will direct attention to certain other explanations made previously.

Backus reported that the teachers of the deaf who participated in her study suggested four kinds of explanation of why stuttering is not often found in individuals with a marked hearing loss. Some of the teachers called attention to the scanning type of speech which is characteristic of the deaf and very hard of hearing. Some conjectured that deaf children are subject to less social pressure about their speech. Others thought that the careful teaching of speech could result in less likelihood of stuttering. Still others thought that it might be because the deaf and hard of hearing are unable to think faster than they speak.

The last suggestion hardly seems to merit serious consideration. In addition to the fact that it involves several assumptions and unknowns, it is a counterpart of two versions of a conjecture that has been advanced to explain the *occurrence* of stuttering among the normally hearing: viz., that a person stutters because he talks faster than he can think, or its inverse, that he stutters because he thinks faster than he can talk. Such explanations are, of course, highly speculative.

In regard to the second and third explanations, it seems very questionable that a deaf person experiences less social pressure about his speech, which is so often difficult to comprehend and many times leads to obvious misunderstandings. Also, although being taught to speak through careful and patient instruction might conceivably be an important factor in generating a better chance for normal fluency than the individual might naturally possess, one must also consider that learning to speak acceptably under such limitations might also be a very frustrating and trying experience. These two explanations are also largely conjectural.

In contrast, the first suggestion is related to direct observation. Moreover, there is a considerable amount of experimentally derived data to support it and give it substance—a substance found in the analysis of other conditions associated with reduced stuttering.

The "scanning" nature of the speech of the severely hearing-impaired is distinguished primarily by the quality of being much slower than the speech of the normal-hearing individual. Various investigators (Hood and Dixon, 1969; Hudgins, 1934; Voelker, 1935, 1937, 1938) consistently have found this to be the most typical feature of the speech of the hearing handicapped. For example, Voelker (1937) reported that only 3 percent of his 98 cases spoke at a normal rate. This slow rate is also pronounced; on the average it is about half the speed of normal speech.

Significantly, this slower rate of speech is expressed through extended duration of phonation. Voelker (1935), for instance, reported that his subjects phonated three times as much as normal-hearing subjects saying the same material. Hood and Dixon found that the average syllable duration in the speech of their subjects was twice as long as in normal speakers. Similar findings are reported in the other sources.

In addition to this basic difference, the speech of the severely hearing-handicapped also shows less variation in pitch and intensity than normal speech. Further, consonants are subordinated, not only through the contrasting predominance of the vowel elements but also by virtue of the fact that many consonants in the speech of the deaf are poorly articulated or actually omitted.

Once again we find, in a seemingly very different type of condition associated with reduced stuttering, the same features revealed repeatedly in the other conditions reviewed: increase in phonation, decrease in rate, and simplification of speech in the form of modulation of both the prosodic contrasts and consonant articulation.

Auditory Masking of Stutterers' Speech

The lower incidence of stuttering among the markedly hearing handicapped has always been assumed to reflect a causal relationship involving hearing acuity. It is possible, of course, that this correlation might be coincidental, or reflect some obscure common cause. However, it is easy to understand why the assumption of a causal functional connection developed and persisted. It does have a certain superficial logic, reflecting the general awareness that speech is in some ways dependent upon hearing.[15] On the other hand, it evidently did not occur to anyone to ask *how* stuttering might be related to hearing deficit. The early work, for example, made no attempt to determine the actual extent of loss in individual cases, nor the nature or etiology of the loss—both of which might have been quite relevant. Subsequent investigation also did not show much interest in considerations of this kind. Rather, it was assumed that stuttering is some function of the *amount* of hearing. Consequently, the next stage of investigation into the relationship between hearing function and stuttering took the form of experimental reduction of hearing level in stutterers with normal hearing through the use of auditory masking.

Actually, the earliest reference to the use of a masking technique was in a publication by Kern (1932), in Germany, who reported finding that stuttering was reduced when a stutterer spoke in the presence of noise produced by beating on a drum. However, his work seems to have remained obscure until mentioned by Cherry, Sayers, and Marland in 1956. Evidently the first formal study investigating the effect of auditory masking on stuttering was not done until more than a decade after the Kern publication, and it was undertaken in reference to the work of Backus, and Harms and Malone. This was a study by Shane, conducted in 1946 but not published until 1955.

Shane's orientation to the investigation of masking effect was consistent with the assumption that stuttering is some function of the amount of hearing. The position she adopted was the one espoused by Wendell Johnson, namely, that stuttering is the result of an overly critical evaluation of one's speech. From this standpoint, the less a stutterer hears of his speech the less basis he should have for making a critical evluation of it. Of course, this position assumes that the auditory channel is the only important avenue through which a stutterer can know he is stuttering. This minimizing of other sources of sensory information reflects both the appeal of the "evaluation hypothesis" and the preoccupation with the role of audition in stuttering.

Shane measured the effect on stuttering of bilateral masking noise delivered at levels of 25 and 95 dB. Her subjects evidenced a significant decrease in stuttering in the condition employing the 95 dB masking but no difference under masking at the 25 dB level. Most of the subjects experienced a very substantial reduction in frequency of stuttering under the high-intensity masking, although only eight of the 25 subjects were completely fluent in this condition.

Even though 20 of the subjects could hear themselves at least a little during the high-level masking, Shane interpreted these findings in terms of altered self-reaction; i.e., when the stutterer is unable to hear himself speak, his anxiety concerning his speech is diminished and he therefore stutters less. She did mention that all subjects reported being aware of stutterings through kinesthetic cues, but interpreted this finding as indicating that auditory cues were clearly the more important.

It is of particular interest that she noted "a marked deterioration of the speech function" under 95 dB masking. Nasality, change in rate, slurring of articulation, and sound substitution and omissions were features listed as reflecting this "definitely decreased control of articulation and voice."

The results of a study by Paruzynski (1951) are of interest mainly for their indication of reduction in stuttering under masking of spontaneous speech; also that the effect of masking can be achieved at a level (unspecified) below 65 dB.

Cherry and Sayers (1956), in their review of several conditions attended by reduced stuttering, presented considerable discussion of the effect of auditory masking. They described some of their own work in which they reported "virtually complete" elimination of stuttering under conditions of bilateral masking. They did not specify the actual dB level of the noise they used, but referred to it as being of an intensity that "approached pain level" and that achieved complete masking of the subject's awareness of the sound of his own speech. Probably because of their primary orientation to the field of telecommunications engineering these authors were concerned almost exclusively with auditory function in speech. They interpreted their findings and observations within a framework of auditory feedback function, and they developed their data as supporting a conception of stuttering as a (auditory) perceptual defect.

Maraist and Hutton (1957) studied the change in stutterers' fluency occasioned by auditory masking at levels of 30, 50, 70, and 90 dB. They found a progressive decrease in stuttering as the intensity of the masking noise increased. It is of some significance that "sizable decreases in the several measures of severity of stuttering" were found to result with progressive increase in level of masking noise beginning at 50 dB. They also noted an increase in speech rate (words per minute) concurrent with the decrease in stuttering. This change, also found in other studies of masked stuttering, is a secondary effect of the decrease in stuttering. This effect is the opposite of what occurs in masking the speech of normal speakers, as we shall see shortly.

In the foregoing studies the masking noise was presented continuously, a procedure assumed to create an experimental analogue of the effect of a hearing loss. The results obtained, which quite consistently showed reduced stuttering with masking and progressive improvement with increased levels of masking, seemed to provide support for the feedback concept of stuttering.

However, Sutton and Chase (1961) conducted an investigation which incorporated a critical modification of this procedure. These authors devised a system using a voice-actuated relay in which delivery of the masking noise was activated by the subject's phonation. The investigators were thus able to create two conditions of contingent masking: one in which the masking noise was presented only while the subject was phonating, and in the other it was present only during the intervals of silence in speech. The effect of each of these two conditions was compared to one in which the masking noise was continuous, as in the earlier studies.

It was found that fluency improved under all conditions of masking. Most significantly, the condition in which noise occurred only during silence was just as effective as the other two masking conditions. With (masking) noise activated only during silence there is, of course, no auditory masking of one's speech. This finding thus raised serious question about the adequacy of the feedback interpretation of stuttering, in that it indicated that improvement in a stutterer's fluency is not due to a masking of auditory feedback. The authors concluded that their results necessitated a reevaluation of the way in which masking noise operates to reduce stuttering.

The Sutton and Chase study was criticized by Webster and Lubker (1968a), but their objections were ably answered by the original authors (Chase and Sutton, 1968). Later, the findings first reported by Sutton and Chase were corroborated by a replication of their study by Webster and Dorman (1970), using single isolated words rather than a continous reading task, which was employed in the original study.

An investigation conducted by Murray (1967) also yielded results consistent with those of Sutton and Chase. Murray compared the effects of continuous white-noise masking with several conditions of intermittent masking. In one of the latter conditions, brief periods of masking were delivered randomly, with from 0 to 9 seconds intervening between these masking pulses. For the remaining two conditions masking was contingent upon the occurrence of stuttering: in one condition the masking was initiated by the subject after he began to stutter; in the other the masking was delivered by the experimenter whenever he observed the beginning of a stutter.

Murray found the continuous masking to be clearly the most effective, but even the condition of random masking resulted in a notable decrease in stuttering. In contrast, the contingent conditions did not have a significant influence on stuttering. That is, masking was not effective when introduced only after the onset of a stutter. The results of the Murray study thus indicate that masking must be operative prior to the initiation of a word attempt in order to produce a beneficial effect on stuttering. The same implication is to be derived from the results of the Sutton and Chase study.

Substantial effort has been made to use auditory masking therapeutically, initially in laboratory or clinic situations where the necessary equipment for generating masking noise was available. While masking typically has quite a dramatic immediate effect, it does not produce much "carry-over" or any very long-lasting residual effect. In combination, these factors encouraged the development of portable masking devices in the expectation that stutterers would be able to make use of the masking effect in ordinary speaking circumstances. Several such devices have been constructed and have figured in a number of reports of their use.

In spite of the enthusiasm that has typically attended these undertakings, the results have generally been discouraging. The interested reader might wish to consult original sources,[16] but a good review of the findings of many of these reports is presented in Van Riper (1973). For our purposes a summary of the essential findings will be sufficient.

The problems inherent in the use of portable masking devices are predominantly a function of difficulties with the method itself, and only secondarily with the portable units, their size, functioning, appearance, etc. The central limitation of masking is that it is tiresome, unpleasant, or annoying. To have a masking noise constantly in one's ears would be understandably disconcerting, and probably intolerable. One would not be able to hear oneself speak, but would not hear much else either. But this impossible situation is not the practically limiting circumstance of the use of masking; stutterers evidently do not adapt to it even on an intermittent, "as needed," basis. In other words, this unnatural stimulus is burdensome even when used part-time.

Aside from the annoyance aspect of masking noise there are other limitations that seriously compromise its expected value. It is very taxing to keep turning it on and off according to whether one is speaking or listening. The alternative, contingent usage, is not very satisfactory either. If one defers use of the noise until a stutter develops, it is then too late for the masking to produce its effect. On the other hand, if one intends to use it only when a stutter is expected, the success rate will not be very high. Despite widespread belief,[17] stutterers are just not that capable of anticipating stutterings.

Certain other problems bear mention. For instance, poor timing in on-off switching interferes with receipt of other's speech as well. Or, the ear-molds reduce hearing acuity even without the noise. There are personal reactions to wearing the units, or to their cosmetic features. Also, the units sometimes elicit inappropriate reactions from other people, such as speaking loudly in the mistaken belief that the wearer is deaf.

In a very real sense, all of the problems attendant upon the effort to use masking therapeutically result from the preconception—and ignorance—of the nature of its effect on stuttering. Van Riper (1973, p. 123) acknowledges this limitation in noting that " . . . there is no real certainty concerning the reason for this effect. The clinician needs to know why he does what he does and it is unfortunate that in this case he cannot be sure."

It is surprising to find that most of the studies investigating the influence of auditory masking fail to mention a very common and quite noticeable phenomenon. A person speaking under conditions of noise will quite naturally speak more loudly. The phenomenon is widely known and has been identified for some time in professional circles as "the Lombard effect," inasmuch as it was first suggested by Lombard (Weiss, 1910) as a test for auditory malingering. The essential feature of this effect is its influence on vocalization, since increased loudness of speech is tantamount to increased vocal intensity. However, other changes in manner of speaking also ordinarily occur under conditions of noise, as we shall see presently.

As one might have expected, some of the literature on auditory masking of stuttering contains reference to an increase in vocal intensity. Cherry and Sayers (1956) mentioned the tendency for subjects to speak more loudly under masking. They discounted increased intensity as the explanation for decreased stuttering, reporting that their subjects were able to maintain improved fluency when instructed to speak quietly under masking. However, their data would hardly seem to provide a fair test—the subjects spoke in this circumstance for only 30 seconds. Parker and Christopherson (1963) also noted the "continual tendency at first to raise the voice" but claimed that with practice a normal loudness level (and presumably continued fluency) can be maintained.

It might well be that loudness *per se* is not responsible for the reduction in stuttering under conditions of noise. However, as indicated above, other adjustments in speaking are induced by masking and these may very well be the important ones. Stromsta (1967) found that progressive decreases in frequency of masking noise below 500 Hz, with intensity of masking held constant, resulted in a progressive increase in vocal pitch and a decrease in stuttering. Certain of the findings of Cherry, Sayers, and Marland (1956) indicate that reduction of stuttering is a function of particular masking effects on voicing; they reported that masking of low frequencies (below 500 Hz) is essential for the fluency-inducing effect, and that masking of bone-conducted transmission is most important. On the other hand, Barr and Carmel (1969) reported a dramatic decrease in stuttering associated with the presentation of individually determined high-frequency narrow-band masking noise, delivered monaurally at the patient's 50 dB sensation level. Selection of the frequency band and the ear to which it would be presented were determined by the combination of these two variables showing the greatest amount of auditory adaptation on the Carhart tone decay test.

Except for determining that stutterers' fluency is improved with auditory masking, research in this area has not investigated other masking-induced changes in the speech of stutterers. Nonetheless, it seems safe to judge that stutterers should evidence the same changes in manner of speaking under masking noise as is found in normal speakers under masking. One might also deduce that it may be such changes in manner of speaking, rather than the altered auditory stimulation, that are responsible for the reduction in stuttering.

Research into the effects of auditory masking on aspects of speech production, utilizing normal speakers, reveals that several changes are induced. Black (1950) found a linear increase in vocal frequency as well as in vocal intensity with progressive increase in loudness level (as measured in loudness level contours) of the masking tone. Atkinson (1952) also reported that the sound pressure level and fundamental frequency of vocal responses increased, in differing ratios, as a function of intensity of the auditory stimulus. Of particular interest in respect to both the Black and Atkinson studies is the fact that the data were obtained on syllables spoken immediately *after* presentation of the masking sound. This finding is of particular relevance in that it is concordant with the results of Sutton and Chase (1961) that masking noise delivered during periods of silence in connected speech is effective in reducing stuttering. Webster and Lubker (1968a) reported a decrease in rate of utterance with increasing levels of masking noise above 65 dB, delivered binaurally. Winchester and Gibbons (1958), using an 80 dB masking noise, found a decrease in speech rate even with monaural masking, although the decrement was more pronounced with binaural masking. Draegert (1951) and Hanley and Draegert (1949) reported a significant increase in phonation/time ratio with binaural masking at "high intensity." Ringel and Steer (1963) also found a significant increase in phonation/time ratio and, as well, a significant increase in mean syllable duration with binaural masking delivered at 94 dB binaurally. Hanley and Steer (1949) found that with increasing levels of binaural masking noise their subjects spoke at successively slower rates and with increased syllable duration. Charlip (1966) found significant increases in (syllable) duration at masking levels beyond 70 dB, even though the subjects' task was simply to repeat continuously the same single-syllable word.

Most of this work has not investigated possible changes in articulation or in modulations of stress contrasts, and so there is little actual evidence available for comment on these features. Only the Ringel and Steer (1963) study included a measure of articulation error; their data indicate an average 47 percent increase with masking, but it was not statistically significant. However, this is sufficient to recall Shane's (1955) notation of a "definitely decreased control of articulation . . ." in her stutterer subjects when speaking under the same level of masking intensity as subjects in the Ringel and Steer study. Quantitative measures of change in articulation and stress contrasts are difficult to make. One might justifiably assume in this case that changes in these two features occur under masking conditions to the extent that these conditions have an effect on speech commensurate with that produced by a natural hearing deficit. However, the most impressive data from the studies of auditory masking effects are those which point to features that have consistently turned up as the salient changes found in conditions that ameliorate stuttering: changes which involve emphasis on phonation.

Stuttering and Delayed Auditory Feedback

The latest stage in constructing the conception of stuttering as a feedback dysfunction derives its support principally from work done with delayed auditory feedback ("DAF"; or, delayed sidetone). Delay in auditory feedback is a procedure that is technically more sophisticated and conceptually more esoteric than auditory masking, features which in themselves have increased its explanatory appeal. It can also have a rather dramatic effect on speech, a factor which also makes it impressive. All these artefacts have had their place in influencing the level of interest in DAF as having explanatory capability.

A number of authors have attempted to explain stuttering as the result of some kind of anomaly in auditory feedback function (Cherry, Sayers, and Marland, 1956; Wolfe and Wolfe, 1959; Mysak, 1960; Gruber, 1965; Butler and Stanley, 1966; Webster and Lubker, 1968; Timmons and Boudreau, 1972). These efforts are special applications of the conception of speech as a type of servo-system. Unfortunately, most of these formulations rely almost exclusively on audition as the important source of feedback information; in fact, in some discussions it is the only source considered. Obviously, these efforts have been influenced substantially by the reports of work on masking, but they have been shaped principally by the interest and activity centering around delayed auditory feedback.

In the last analysis we are interested here in the matter of delayed auditory feedback as another of those conditions that has an ameliorative influence on stuttering. But the relationship of DAF to stuttering is not as straightforward as that between stuttering and hearing loss, or stuttering and auditory masking. In fact, curious inconsistencies are to be found in the relevant literature and these inconsistencies, in particular, require some breadth of preliminary discussion so that we might better understand the proper place of DAF in relation to stuttering.

The effects of DAF on normal speakers were originally seen as presenting an experimental analogue of stuttering and, indeed, many authors continue to view DAF as the model by which stuttering is to be explained. Not until sometime later was it discovered that DAF actually had a salutary effect on stuttering. This effect has been found with such regularity that DAF has been used often as a therapy procedure. However, this frequently recorded evidence that delayed auditory feedback *reduces* stuttering seems not to have disturbed the stance of those who see in DAF an explanation for the *cause* of stuttering.

The original reference to delay in auditory feedback appeared as a letter to the editor of the *Journal of the Acoustical Society of America* (Lee, 1950b). It reported certain unique effects on speech that the writer had been prompted to investigate after the phenomenon had been discovered rather casually during the course of adjusting some electronic equipment. In his discussion of the effects, Lee made reference to *Cybernetics*, the book by Norbert Weiner that is the modern font of thinking about servo-systems. In particular, he mentioned Weiner's example of an electronic circuit oscillating with feedback, and he went on to suggest that oscillation and stutter are analogous.

In some respects the implications to be derived from the effects of delayed auditory feedback did not constitute a basis for corroborating or extending certain notions about the significance of audition in stuttering. In particular, the implications of DAF would not encourage elaboration of the view that audition provides the vehicle for negative self-evaluation. The findings could be interpreted in a manner consistent with the claims that stuttering and normal disfluency are continuous and simply a matter of degree and that stuttering is "learned behavior." Of course, the findings also constituted additional evidence for viewpoints which simply held that stuttering is in some way related to hearing function.

The conceptual climate within the profession was therefore generally receptive to the implications drawn by Lee with respect to the significance of DAF-induced phenomena for an understanding of stuttering. Clearly, Lee's reports indicated a similarity between certain speech characteristics he observed in some individuals speaking under DAF and the type of speech acts usually identified as stuttering. In his second publication Lee (1950a) also mentioned stuttering, referring to " . . . the artificially induced stuttering which occurs . . ." and he used the term "artificial stutter" as the title of his subsequent article (Lee, 1951). Since he used the word "artificial," he evidently did not intend to suggest that the two phenomena were identical in nature. However, the reference did suggest that the observable features were the same, and this then permitted the inference that the mechanism of their generation is the same. This inference has appeared repeatedly in the subsequent literature and in fact has too often been discussed as though having an established validity.

Contradictions in the stuttering analogue.—Lee observed something in the speech of some of his subjects when speaking under DAF that prompted him to describe it as "stuttering." From his own account it is clear that this "something" was the occurrence of syllable repetitions: he presented as an example of "stuttering errors" the observation that under delayed sidetone a speaker may say *aluminum-num* (Lee, 1950a; 1951). It is understandable that Lee might have thought of this as stuttering. In Chapter 4 we identified syllable repetitions as one class of the distinctive features of stuttering. Furthermore, syllable repetitions are a type of disfluency most used by lay persons in making judgments of stuttering (Boehmler, 1958; Giolas and Williams, 1958; Sander, 1963; Williams and Kent, 1958).

While it is understandable that Lee might have made this judgment, it is incredible that persons presumably knowledgeable about stuttering should have accepted it. There is extensive documentation that actual stuttering occurs either on the first syllable of a word or on a stressed syllable. In the particular example given by Lee—aluminum—actual stuttering will occur either on the first syllable or on the second, but not on the fourth. The form of syllable repetition noted by Lee is thus not the same as syllable repetition in stuttering. Anyone familiar with the occurrence of syllable repetition under DAF will recognize that it is invariably of this "addition" character epitomized in Lee's example. It is equally important to note that even this kind of syllable repetition does not occur often under DAF.

In other respects, too, Lee's observations were not consistent with what we know to characterize the phenomenal features of stuttering. For instance, Lee (1951) reported that he found no instances of phoneme repetition as an effect of DAF. This is consistent with the findings of other studies of DAF influence on speech. In only one report (Fairbanks and Guttman, 1958) is there a definite identification of phoneme repetitions, and these were discussed by the authors as "additions," suggesting that if phoneme repetitions occur in speech under DAF they also occur, like syllable repetitions under DAF, at the ends of words. Of course, the sound repetitions of stuttering are only found in the same locations as are the syllable repetitions of stuttering, so the contrast is identical.

Lee did not mention occurrence of abnormal prolongations or instances of any ancillary or accessory features. On the other hand, certain investigators have referred to "blocking" and suggestions of struggle behavior reminiscent of actual stuttering. However, certain very necessary qualifications of such reports need to be made. First, such happenings occur rarely, and they are idiosyncratic to certain subjects. Second, suggestion of "struggle" apparently occurs only when a subject attempts to resist the predominant influence of DAF, which is to slow speech rate. Third, at least some of what has been interpreted as "blocking" might well be a pausing such as described by one of Beaumont and Foss' (1957) subjects as "allowing my ears to catch up with my voice."

There are other cogent bases for serious doubt that stuttering and certain effects of delayed sidetone are similar. One very clear-cut distinction is to be made in terms of the circumstances necessary for their occurrence. Any disfluency that is the product of delayed sidetone can only occur after speech has begun. In contrast, actual stuttering very often occurs in the attempt to initiate speech.

Another major contradiction is supplied in the results of some experimentation undertaken with the express purpose of comparing stuttering and the speech characteristics induced by DAF. Neelley (1961) had stutterers and nonstutterers read aloud in normal conditions and under delayed sidetone. Recordings of these samples were then appraised by a group of independent listeners and by the stuttering subjects themselves.

Several very significant results evolved from this study. First, Neelley found that the independent listeners were readily able to distinguish samples of the usual speech of stutterers from the speech of nonstutterers speaking under delay. Second, the listeners could also distinguish between samples of the stutterers' speech under normal conditions and under DAF. Third, the DAF speech samples of both groups received comparable ratings from these judges in rating them on a nine-point scale of "speech disturbance," suggesting that the listeners perceived the extent of speech disturbance to be essentially the same in both groups, i.e., that DAF produced similar effects on the speech of stutterers and nonstutterers. Fourth, the stutterers themselves reported recognizing differences between their usual stuttering and their speech under DAF. These findings led Neelley to conclude that:

> The hypothesis that stuttering may be somehow related to delay in auditory feedback, on the ground that speech produced under conditions of delayed auditory feedback appears to behave like stuttering, to sound like stuttering, and to be an experience like stuttering, is not supported by the findings of this experiment.

Neelley's findings have constituted a substantial threat to the feedback interpretation of stuttering. A seemingly damaging criticism of Neelley's work, made by Yates (1963), has been cited sufficiently often that it deserves examination. Yates contended that Neelley's findings are "totally irrelevant to the issue whether speech behavior under DAF is determined by the same factors which maintain stammering behavior. The two groups are in no way meaningfully comparable in these respects." He goes on to claim that they are not comparable because the experience of DAF is a first-time adjustment for normal speakers whereas the stutterers have presumably spent many years making adjustments to the perceptual defect, if there is one. But, Neelley's results are at least as relevant as is the issue itself. Yates has overlooked the very basic fact that the whole idea of explaining stuttering as a kind of delay dysfunction would not have developed if Lee had not suggested the plausible similarity between these very phenomena, *long-term stuttering* and certain limited aspects of *first-time effect* of delay on normal speech. This is the fountainhead and nexus of the whole issue, and it was to this that Neelley's research was addressed. His study simply raised the question of whether the two phenomena are comparable. It would be logically more defensible to pursue investigation into possible factors of a common *source* for stuttering and DAF effects on normal speech if, in fact, there were at least some credible evidence to support the assumption of similarity in the *phenomena*. Neelley's conclusions make no claim about the nature or the existence of underlying factors; they simply reflect his findings, which indicate very clearly and consistently that the belief in a similarity of the two phenomena is ill-founded.

These findings are tantamount to corroboration of the preceding discussion regarding the lack of adequately developed criteria for the specification of stuttering. Errors in identification and subsequent erroneous expansions are encouraged by such limitations.

Neelley's results are not alone in indicating that DAF has a comparable effect on the speech of stutterers and nonstutterers. Ham and Steer (1967), Logue (1962), Nissel (1958), and many others have reported similar findings. A study of Baccara (1955) yielded results of particular relevance to this issue. He obtained EEG tracings from six stutterers and six nonstutterers speaking under normal conditions and under DAF. He found the tracings from both groups to be comparable in each of the conditions, but that in both groups the amplitude of the potentials increased under DAF.

Incidentally, another criticism by Yates—that Neelley used only one delay time—is nullified by the findings from many different sources that similar effects of delay are produced by a wide variety of delay intervals.

Undoubtedly the most powerful contradiction of the belief in a commonality between stuttering and the effects of DAF is posed by the evidence that most often stutterers show substantial improvement in fluency when speaking under delayed sidetone (Adamczyk, 1959; Chase,

Sutton, and Rapin, 1961; Gross and Nathanson, 1967; Goldiamond, 1965, 1966; Lotzman, 1961; Neelley, 1961; Ryan, 1968; Soderberg, 1967, 1969). Some investigators (Chase *et al.*, 1959; Lotzman, 1961) report finding individual differences among stutterers in speaking under DAF, with some stutterers showing less improvement than others. Apparently certain delay times are more crucial, or more specific, for some stutterers, but these variables have not been sufficiently well investigated. In fact, the very important variable of the intensity of the DAF signal is too frequently ignored in the relevant research and discussions.

In rare instances DAF has been reported to decrease the fluency of stutterers. Whether this effect is primarily a certain kind of disfluency, an admixture of disfluency forms, or an exacerbation of stuttering is not adequately documented in the reports.[18]

Other limitations of the feedback conception.—The foregoing contradictions are intrinsic to the error of drawing an analogy between stuttering and DAF speech, and they carry considerable weight in indicating that auditory feedback dysfunction does not provide an acceptable explanation of stuttering. A number of other substantive considerations indicate that auditory feedback dysfunction does not offer a very credible explanation of stuttering.

Two serious limitations of the conception become clearly evident. First, its formulation is couched in three very tenuous assumptions. One is that audition is the principal source of feedback control in speech. Another is that all features of oral expression are some immediate function of auditory input. The third, less obscure and more ingenuous, is that since stuttering is influenced by modifications in audition it must therefore be the result of certain alterations in auditory function.

Second, the reasoning involved in developing the conception ignores certain very relevant and important points which either remain completely unexplained by the feedback notion, are beyond incorporation into it, or are patently contradictory to it.

Certainly, learning to speak normally depends on being able to hear and a reasonably intact auditory sensory system is requisite to the development of normal speech. Certain kinds of defective speech are the result of anomalies in the auditory system; the speech of the deaf and the hard of hearing is symptomatic of their auditory limitations. Sometimes the relationship between the quality of the defective speech and particulars of the hearing dysfunction may be fairly specific, e.g., the lack of good fricative sounds as a function of hearing loss in the high frequencies. This relationship is sufficiently reliable that a provisional diagnosis regarding the nature of the hearing disability might be made from careful assessment of the individual's speech. But this capability should not encourage the assumption that any speech defect that has no discernible physical basis is then explicable in terms of some form of auditory dysfunction. A particular case in point is provided in the so-called functional articulation defects. The relation between articulation error and hearing function is both technically and conceptually much simpler than any hypothetical relation between stuttering and hearing function, yet much research has shown that there are no specifically relevant auditory limitations associated with "functional" articulation defects (see Winitz, 1969, pp. 180–198).

The fact that the ordinary speech of normal speakers can be notably affected by alterations in auditory input is instructive for certain purposes and permits inferences of a certain level. But the inferences should be consistent with the direction of the evidence. It seems that inferences drawn from observations of certain speech changes induced by modifications in auditory input have failed to recognize that the alterations in speech are more compensatory than disordered. For example: the normal reaction a person makes when speaking under conditions of noise is to increase his vocal intensity—the Lombard effect. It is a compensation in kind, an adjustment in volume made to a change in volume. Similarly, the predominating adjustment made to the impress of delayed auditory feedback is to speak more slowly—an evident effort to compensate for a distortion in the temporal dimension. There are other examples. For instance, Peters (1955, 1956) has shown that an increase in speech intelligibility results from filtering of particular frequencies or introduction of specific competing auditory stimuli.

Certain well-documented matters in our knowledge of stuttering are not in any way accommodated by an auditory feedback conception. Foremost among these is the fact that stuttering often occurs in the effort to initiate speech, and in such instances auditory feedback is not operative. Other "position effects" in stuttering also would be difficult to explain by the auditory feedback hypothesis, such as the occurrence of stuttering in word-initial position and the relatively greater incidence of stuttering on words early in phrases or sentences.

Other facts about stuttering which reflect some link to certain formal and linguistic properties of words and word combinations also defy satisfactory explanation by a feedback concept. For instance, substantial evidence indicates that stuttering is a function of the length of a word. It is also related in some manner to the phonetic structure of words, at least in terms of consonant-vowel dichotomy in word-initial position. Stuttering is also a function of the familiarity and usage of a word, and it is clearly related to the grammatical class to which the word belongs.

Without attempting to develop the matter at any length, it should be noted that a delayed auditory feedback model of stuttering is also contradicted by our knowledge of coarticulation effects in speech (see, e.g., Kozhevnikov and Chistovich, 1965).

The auditory feedback hypothesis also does not provide any kind of explanation for the ameliorative effects on stuttering of such circumstances as singing, choral speaking, rhythm, etc. In the case of the rhythm effect itself, recall that the salutary influence can be induced through visual or tactual modalities as well as through audition. It would be very difficult to structure an explanation, based on modification of auditory feedback function, that could account for the effect of any of these conditions.

Several other facets of stuttering remain beyond incorporation into a feedback model. For instance, the phenomenon of expectancy, reported by some stutterers, does not fit the model of a feedback loop. Also, the intermittency and periodicity of stuttering under ordinary circumstances, the adaptation effect, and the so-called consistency effect in laboratory conditions are not accountable by auditory feedback unless the explanation is buttressed by supplementary explanations which are themselves conjectural.

It should be acknowledged that results of some research have suggested certain irregularities in auditory function among stutterers. For example, Rousey *et al.* (1959) reported the sound-localization ability of stuttering children to deviate from that of normal youngsters and from children with other problems. Asp (1965) also found anomalies of auditory localization in stuttering youngsters as compared to normally speaking children. Tomatis (1954a, 1954b) claims evidence for disturbed auditory dominance among stutterers, and Curry and Gregory (1967, 1969) have reported similarly suggestive findings. Onufrak (1973) found stutterers to be inferior to, and more variable than, nonstutterers in identifying the locus of "clicks" embedded in recorded speech samples.

However, such findings should not precipitate much excitement regarding their potential contribution to an auditory feedback interpretation of stuttering; they are all encumbered by qualifications which limit their implications. Certainly, their relevance to on-line auditory control function is remote. In the last analysis, they may be simply correlative, providing separate additional evidence of subtle malfunction somewhere in the central nervous system.

There are other, even more broadly based reasons for doubting that the auditory feedback conception of stuttering has any real substance. Careful considerations of the role of audition in speech suggest that its on-line contribution to speech regulation may be quite subsidiary.

Some time ago Hudgins (1934), who worked extensively with the speech of the deaf, commented on the evidence that all aspects of speech production are relatively independent of auditory function in their immediate expression:

> . . . the chest-abdominal coordinations involved in the normal phrasing movements, the proper functions of the consonants in syllables, and the normal speech rhythms are not dependent upon hearing. They are similar to other types of skilled movements in that they may be controlled by cues from the movements themselves (kinesthesia). We have seen how subjects who lost their hearing after they had learned to speak continue to use the normal speech coordinations although they never hear the sounds which these coordinations produce. Indeed, those who are "congenitally" deaf learn a certain type of speech coordination and use it in spite of the fact that they never hear the sounds.

Dedo (1968) points out that phonation is not dependent upon auditory feedback control[19] and that even the control of pitch is not exclusively auditory, as evidenced by the fact that singers can begin a song at the right note and key, i.e., on pitch.

The foregoing considerations regarding DAF and stuttering are of great importance to stuttering theory, but they also have substantial significance for stuttering therapy and management. They provide overwhelming evidence that the significance of DAF for stuttering therapy does not focus in the auditory function per se.[20] The practical implication of this evidence is that therapy should not rely upon, let alone emphasize, modification of audition as the therapy technique. In sum, no form of intervention in auditory function should be considered, in itself, an adequate or appropriate means of treating stuttering. In final form, this means that the projected aspiration to develop a portable DAF apparatus is groundless and misguided, and that the suggestion of surgical intervention is not only more ridiculous but unprincipled as well.[21]

Channels of the salutary effect of DAF.—Material in the preceding section has identified the inadequacy of feedback explanations of the salutary influence of delayed sidetone on stuttering. Another interpretation, developed by Goldiamond (1965, 1966), is equally inadequate. Because this formulation has been accepted so uncritically yet enthusiastically some effort should be made here to reveal its serious limitations.

Goldiamond attempted to explain the fluency enhancing effect of DAF with the language of operant learning, by which the change in fluency is attributed to a program of differential reinforcement. In this scheme DAF was assumed to be "aversive" and to constitute negative reinforcement of the stuttering. Fluency, of course, would be positively reinforced (by agents of *ad hoc* construction). How DAF acquired the property of aversiveness and how it functioned as a negative reinforcement were never made clear. The means by which DAF could differentially affect stuttering, but not fluency, during the course of its continuous involvement with ongoing speech remained a persisting, but unattended, mystery. Further, there was no specification of what was supposedly receiving the presumed positive reinforcement—other than "fluency" or "a novel pattern," which of course tells nothing. The vagueness of all the critical features, in particular, reflects the speculativeness of the whole scheme. In effect, it is an explanation without essential substance, which reveals a perfunctory use of learning principles and a superficial familiarity with stuttering.

It would seem that the most reasonable approach to achieving an understanding of how delayed auditory feedback improves fluency is to take note of the actual effects on speech that are routinely induced by the condition. As in the case of our previous analysis of the effects of masking, assessment of the influence of DAF on stuttering can be implemented through identifying certain of the fundamental effects which delayed sidetone produces on normal speech.

The most commonly reported effect of DAF is a general slowing down of speech (Agnello, 1970; Atkinson, 1953; Attanasio, 1962; Beaumont and Foss, 1957; Black, 1951; Bayer and Garwood, 1963; Brokaw, Singh, and Black, 1966; Butler and Galloway, 1957; Chase and Guilfoyle, 1962; Chase *et al.*, 1959; Chase, Sutton, and Rapin, 1961; Davidson, 1959; Fairbanks, 1955; Fairbanks and Guttman, 1958; Hanley and Tiffany, 1954; Kodman, 1961; Lee, 1950a, 1950b, 1951; McCroskey, 1958; Melrose, 1954; Peters, 1954; Rawnsley and Harris, 1954; Spilka, 1954; Tiffany and Hanley, 1952, 1956). The regularity with which this effect is found prompts recall of Lee's (1951) prophetic remark that " . . . while the artificial stutter is the most striking reaction it is the less spectacular speed governing effect which probably will provide the most useful information."

It is of considerable significance that this "slowing down" is expressed primarily in syllable duration and phonation time. For example, Black (1951) found phrase duration to increase as a function of delay time. He noted that even the shortest delay produced a measurable increase in duration, with a discrete increment at 0.06 seconds and a generally linear trend to a maximum at 0.18 seconds. Atkinson's (1953) findings were consistent with those reported by Black. Fairbanks (1955) also found total sentence duration and mean duration of phonation time to show a linear trend of increase, much like that reported by Black. Spilka (1954) reported an increase in both syllable duration and percent phonation time. Rawnsley and Harris (1954), from a spectrographic analysis of the same phrases spoken normally and under delayed sidetone, observed several differences in the speech of all three subjects when speaking under delay: increased duration, emphasis on most sounds, vowel distortion, and slurring across stop gaps. Agnello (1970) studied the effects of DAF on different phoneme classes and found that the general prolongation effect is clearly associated with the vocalic features of the speech signal. Figure 8:3 illustrates these effects.

Increase in vocal intensity is another common effect noted by most investigators (Atkinson, 1953; Black, 1951; Chase, Sutton, and Rapin, 1961; Fairbanks, 1955; Lee, 1951; Melrose, 1954; Rawnsley and Harris, 1954; Spilka, 1954). Fairbanks (1955) and Davidson (1959) have reported changes in vocal pitch as an effect of delayed sidetone. Several authors (Black, 1951; Fairbanks, 1955; Fairbanks and Guttman, 1958; Rawnsley and Harris, 1954) have mentioned articulatory errors or consonant slurring.

These numerous investigations of the influence of DAF on the speech of normally fluent individuals reveal the same predominant features uncovered in our analyses of all the other conditions known to have a salutary effect on stuttering. Once more we find the primary feature to be emphasis on phonation. Again, it is expressed primarily in slowing down as developed through extended syllable duration.[22]

Particularly in view of the dramatic regularity with which these features are found to be prominently operative in all the conditions known to ameliorate stuttering substantially, we are compelled to deduce that these are the agents by which the fluency of stutterers is improved.

Our consideration of all the ameliorative conditions has consistently provided grounds for this deduction through analysis and rational inference. In the case of delayed auditory feedback we have, in addition, confirming evidence in data obtained from use of DAF with stutterers. As noted earlier, the findings of several studies reveal that delayed auditory feedback produces the same effects in stutterers as in normal speakers. Of particular pertinence to our immediate discussion, several sources (Ham and Steer, 1967; Logue, 1962; Lotzman, 1961; Soderberg, 1959) have identified slowing down as the salient aspect of the DAF influence on the speech of stutterers. Findings which evolved from therapeutic efforts with DAF have provided even greater assurance of the central agency of slowing down. Delayed auditory feedback was tried as a therapy technique simply because the first investigations of it with stutterers showed that it had a salutary effect on stuttering. The theoretical explanations for why it "worked" were attached later. However, recognition of the role played by slowing down eventually became undeniable. Gross and Nathanson (1967) actually instructed their patients to speak in a "slow, blending pattern," though using DAF. Goldiamond acknowl-

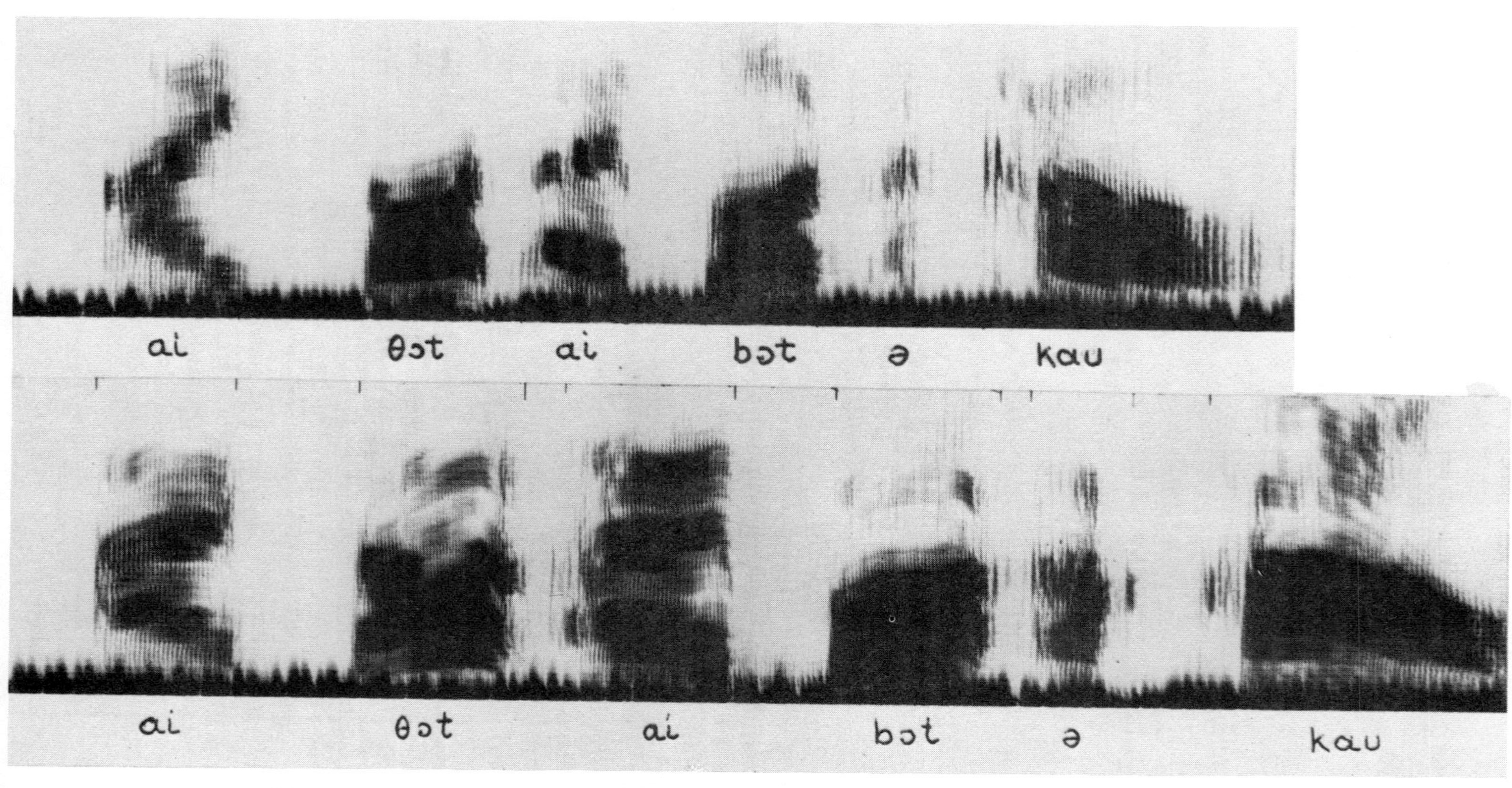

Figure 8:3 *Sonograph tracings of the same phrase spoken normally (top sample) and under delayed auditory feedback (lower sample).*

edged that when stutterers were instructed simply to prolong their speech the results were equivalent with those obtained under DAF.[23] Soderberg (1968) discussed "establishing a slow or prolonged-fluent pattern" as the focal process in DAF-assisted therapy.

SUMMARY

In contrast to the extensive range of material covered in this chapter, it is possible to provide a very succinct summary statement. Distillation of this wealth of material relating to conditions having a substantial salutary effect on stuttering reveals as the principal agent of each effect an induced emphasis on phonation, implemented most effectively by increase in duration,[24] expressed (at least experientially at this point) through "slowing down," and commonly involving modulation of stress contrasts; in brief, changes in prosodic expression.

While the summary may be succinct, other lengthier comments are in order. I am sure that many persons in the field of stuttering, especially within the United States, will greet the analysis developed in this chapter with chagrin—if not outright rejection. I can appreciate that the denouement of this inquiry is not sufficiently exotic for many tastes, and for others it represents a clear-cut refutation of favored beliefs—which will not fade easily.

In some respects I can understand that it may be disappointing and even deflating to struggle through the seemingly inscrutable mysteries of stuttering only to discover something as apparently simple as we have identified here, particularly since it contains a semblance of matters that have previously been rejected many times. But the truth often hides in simple places, which is part of what makes it difficult to find. At the same time, this apparent simplicity may well mask an underlying complexity of which we can be only dimly aware.

There is something of a case to be made in respect to the matter of "slowing down" as a method of stuttering therapy. As mentioned in an earlier chapter, slowing down has been well repudiated within the profession, yet on questionable and quite limited grounds. Reviewing the evidence reviewed in this chapter, one would seem forced to consider seriously that there should be something really substantial in the method of slowing down. There is corroborating evidence from other sources. In our review of stuttering remission in Chapter 5 "slowing down" stood out as an explanation for recovery given repeatedly—by predominantly lay people. From another direction, slowing down has been used very often in the past as a principal therapy method, and it continues to be advocated by certain professional as well as lay persons (cf. Bender, 1944; Bocks, 1967; Curlee and Perkins, 1969; Wilton, 1950). Somewhat independent of the use of slowing down as a therapy method, the technique of prolonging vowel sounds has itself had a place in stuttering therapy for a long time.

There is no intention here to claim that simply reducing the rate of speech constitutes all that is necessary for the treatment of stuttering. The evidence revealed in our analysis of ameliorating conditions clearly indicates that reduced rate, in and of itself, is not likely to represent the crux of the ameliorative effect that is associated with it. But it is equally clear that in some way reduced rate participates positively in the induction of fluency.

Within the profession there are some vigorous negative reactions to the use of slowing down as a therapy method, with the associated claim that it is valueless. But most of the evidence contradicts this claim. I too have heard from time to time that slowing down "doesn't work," but I have gradually come to suspect that there may be something wrong with the conditions or the manner of its use in the case of those who claim it is useless. I have the same suspicion regarding the repudiation of voluntary prolongation as a therapy technique. My suspicions quickly turn to matters of the motivation, commitment, and application of the stutterer for whom these efforts "don't work," particularly when considering the success reported by many persons, some of them very unsophisticated, who have employed identical or similar techniques. It should be recalled that in most of these accounts of success, for which such information is available, one also found such ingredients as dedication, application and persistence.

There are other considerations. Foremost among these is that perhaps where we find report of successful use of "slowing down" there has been inadvertent but adequate implementation of the principles summarized at the beginning of this section. Effective exploitation of these principles in a structured therapy program requires not only their identification but also an adequate appreciation of the context in which they should be implemented. We will consider this "context" in the next chapter, and relate it to the principal feature distilled in this chapter—the importance of phonatory modulation.

Notes

1. The notable exceptions being the conditions of hearing loss, auditory masking, and delayed auditory feedback.

2. *Websters New World Dictionary of the American Language*, 1966.

3. The marked increase in vowel duration is impressive even in this sample, which, produced by a trained singer, probably has less pronounced vowel-consonant difference than is usually produced by an untrained singer. In fact Vennard and Irwin, noting that the quality of articulation was a critical element in the study, called attention to the fact that this singer's diction in this particular selection had been assessed and praised widely by professional critics.

4. Singing; whispering; "sing-song"; speaking to a metronome, to an arm swing; speaking slowly, rapidly, softly, loudly, in a high pitch; and the two chorus conditions.

5. For one condition (nonsense syllables read by a stutterer accompanist) significance was at the .05 level; the rest of the conditions produced significance beyond the .01 level.

6. They assumed that "The accompanist reads at a regular rate, . . ."

7. Evidently this reference was to many more than the 54 individuals who constituted the subject sample in the work cited.

8. That is, perception in terms of features of the speech signal, as contrasted to the meaning of "perception" intended, for example, in the work of Johnson or Barber or Bloodstein where the meaning of perception has to do with *self*-perception, qualitative and subjective judgment and appraisal of the self-image, etc.

9. I have observed this to happen where "subject" and "accompanist" were not peers (as in the study discussed above); for instance, when a therapist asks a patient to read something with her.

10. Actually, there is reason to judge that not all of these articles represented separate investigations.

11. The author has observed this tendency in himself and others, when using shadowing either for demonstration or therapeutic purposes.

12. It so happens that a speaker of English is actually induced to emphasize the pattern that is central to the prosody of his language, which is a process of moving from one major stress to another (see, for instance, Sanderson, 1966, p. 23; or Smalley, 1964, p. 159).

13. The criterion of 85 percent was set arbitrarily by the present author.

14. A similar conjecture was advanced earlier by Waltz and Vogt (1932) on the basis of their finding of mild hearing loss in some stutterers as well as in individuals with other speech defects. On the assumption that hearing loss and lack of auditory training are "generally known" to be responsible for "a high percentage of other speech defects" they suggested that audition might be in some way connected with the onset of stuttering.

15. As a point of contrast we might note Weinberg's (1964) finding that stuttering occurs much more frequently (1.5%) among the blind and partially sighted than in the general population. This result has not prompted a widespread assumption that stuttering is somehow due to diminished visual capability. The significance of this correlation remains undetermined, but in this case it seems more "natural" to look for other causes. (Some of Weinberg's data suggest, in fact, that the explanation might lie in the fact that a third of these stutterers had "other problems" such as "slow learner," "retarded," and "neurologically disordered.")

16. Klein, 1967; MacCulloch, *et al.*, 1970; Mooney, 1966; Narlock, 1969; O'Sullivan, 1967; Parker and Christopherson, 1963; Perkins and Curlee, 1969; Razdol'skii, 1965; Trotter and Lesch, 1967; Van Riper, 1965.

17. The idea that stutterers can predict their stutterings has been appealing and intriguing. It also has been contended so frequently that it has gained acceptance as a regular, essentially ubiquitous, occurrence among stutterers. Actually, fairly extensive research on the matter reveals that stutterers vary considerably in their ability to predict stutterings, and that on the average they do not do very well. (Cf. Wingate, 1973.)

18. I am aware of only two sources reporting this effect. Lotzman (1961) describes the resulting speech as "nervous and hurried and has obvious resemblances to clutterings." Soderberg (1969) reports a personal communication from Chase mentioning "increased stuttering," which might only mean more (unspecified) repetitions.

19. Stromsta (1959) and Homann (1964) reported experimental blockage of a sustained vowel by instrumentally distorted sidetone under certain conditions. The significance of these findings for the role of audition in speech control function remains unclear.

20. This might seem contrary to some reports (see Soderberg, 1969) of variability in reaction to DAF among some stutterers which appears to be some function of delay interval and perhaps level of stuttering severity. However, as Soderberg noted, the reported variability might be an artefact of differences in amplification employed. Studies reporting such variability have not been careful about the dimension of feedback intensity, which other work has shown to be very important—as one might judge in view of the findings from auditory masking.

21. I have heard recently that several stutterers have followed the recommendation, made by a professional person in the field, that they undergo surgical resection of the stapedius muscle, on the assumption that the so-called "auditory reflex" is the cause of their stuttering. In view of all the negative evidence regarding auditory function in stuttering, and particularly the flimsy, presumptive connection drawn between stuttering and the action of the stapedius, a recommendation of this kind is incredibly irresponsible.

22. Some evidence also suggests the effect of modulation of stress contrasts and minimization of consonant articulation, although this is not as clear-cut here as in a number of the other conditions.

23. Reported by Soderberg (1968) as a personal communication. He also mentioned that in the early stage of Goldiamond's therapy method, patients' speech was paced electrically at 25 words per minute. This is a very much slower beginning rate than any reported in the use of rhythm.

24. By implication, duration of syllable nuclei, since these represent the major phonatory aspect of speech.

References

Adamczyk, B. Anwendung des apparatus fur dïe erzeugung von kunstlichem widerhall bei der behandlung des stotterns. *Folia Phoniat.*, **11**, 216–218, 1959.

Agnello, J. G. Durational differences in speech production under normal and delayed auditory feedback. *Sp. Monogr.*, **37**, 195–198, 1970.

Appelman, D. Ralph. *The Science of Vocal Pedagogy*, Univ. of Indiana Press, Bloomington, 1967.

Asp, C. W. An investigation of the localization of interaural stimulation by clicks and the reading times of stutterers and nonstutterers under monaural sidetone conditions. *De Therapia Vocis et Loquelae*, **I**, **B-24**, 353–356, 1965.

Atkinson, C. J. Vocal responses during controlled aural stimulation. *J. Speech Hearing Dis.*, **17**, 419–426, 1952.

———Adaptation to delayed sidetone. *J. Speech Hearing Dis.*, **18**, 386–391, 1953.

Attanasio, F. G. Duration of oral reading times and sound pressure levels under conditions of delay and intensity of sidetone transmission. *Speech Monogr.*, **24**, 85, 1962.

Baccaro, P. M. A comparative study of cortical potentials of stutterers and nonstutterers under normal reading and delayed speech feedback conditions. M. A. thesis, Univ. of Mississippi, 1955.

Backus, O., Incidence of stuttering among the deaf. *Ann. Otol. Rhinol. Laryng.*, **47**, 632–635, 1938.

Barber, V. Studies in the psychology of stuttering XV. Chorus reading as a distraction in stuttering. *J. Speech Dis.*, **4**, 371–383, 1939.

Barr, D. F. and N. R. Carmel. Stuttering inhibition with high-frequency narrow-band masking noise. *J. Audit. Res.*, **9**, 40–44, 1969.

Beaumont, J. T. and B. M. Foss. Individual differences in reacting to delayed auditory feedback. *Brit. J. Psychol.*, **48**, 85–89, 1957.

Bender, J. F. Do you know someone who stutters? *Scientific Monthly*, **59**, 221–224, 1944.

Black, J. W. Some effects upon voice of hearing tones of varying intensity and frequency while reading. *Sp. Monogr.*, **17**, 95–98, 1950.

———The effects of delayed sidetone upon vocal rate and intensity. *J. Speech Hearing Dis.*, **16**, 56–60, 1951.

Bloodstein, O. Conditions under which stuttering is reduced or absent: A review of the literature. *J. Speech Hearing Dis.*, **14**, 295–302, 1949.

———A rating scale study of conditions under which stuttering is reduced or absent. *J. Speech Hearing Dis.*, **15**, 29–36, 1950.

Bluemel, C. S. *Stammering and Cognate Defects of Speech*, G. E. Stechert, New York, 1913.

Bocks, V. D. *Freedom from Your Stammer*, Modern Publications, London, 1967.

Boehmler, R. M. Listener responses to non-fluencies. *J. Speech Hearing Res.*, **1**, 132–141, 1958.

Boomsliter, P. C. and G. S. Hastings, Jr. The "instant" of the syllable. *J. Acoust. Soc. Am.*, **49**, 104, 1971.

Boyer, E. L. and V. P. Garwood. Effects of delayed sidetone and speech content on elapsed reading time. *J. Commun.*, **12**, 44–50, 1963.

Brokaw, Sonia P., S. Singh, & J. W. Black. The duration of speech in conditions of delayed sidetone. *Sp. Monogr.*, **33**, 452–455, 1966.

Brown, S. F. From one stutterer to another. In *To The Stutterer*, Speech Foundation of America Publication # 9, 63–65, 1973.

Butler, R. A. and F. T. Galloway. Factorial analysis of the delayed feedback phenomenon. *J. Acoust. Soc. Am.*, **29**, 632–635, 1957.

Butler, R. R., Jr. and P. E. Stanley. The stuttering problem considered from an automatic control point of view. *Folia Phoniat.*, **18**, 33–44, 1966.

Charlip, W. S. Some effects of random noise upon selected speech parameters. M. S. thesis, Purdue Univ., 1964.

Chase, R. A. and G. Guilfoyle. Effect of simultaneous delayed and undelayed auditory feedback on speech. *J. Speech Hearing Res.*, **5**, 141–151, 1962.

———S. Harvey, S. Standfast, Isabelle Rapin, and S. Sutton. Comparison of the effects of delayed auditory feedback on speech and key-tapping. *Science*, **129**, 903–904, 1959.

———S. Sutton, and Isabelle Rapin. Sensory feedback influences on motor performance. *J. Audit. Res.*, **3**, 212–224, 1961.

———and S. Sutton. Reply to: Masking of auditory feedback in stutterers' speech. *J. Speech Hearing Res.*, **11**, 222–223, 1968.

Cherry, E. C. *On Human Communication*, M.I.T. Press, Cambridge, 1957.

———Some experiments on the recognition of speech, with one and two ears. *J. Acoust. Soc. Amer.*, **25**, 975–979, 1953.

———B. M. Sayers, and Pauline Marland. Experiments on the complete suppression of stammering. *Nature*, **176**, 874–875, 1955.

———B. M. Sayers, and Pauline Marland. Experiments upon the total inhibition of stammering by external control, and some clinical results. *J. Psychosom. Res.*, **1**, 233–246, 1956.

———B. M. Sayers, and Pauline Marland. Some experiments on the total suppression of stammering. *British Psychol. Soc. Bull.*, **30**, 43–44, 1956.

Curlee, R. F. and W. H. Perkins. Conversational rate control therapy for stuttering. *J. Speech Hearing Dis.*, **34**, 246–250, 1969.

Curry, F. K. W. and H. H. Gregory. A comparison of stutterers and nonstutterers on three dichotic tasks. *Program of 43rd Annual Conv.*, Am. Sp. Hearing Assn., 109, 1967.

———The performance of stutterers on dichotic listening tasks thought to reflect cerebral dominance. *J. Speech Hearing Res.*, **12**, 73–82, 1969.

Davidson, G. D. Sidetone delay and reading rate, articulation and pitch. *J. Speech Hearing Res.*, **2**, 266–270, 1959.

Dedo, H. H. Discussion of papers, pp. 202–203 of "Sound production in man." *Annals New York Acad. Sciences*, **155**, 1–381, 1968.

DeLattre, P. Vowel color and voice quality: An acoustic and articulatory comparison. *Nat'l. Assn. Tchrs. Singing Bull.*, **15**, 4–7, 1958.

Draegert, G. Relationships between voice variables and speech intelligibility in high level noise. *Speech Monogr.*, **18**, 272–278, 1951.

Eisenson, J. and C. Wells. A study of the influence of communicative responsibility in a choral speech situation for stutterers. *J. Speech Dis.*, **7**, 359–362, 1942.

Fairbanks, G. Selective vocal effects of delayed auditory feedback. *J. Speech Hearing Dis.*, **20**, 333–346, 1955.

———and N. Guttman. Effects of delayed auditory feedback upon articulation. *J. Speech Hearing Res.*, **1**, 12–22, 1958.

Giolas, T. G. and D. E. Williams. Children's reactions to nonfluencies in adult speech. *J. Speech Hearing Res.*, **1**, 86–93, 1958.

Goldiamond, I. Operant analysis in control of stuttering. *Program of 42nd Annual Convention*, Am. Sp. Hearing Assn., 54, 1966.

———Stuttering and fluency as manipulatable operant response classes. In Krasner, L. and L. Ullmann (Eds.), *Research in Behavior Modification: New Developments and Implications*, Holt, Rinehart, and Winston, New York, 1965.

Gross, M. S. and S. N. Nathanson. A study of the use of a DAF shaping procedure for adult stutterers. *Program of 43rd Annual Convention*. Am. Sp. Hearing Assn., 39, 1967.

Gruber, L. Sensory feedback and stuttering. *J. Speech Hearing Dis.*, **30**, 378–380, 1965.

Gutzmann, H. *Sprachheilkunde. Das Stottern und Seine Grundliche Beseitigung.* Berlin, 1912.

Ham, R. and M. D. Steer. Certain effects of alteration in auditory feedback. *Folia. Phoniat.*, **19**, 53–62, 1967.

Hanley, C. N. and W. R. Tiffany. An investigation into the use of electro-mechanically delayed sidetone in auditory testing. *J. Speech Hearing Dis.*, **19**, 367–374, 1954.

Hanley, T. and G. Draegert. Effects of level of distracting noise upon speaking rate, duration and intensity. Tech. Report SDC 104-2-14. Contract N 60 ri 104. T.C.II, 1949.

Hanley, T. D. and M. D. Steer. Effect of level of distracting noise on speaking rate, duration, and intensity. *J. Speech Hearing Dis.*, **14**, 363–368, 1949.

Harms, M. A. and J. Y. Malone. The relationship of hearing acuity to stammering. *J. Speech Dis.*, **4**, 363–370, 1939.

Homann, H. W. W. Experimentally induced blockage of a sustained vowel by nonlinear distortion of sidetone. *Speech Monogr.*, **31**, 233, 1964.

Hood, R. B. and R. F. Dixon. Physical characteristics of speech rhythm of deaf and normal-hearing speakers. *J. Commo. Dis.*, **2**, 20–28, 1969.

Hudgins, C. V. A comparative study of the speech coordination of deaf and normal subjects. *Ped. Sem. & J. Genet. Psychol.*, **44**, 3–48, 1934.

Johnson, W. and L. Rosen. Studies in the psychology of stuttering. VII Effect of certain changes in speech pattern upon frequency of stuttering. *J. Speech Dis.*, **2**, 105–110, 1937.

Kelham, R. and A. McHale. The application of learning theory to the treatment of stuttering. *Brit. J. Dis. Commun.*, **1**, 114–118, 1966.

Kern, A. Der einflusz des horens auf das stottern. *Arch. Psychiat.*, **97**, 429–449, 1932.

Klein, M. E. Anti-stuttering device and methods. United States Patent No. 3,349,179, Oct. 24, 1967.

Kodman, F. Controlled reading rate under delayed speech feedback. *J. Audit. Res.*, **3**, 186–194, 1961.

Kondas, O. The treatment of stammering in children by the shadow method. *Behav. Res. Ther.*, **5**, 325–329, 1967.

Kozhevnikov, V. A. and L. A. Chistovich. *Speech: Articulation and Perception.* U. S. Dept. of Commerce, Joint Publications Research Service, 1965.

Lee, B.S. Effects of delayed speech feedback. *J. Acoust. Soc. Amer.*, **22**, 824–826, 1950a.

———Some effects of sidetone delay. *J. Acoust. Soc. Amer.*, **22**, 639–640, 1950b.

———Artificial stutter. *J. Speech Hearing Dis.*, **16**, 53–55, 1951.

Logue, L. The effects of temporal alterations in auditory feedback upon the speech output of stutterers and non-stutterers. Master's thesis, Purdue Univ., 1962.

Lotzmann, V. G. Zur anwendung variierter verzogerungszeiten bei balbuties. *Folia. Phoniat.*, **13**, 276–312, 1961.

MacCulloch, M. G., R. Eaton, and E. Long. The long term effect of auditory masking on young stutterers. *British J. Dis. Commun.*, **5**, 165–173, 1970.

Maclaren, J. The treatment of stammering by the Cherry-Sayers method: Clinical impressions. In Eysenck, H. J. (Ed.), *Behavior Therapy and the Neuroses*, Pergamon, Oxford, 1960.

Maraist, J. A. and C. Hutton. Effects of auditory masking upon the speech of stutterers. *J. Speech Hearing Dis.*, **22**, 385–389, 1957.

Marland, Pauline. "Shadowing"—A contribution to the treatment of stammering. *Folia. Phoniat.*, **9**, 242–245, 1957.

McCroskey, R. L., Jr. The relative contribution of auditory and tactile cues to certain aspects of speech. *Southern Sp. J.*, **24**, 84–90, 1958.

Melrose, J. The temporal course of changes in the amount of vocal disturbance produced by delayed auditory feedback. Doctoral dissertation, Univ. of Illinois, 1954.

Mooney, Mary J. The effectiveness of auditory masking in the mitigation of stuttering. M. S. thesis, Marquette Univ., 1966.

Murray, F. P. The effects of variably presented masking noise upon the speech of stutterers. Doctoral dissertation, Univ. of Denver, 1967.

Mysak, E. D. Servo theory and stuttering. *J. Speech Hearing Dis.*, **25**, 185–195, 1960.

Narlock, Sister Marcella M. The effect of the stutter aid on the conversational speech of the stutterer. M. S. thesis, Marquette Univ., 1969.

Neelley, J. N. A study of the speech behavior of stutterers and nonstutterers under normal and delayed auditory feedback. *J. Speech Hearing Dis., Monogr. Suppl.*, **7**, 63–82, 1961.

Nessel, E. Die versogerts sprachruckklopplung (Lee effect) bei der stotterern. *Folia Phoniat.*, **10**, 199–204, 1958.

Onufrak, J. A. Stutterer's and nonstutterer's location of clicks superimposed on sentences of various types. Ph.D. dissertation, State Univ. of New York at Buffalo, 1973.

O'Sullivan, Jane E. Long-range clinical use of the Zenith stutter aid and its effect on the frequency of occurrence of stuttering. M. S. thesis, Marquette Univ., 1967.

Parker, C. S. and F. Christopherson. Electronic aid in the treatment of stammer. *Med. Electron. Biol. Engng.*, **1**, 121–125, 1963.

Paruzynski, T. A study of the speech behavior of stutterers under the influence of circumstances created by inhibiting auditory and visual sensation. Master's thesis, Marquette Univ., 1951.

Pattie, F. A. and B. B. Knight. Why does the speech of stutterers improve in chorus reading? *J. Abnorm. Soc. Psychol.*, **39**, 362–367, 1944.

Perkins, W. H. and R. F. Curlee. Clinical impressions of portable masking unit effects in stuttering. *J. Speech Hearing Dis.*, **34**, 360–362, 1969.

Peters, R. W. The effect of acoustic environment upon speaker intelligibility. *J. Speech Dis.*, **21**, 88–93, 1956.

———The effect of filtering of sidetone upon speaker intelligibility. *J. Speech Dis.*, **20**, 371–375, 1955.

———The effect of changes in sidetone delay and level upon rate of oral reading of normal speakers. *J. Speech Hearing Dis.*, **19**, 483–490, 1954.

Rawnsley, Anita I. and J. A. Harris. Comparative analysis of normal speech and speech with delayed sidetone by means of sound spectrograms. *U.S.N. Submar. Res. Lab. Rep.*, **13**, (9), No. 248, 1954.

Razdol'skii, V. A. State of speech of stammerers when alone. *Zhurnal Nevropatologii i Psikhiatrii imeni S. S. Korsakova*, **65**, 1717–1720, 1965.

Robinson, F. B. *Introduction to Stuttering*. Englewood Cliffs: Prentice Hall, 1964.

Rousey, C. L., C. P. Goetzinger, and D. Dirks. Sound localization ability of normal, stuttering, neurotic and hemiplegic subjects. *AMA Arch. Gen. Psychiat.*, **1**, 640–645, 1959.

Ruigel, R. L. and M. D. Steer. Some effects of tactile and auditory alterations on speech output. *J. Speech Hearing Res.*, **6**, 369–378, 1963.

Ryan, B. P. The establishment, transfer, and maintenance of fluent speaking and reading in a stutterer using operant technology. *Program of the 44th Annual Convention*, Am. Sp. Hearing Assoc., 132, 1968.

Sander, E. K. Frequency of syllable repetition and "stutterer" judgments. *J. Speech Hearing Dis.*, **28**, 19–30, 1963.

Sanderson, P. *Key English*, Pergamon, New York, 1966.

Sergeant, Russell L. Concurrent repetition of a continuous flow of words. *J. Speech Hearing Res.*, **4**, 373–380, 1961.

Shane, Mary Lou S. Effect on stuttering of alteration in auditory feedback. In Johnson, W., (Ed.), *Stuttering in Children and Adults*, Univ. of Minnesota Press, Minneapolis, 1955, Chapter 22.

Smalley, W. A. *Manual of Articulatory Phonetics*, Ann Arbor, Cushing-Malloy, 1964.

Soderberg, G. A. A study of the effects of delayed auditory sidetone on four aspects of stutterers' speech during oral reading and spontaneous speaking. Doctoral dissertation, Ohio State Univ., 1959.

———Delayed auditory feedback and the speech of stutterers: A review of studies. *J. Speech Hearing Dis.*, **34**, 20–29, 1969.

———Delayed auditory feedback and stuttering. *J. Speech Hearing Dis.*, **33**, 260–266, 1968.

Spilka, B. Some vocal effects of different reading passages and time delays in speech feedback. *J. Speech Hearing Dis.*, **19**, 34–47, 1954.

Stromsta, C. Experimental blockage of phonation by distorted sidetone. *J. Speech Hearing Res.*, **2**, 286–301, 1959.

———The effects of altering the fundamental frequency of auditory masking on the speech performance of stutterers. *Tech. Rept. of Public Service Grant No. B-1331*, Ohio State Univ., 1967.

Sundberg, J. Formant structure and articulation of spoken and sung vowels. *Folia Phoniat.*, **22**, 28–48, 1970.

Sutton, S. and R. A. Chase. White noise and stuttering. *J. Speech Hearing Res.*, **4**, 72, 1961.

Tiffany, W. R. and C. N. Hanley. Delayed speech feedback as a test for auditory malingering. *Science*, **115**, 59–60, 1952.

———and C. N. Hanley. Adaptation to delayed sidetone. *J. Speech Hearing Dis.*, **21**, 164–172, 1956.

Timmons, Beverly A. and J. P. Boudreau, Auditory feedback as a major factor in stuttering. *J. Speech Hearing Dis.*, **37**, 476–484, 1972.

Tomatis, A. Recherches sur la pathologie du begaiement. *J. Franc., O.R.L.*, **3**, 384, 1954a.

———Role directeur de l'oreille dan le determinisme des qualities de la voix normale (parlee et chantee) et dans la genese de ses troubles. *Act. Oto-Rhino-Laryngol*, 1954b.

Trotter, W. D. and M. M. Lesch. Personal experiences with a stutter-aid. *J. Speech Hearing Dis.*, **32**, 270–273, 1967.

Van Riper, C. Clinical use of intermittent masking noise in stuttering therapy. *Asha*, **7**, 381, 1965.

———*The Treatment of Stuttering*, Prentice-Hall, Englewood Cliffs, 1973.

Vennard, William. *Singing: The Mechanism and the Technique*, Edwards Bros., Ann Arbor, 1949.

———and J. W. Irwin. Speech and song compared in sonagrams. *Nat'l. Assn. Tchrs. Singing Bull.*, **23**, 18–23, 1966.

Voelker, C. H. A preliminary stroboscopic study of the speech of the deaf. *Am. Annals Deaf*, **80**, 243–259, 1935.

———An experimental study of the comparative rate of utterance of deaf and normal hearing speakers. *Am. Annals Deaf*, **83**, 274–284, 1938.

———An objective study of the comparative number of speech sounds spoken per minute by the deaf and the normal. *Ann. Otol. Rhinol. Laryngol.*, **46**, 471–476, 1937a.

Voelker, E. S. and C. H. Voelker. Spasmophemia in dyslalia cophotica. *Ann. Otol. Rhinol. Laryng.*, **46**, 740–743, 1937b.

Walton, D. and D. A. Black. The application of learning theory to the treatment of stammering. *J. Psychosom. Res.*, **3**, 170–179, 1958.

———and M. D. Mather. The relevance of generalization techniques to the treatment of stammering and phobic symptoms. *Behav. Res. Ther.*, **1**, 121–125, 1963.

Waltz, R. H. and A. N. Vogt. The relations between speech defects and hearing ability. *Proc. Amer. Sp. Corr. Assn.*, **2**, 74–76, 1932.

Webster, R. L. and M. F. Dorman. Decrease in stuttering frequency as a function of continuous and contingent forms of auditory masking. *J. Speech Hearing Res.*, **11**, 219–223, 1968.

———and B. B. Lubker. Masking of auditory feedback in stutterers' speech. *J. Speech Hearing Res.*, **11**, 221–222, 1968a.

———Interrelationships among fluency producing variables in stuttered speech. *J. Speech Hearing Res.*, **11**, 754–766, 1968b.

Weinberg, B. Stuttering among blind and partially sighted children. *J. Speech Hearing Dis.*, **29**, 322–326, 1964.

Weiss, M. Rapport sur un travail du Doctor Lombard, intitule: Contribution a la semeiologie de la surdite. Un nouveau signe pour en deboiler la simulation. *Bull. Acad. Med.*, Paris, **64**, 127–130, 1910.

Williams, D. E. and Louise R. Kent. Listener evaluations of speech interruptions. *J. Speech Hearing Res.*, **1**, 124–131, 1958.

Wilton, C. *How to Overcome Stammering*, Harper & Row, New York, 1950.

Winchester, R. A. and E. W. Gibbons. The effect of auditory masking upon oral reading rate. *J. Speech Hearing Dis.*, **23**, 250–252, 1958.

Wingate, M. E. Change of speech performance in choral reading. Unpubl. res.

———Expectancy as basically a short term process. *J. Speech Hearing Res.*, **18**, 31–42, 1975.

Winitz, H. *Articulatory Acquisition and Behavior*, Appleton-Century-Crofts, New York, 1969.

Wolfe, A. A. and E. G. Wolfe. Feedback processes in the theory of certain speech disorders. *Speech Path.*, **2**, 48–49, 1959.

Yates, A. J. Recent empirical and theoretical approaches to the experimental manipulation of speech in normal subjects and in stammerers. *Behav. Res. Therapy*, **1**, 95–119, 1963.

III

THERAPY: THE OBJECTIVE AND THE APPROACH

9

THE BASIS OF THERAPY

In the analysis of stuttering developed in Chapter 4 elemental repetitions and prolongations were identified as the unique features that characterize stuttering in a descriptive and denotative sense. We also noted that extending the analysis would enable us to identify the essence of stuttering in the functional or performance sense. That is, further refinement would yield specification of the nature of an instance of stuttering.[1]

THE NATURE OF A STUTTERING EVENT

We can achieve a major simplification in understanding stuttering by considering the elemental features as the distinctive "markers" of a stutter. It is a mistake to consider them to *be* the stuttering. They are more properly understood as marking an event which is the essence of stuttering. This event is a failure in phonetic transition, i.e., a failure to move smoothly to the next phoneme in the required sequence. "Failure" is only a superficial description of what actually happens. The fact that the speaker does not move forward in spite of clear intention to do so makes it appropriate to view the failure as *inability* to continue in the phonetic sequence.

Isolating transition failure as the essential event in an occurrence of stuttering resolves some of the problems encountered in the issue of identifying stuttering. Elemental repetitions and prolongations are the most obvious markers of the occurrence of stuttering, their unique nature clearly characterizing the interference in speech flow. Other kinds of disfluency may sometimes mark an instance of stuttering, provided there is evidence of the inability to move forward. For instance, a repetition of a long word or a phrase, if it occurs as an evident adjustment[2] to an inability to move forward, can also serve to mark a stuttering event. The following examples provide illustration of such different markers of a stutter occurring in the word "paper" as it might appear in the sentence, "I saw it in the daily paper."

	locus of stutter
1	aĩ sɔ ĩt ĩn ðə deilĩ p-p-p-peipɚ
2	aĩ sɔ ĩt ĩn ðə deilĩ pə pə pəeipɚ
3	aĩ sɔ ĩt ĩn ðə deilĩ p . . . . . .eipɚ
4	aĩ sɔ ĩt ĩn ðə deilĩ pəəəəeipɚ
5	aĩ sɔ ĩt ĩn ðə deilĩ deilĩ peipɚ
6	aĩ sɔ ĩt ĩn ðə deilĩ ĩn ðə deilĩ peipɚ

Note that in each case the actual stutter occurs at the same locus.

The fact that markers may be disfluencies other than the readily perceived elemental repetitions or prolongations does not modify the significance of these unique features. They remain the distinctive, the most evident, and the most frequent markers of the inability to continue smooth forward movement.

Difficult Sounds and Words

Traditionally stuttering has been thought to occur "on" certain sounds—those sounds which appear to express clearly the obvious breakdown in fluency, for example, the /p/ phoneme in the examples above. Therapists and some older stutterers refer to these as "difficult sounds," the implication being that there is something about these sounds that constitutes the focus of the stutter. The equally common reference to "difficult words" is simply another way of expressing the same conception, since the reportedly difficult words are ones that contain (usually begin with) a difficult sound.

A considerable amount of research investigating phonetic factors in stuttering has proceeded in reference to this conception of difficult sounds (see Brown, 1938; Bryngelson, 1955; Hahn, 1942; Johnson and Brown, 1935; Soderberg, 1962; Taylor, 1966a, 1966b). The most regular finding in this research has been that consonants are stuttered more frequently than vowels, a finding consistent with other less formal investigations and many casual reports. However, discussions of this finding have not always noted the important qualification that, in English at least, many more words begin with consonants than with vowels.[3]

There is some suggestion in these research data of a rank order of difficulty of sounds. However, the import of this possibility has remained very indeterminate because, again, certain important qualifications—such as the frequency of various positional occurrences of the different sounds—have not been considered.

It is easy to see how the idea of difficult sounds developed. Undoubtedly it was occasioned by the perceived prominence of these sounds in the instance of the stuttering occurrence. However, there is good reason to conclude that this prominence has been misleading. There is ample evidence to indicate that it is not something about the sounds themselves that constitutes the problem,[4] but that the difficulty must lie elsewhere.

First, the research investigating difficult sounds has not yielded very encouraging results. As noted above, the finding of substantially more stuttering on consonants than vowels has probably reflected an artefact of phoneme occurrence; and the report of a rank order of difficulty among either consonants or vowels is questionable for similar reasons. Second, the research has not uncovered any general factor of phonetic difficulty; i.e., there are no particular sounds more frequently associated with stuttering among even a majority of stutterers. Third, while there is some suggestion that for certain individuals stuttering tends to occur relatively more often in association with certain sounds, such occurrence is recognized to be quite variable.

The latter finding can be readily corroborated by any clinician. Even among those stutterers who do claim to have difficult sounds, careful observation will detect many instances in which these sounds are spoken without associated stuttering.

There is another, more universally based, contradiction to this traditional notion of difficult sounds. No matter what the particular sound in question might be, the possibility of it being associated with stuttering is completely qualified by where it occurs. Thus, a sound *may* be associated with stuttering if it occurs in a syllable-initial (mostly word-initial) position. In contrast, it *will not* be associated with stuttering when it occurs in a syllable-final position. For example, in respect to the following sample words, even a stutterer who claims specific difficulty with /t/ and /k/ only *may* give evidence of trouble at position 1, but he *will not* have trouble at position 2.

	1 2
tack	/tæk/
cat	/kæt/
tackle	/tækl/
cattle	/kætl/

These samples could be multiplied indefinitely, with any phoneme selection. This is a particularly important fact about stuttering that has not received adequate recognition. It indicates that, whether or not a particular sound may have features in its articulatory structure that are potentially troublesome, the *locus* of the sound is the really important factor in its association with stuttering. We will have more to say about this presently.

A further basis for repudiating the traditional view of difficult sounds can be derived from a careful consideration of actual instances of the purported stuttering "on" difficult sounds. For example, in the illustration presented earlier (p. 254) the /p/ phoneme would be identified as the difficult sound. Considering first the repetition of /p/ (item **1**), it should be evident upon reflection that the speaker is not really experiencing difficulty with this sound. Actually, he is making it very well—the deviance is that he is making it excessively and is not moving into the next sound. In actuality, then, the difficulty must involve the following sound.

In the silent prolongation of a sound (item **3**) the speaker seems blocked "on" the sound because he appears to remain fixed in the (actually appropriate) articulatory posture for it. Here too, however, the trouble is not "on" the sound in prominence, but in moving into the following sound.

With audible prolongation (item **4**) the prolongation clearly involves the next sound, not the initial one.

The reader may have noticed that our examples have featured consonants rather than vowels in the initial position. We will consider the matter of initial vowels presently; discussion of initial consonants requires prior consideration. Our examples have featured consonants in the initial position for two reasons. First, this represents a phonetic fact of English—that most words do begin with consonants (see fn 3). Second, it also serves to highlight the fact that there *is* a distinction to be made between consonants and vowels with regard to their association with stuttering. The disctinction, however, is diametrically opposite to that made in the traditional view of "difficult" sounds.

The Focus of Difficulty

It will be noted that in the examples given, which represent the vast majority of instances in stuttering occurrence, the "following" sound is invariably a vowel. The analysis developed here thus reveals that the focal disturbance in stuttering involves *vowels* and not consonants.

There is further evidence of the validity of this analysis. Not infrequently a consonant *blend* will be associated with a stuttering event, such as in the word "stutter" for example. An elemental repetition here will find both consonants of the blend figuring in the repetition; e.g., st-st-stutter. The same phenomenon can be observed with words having an initial blend of three consonants; e.g., str-str-strike.

Another indication that the essential problem in stuttering lies with the vowels is the frequent (inappropriate) preliminary occurrence of what is called the neutral vowel, appearing as either a repetition or prolongation, in place of the "target" vowel that the system should achieve and is evidently seeking (examples **2** and **4**, page 254). The appropriate vowel is not "actualized" by the speaker's effort.

In those instances in which stuttering is associated with a vowel (rather than a consonant) in initial position, one will regularly find evidence of difficulty in "actualizing" or "developing" the vowel, i.e., in achieving the configuration of the vowel which fully distinguishes it.[5] Again, this difficulty in developing the vowel is often signalled by the inappropriate preliminary occurrence of the neutral vowel, as well as other evidence of difficulty in "realizing" the appropriate vowel form.

Actually, there is very good reason to deduce that it is incorrect to speak of the "neutral vowel" in respect to the occurrence of this "sound" in stuttering. The circumstances of its occurrence suggest that it is neither linguistically nor communicatively significant.[6] It seems more correct to describe such occurrences of this sound as an abortive verbal gesture. Perceptually it may appear to be a phoneme, but productively it would seem to simply signify defective integration in the system. It gives evidence that execution of the intended vowel is not proceeding as it should. In essence this "sound" reveals that the phonatory aspect of the intended vowel has only been initiated but that it is not being developed or coordinated with proper oral shaping.

The Relevance of Position

We should recall at this point that the factor of position figures prominently in the locus of stuttering. Stuttering occurrence is clearly associated with initial position—to some extent with respect to word position in phrases and sentences, but predominantly in regard to the initial syllable of words. On close inspection this relationship (stuttering and word-initial position) turns out to be another artefact. Again, it is an artefact that masks a very important feature of stuttering. The predominant occurrence of stuttering in word-initial position appears simply to reflect the fact that most English words are stressed on the first syllable.[7] Therefore, the predominant occurrence of stuttering in word-initial position[8] means simply that stuttering is associated primarily with verbal stress. The validity of this inference is corroborated by ample evidence (see below) that stuttering is clearly associated with the stressed syllable whatever its position in a word.

The Central Element

The concurrence of stuttering and verbal stress is one of the most neglected facts of stuttering. Brown (1938) discovered this relationship many years ago; in fact, his data indicated a striking concurrence of stuttering and stressed syllables. However, Brown was much more interested in the suggestive evidence that grammatical factors were determinative in stuttering, and he ignored his impressive findings regarding the evident role of linguistic stress. Subsequent interest within the profession followed Brown's emphasis on grammatical features, until a few years ago when the present author became persuaded of the importance of prosodic factors in stuttering. Research (Wingate, 1967a, 1967b) again suggested the significance of verbal stress in stuttering. More recently, Hejna (1972) and Wingate (1972) have presented further compelling evidence of the concurrence of stuttering and stress in connected speech.

So, stuttering locus is clearly a function of linguistic stress; it occurs almost exclusively in association with stressed syllables. Linguistic stress is expressed through phonatory changes; the locus of stress expression is in the syllable nucleus; and the syllable nucleus is almost invariably a vowel. In other words, linguistic stress is expressed via vowels (or diphthongs; the distinction is not material here).

In identifying stuttering as a transition failure, the transition in focus is the movement into a stressed vowel, i.e., the activity necessary to "develop" a stressed vowel. Sometimes the required transition is from a position of rest (as when a word begins with a vowel); more often it is a movement from another speech gesture (as when a word begins with a consonant). In contrast, it is highly significant that stuttering is not associated with the transition *from* a position of stress, viz., the consonant immediately following a stressed vowel is never involved in a stutter. Also, stuttering does not occur on closely following vowels of lower stress; the next occurrence of stuttering will involve another vowel bearing stress prominence.[9]

One of the more widely acknowledged facts of stuttering is that it occurs much more frequently in connected speech than in the speaking of isolated words or short phrases. This fact has been subjected to several interpretations which seek an explanation in terms of certain differences between the two circumstances; for example, that connected speech involves more "propositionality" than speaking isolated words. However, a simpler account of why there is more stuttering in connected speech would emphasize a commonality of spontaneous speech and the speaking of words and phrases.

We know that in both connected speech and in the speaking of isolated words stuttering occurs on stressed syllables. Now, it is readily evident that stress patterns are extended and more complicated in connected speech than in speaking isolated words or brief phrases. There is, then, in connected speech increased expression of the feature with which stuttering is most regularly associated. It would follow that the more frequent occurrence of stuttering in connected speech is a clear reflection of the influence of linguistic stress.

INTEGRATION

Fundamentally speech is an undulating vocalized sound, a more-or-less continuous tone that evidences substantial changes in its various aspects while being produced. Within certain qualifications, these changes are referred to as the prosody of speech.

Identification of prosody as structurally fundamental to speech is corroborated by the evidence that it is developmentally fundamental as well. It is the dimension of verbal communication to which the infant first responds with evidence of comprehension, and it is also the first approximation of verbal communication of which he is capable. Vowels are the earliest modification of this sound and they continue to constitute its linguistically meaningful shapes. Further, and most importantly for our interest, it is through the vowels that the undulations in the stream of sound (i.e., its prosody) are expressed.

Discussion in this chapter has centered around two major points relating stuttering to specific features of speech: (a) stuttering occurs in vowels, and (b) stuttering is almost exclusively associated with syllables bearing major stress. We have not yet related these two items to each other, but this is easily done. The two points meld together through the interrelationship that exists among vowels, syllables, and stress; namely, vowels are the nuclei of all stressed syllables, and it is through vowels that linguistic stress is expressed.

We have now arrived at what is, for the immediate future at least, the ultimate refinement in identifying the phenomenal nature of stuttering: it is a prosodic defect. Stuttering occurs when undulations in the vocal sound are moving toward crests of relative prominence. Stuttering is, then, an intermittent disorder of actualizing stress increase.

There are several variables involved in effecting changes in stress, the most prominent of which are pitch, intensity, and duration. The relative importance of these variables in the instance of stuttering is presently unknown and remains a matter to be pursued in continued research. However, we know that the "final end product" of these variables (i.e., stress, or prosodic variation) is associated in a unique and consistent manner with stuttering occurrence. This knowledge, of itself, provides a significant, substantive rationale for a treatment program. However, confidence in the use of this knowledge is augmented significantly by other substantive support, which we encountered earlier.

The reader is reminded of the analysis developed in the preceding chapter. From the extensive literature dealing with conditions that have a salutary effect on stuttering we extracted a common principle: amelioration of stuttering is implemented through prosodic modification, the major features of which were (a) emphasis on phonation and (b) modulation of stress contrasts.

Thus, analysis of the nature of stuttering, as culminated in this chapter, and the previous analysis of the factors that ameliorate stuttering, converge on a single focus: the prosodic aspects of speech.

It follows from the analyses developed here that the problem faced in working with stuttering is one of dealing with control of vocalization as it figures in the expression of stress and stress contrast; specifically, with those actions involved in effecting increases in stress. This identifies the objective of therapy; it also delineates the character of therapy strategies, which we will consider in the next chapter.

Notes

1. There is no attempt here to imply the nature of stuttering in an etiologic sense. The objective is simply to isolate the nexus of the act of stuttering, as an event. At the same time, the analysis which unfolds does clearly suggest directions in which to explore the matter of etiology.

2. Evidence of such adjustment is supplied in the kind of cues reviewed earlier (pp. 45, 47), e.g., visual signs, inappropriate locus of the repetition, etc.

3. A composite analysis (Wingate, 1973) of four lists of the 1,000 most frequently occurring words used in speaking reveals that, as an average, 81 percent of the listed words begin with consonants. This figure may be slightly inflated since certain words used repeatedly begin with vowels. For instance, data reported by French, Carter, and Koenig (1930) indicated that 67.2 percent of words appearing in conversations had initial consonants.

4. This misidentification of what is difficult also subverts those explanations of stuttering occurrence that account for stuttering in terms of a reaction to a *perceived* difficulty of sounds. That is, the perception of difficulty cannot be an adequate explanation since the sound perceived as difficult is not where the stutter occurs.

5. It may be appropriate, then, to speak of stuttering "on" an initial sound when that initial sound is a vowel.

Another matter meriting consideration is that the reports of more frequent stuttering on consonants might indicate that vowels are easier to produce when not preceded by a consonant. That is, it may be easier to produce a vowel as an initial sound than to shift from the articulation of a consonant to the production of a vowel. Of course, in either case the actual difficulty is still in developing the vowel, but the matter deserves further investigation.

6. For comparison, the meditative "uh" has communicative significance.

7. Trnka's (1966) analysis of the 100,000 words in Dewey's work reveals that monosyllabic and initially stressed bisyllabic words comprise 70.3 percent of all words. A similar analysis of Voelker's (1942) list of the 1,000 most frequently occurring words yields a comparable figure (73.5 percent). Further analysis of Voelker's list indicates that 81 percent of all the words in his sample are monosyllables or are stressed on the first syllable. The distribution of stress patterns in 5,800 English words analyzed by Delattre (1963) is very comparable to the pattern for Voelker's list. In effect, then, the available evidence indicates that less than 20 percent of English words have primary stress on other than the first syllable.

8. As noted earlier (p. 229ff) this fact supplies a simple criterion for distinguishing a stutter from a disfluency that might be thought to resemble it. For instance, a repetition involving a final unstressed syllable is just not distinctive of stuttering.

9. Occasionally stuttering will be observed to involve an unstressed vowel immediately preceding a syllable bearing stress prominence. This observation does not seem to contradict the salience of linguistic stress in the stuttering event. It seems reasonable to hypothesize that in such cases coarticulatory planning for the adjustments necessary to express stress is slightly premature.

References

Brown, S. F. A further study of stuttering in relation to various speech sounds. *Quart. J. Speech*, **24**, 390–297, 1938.

———Stuttering with relation to word accent and word position. *J. Abn. Soc. Psychol.*, **33**, 112–120, 1938.

Bryngelson, B. A study of the speech difficulties of thirteen stutterers. In Johnson, W., (Ed.). *Stuttering in Children and Adults*, Univ. of Minnesota Press, Minneapolis, 1955, Chapter 36.

Delattre, P. Comparing the prosodic features of English, German, Spanish, and French. *Internat'l Review Applied Linguistics*, **1**, 193–210, 1963.

French, N. R., C. W. Carter, and W. Koenig. The words and sounds of telephone conversations. *Bell Syst. Tech. J.*, **9**, 290–324, 1930.

Hahn, E. F. A study of the relationship between stuttering occurrence and phonetic factors in oral reading. *J. Speech Dis.*, **7**, 143–151, 1942.

Hejna, R. F. The relationship between stress or accent and stuttering during spontaneous speech. *Asha*, **14**, 479, 1972, (abstr.)

Johnson, W. and S. F. Brown. Stuttering in relation to various speech sounds. *Quart. J. Speech*, **21**, 481–496, 1935.

Soderberg, G. A. Phonetic influences upon stuttering. *J. Speech Hearing Res.*, **5**, 315–320, 1962.

Taylor, I. K. The properties of stuttered words. *J. Verb. Lrng. Verb. Behav.*, **5**, 112–118, 1966a.

———What words are stuttered? *Psychol. Bull.*, **65**, 233–242, 1966b.

Trnka, Bohumil. *A Phonological Analysis of Present Day Standard English*, Univ. of Alabama Press, University, Alabama, 1966.

Voelker, C. H. The one thousand most frequent spoken words. *Quart. J. Sp.*, **28**, 189–197, 1942.

Wingate, M. E. Slurvian skill of stutterers. *J. Speech Hearing Res.*, **10**, 844–848, 1967a.

———Stuttering and word length. *J. Speech Hearing Res.*, **10**, 146–152, 1967b.

———Symposium on linguistic-motor determinants of stuttering. Paper presented at the annual convention, Am. Sp. Hearing Assn., Nov. 1972.

———The structural character of the most commonly occurring words, Unpubl., 1973.

10

THE FORM OF THERAPY

This chapter considers procedures found indifferent approaches to stuttering therapy with a view to isolating certain recurring features that might reflect universal principles. The discussion will be developed in reference to two rather comprehensive points that are especially significant to an appreciation of fundamental processes in stuttering therapy. One deals with the matter of cognitive function in stuttering therapy; the other centers in a distinction between two basic forms of therapeutic effort.

COGNITIVE PROCESS

All current stuttering therapies are based on cognitive function. That is, the direct therapy of stuttering is a conscious teaching process in which both patient and therapist: (a) recognize that remediation of the problem is being attempted, and (b) are aware of the immediate therapy activity and, in most cases, of its objective.

In most approaches to stuttering therapy this point is not denied, but it is not regularly given sufficient recognition. At least some advocates of "operant" approaches to stuttering modification evidently like to believe otherwise (see below).

It is precisely because stuttering therapy is typically a cognitive process that dealing with the very young stutterer has presented such a formidable problem, particularly in this country. On the one hand, there has been a massive reluctance to deal openly with stuttering in the young child. This reluctance reflects (a) the questionable assumption that the child is unaware of the problem and (b) the inordinate fear that bringing the matter to the child's awareness will either activate or exacerbate the stuttering.[1] On the other hand, the alternative of dealing openly with the problem is beset by great uncertainty and reservation regarding what one might realistically expect to teach little children about modifying their stuttering. This reservation seems to assume that the therapy must be a formal didactic process comparable to that utilized with adults—an understandable assumption since most direct therapy measures have developed in work with older stutterers.

The adjustment to this dilemma has found expression in various forms of ineffectual or dubious approaches. One of these is to take the presumably "safe" recourse of working with the parents. This is consistent with the commonly held belief that parents "have a part" in the child's stuttering, meaning that they have caused it or at least exacerbate it. Frequently then, parents receive counseling with the objective of having them "realize" how their relationship with the child is a source of his problem. (We will have more to say about this matter in Chapter 12). Sometimes the counseling is of a more mundane character, in which the parents are given advice about everyday circumstances that may influence the occurrence of their child's stuttering. Certain of these suggestions may well have some benefit (such as: to modify living circumstances that are obviously overstimulating), but many of the recommendations are of very questionable value (for example: advising the parent to read to the child, or to ignore the stuttering, or to listen for his normal nonfluencies, etc.).

Another dimension of ineffectual adjustment to the problem is represented in "playing games," "just talking," reading aloud, building models and other similar activities. The poor results obtained by these means of dealing with the problem attest well to their inutility. Such activities do not really constitute therapy for stuttering.[2]

In terms of the way it is typically handled in the United States, and certain locales in other countries, the management of stuttering in the young child thus assumes the proportions of the special case; i.e. the problem (stuttering) is handled very differently in younger children. However, some European approaches to dealing with stuttering in young children are not beset by such a dilemma and do approach the stuttering directly. These methods clearly involve cognitive function and we will take note of some of them later in this chapter.

The major point to be made at this juncture is that the central activity in stuttering therapy is assisting the patient to improve his coordination of certain motor functions involved in the act of speaking. In essence, the process is skill training of a special kind, and typically the patient's understanding and active effort are involved.[3]

TWO FORMS

The second point to be considered is that most stuttering therapies[4] assume one of two forms. This feature is seldom acknowledged, yet it is a matter of particular relevance to an understanding of stuttering therapy.

A therapy approach will either (a) focus on stuttering, or (b) concentrate on speaking without stuttering.

Focus on Stuttering

Therapy of this form is concerned principally with instances of stuttering, i.e., attention is focused on those actions of the speech apparatus that evidently constitute stuttering events. The principal therapy effort is directed at modifying the various aspects of these events, with the objective of at least minimizing both the frequency with which they occur and the extent of involvement when they do occur.

There are two major subcategories under this general classification. One category includes a group of methods that might be best described as "reconstructive" treatment which have been in use for some time, especially in this country. The other category consists of the so-called "operant" approaches, which have become popular only recently. There are certain important differences between these two subtypes, in spite of certain similarities and a common focus. At the same time, as we shall see presently, both of these categories have certain features in common with the therapies of the second form, in spite of the major difference in basic focus.

"Reconstructive" therapy—This type of stuttering therapy has been most widely used in this country within the present century, particularly since the development of speech pathology as a profession. There are several variants[5] of this approach, but all have the common aim of teaching the stutterer how to modify his stuttering. Some of the therapies of this type have as their objective the elimination of stuttering. Others have the more modest goal of reducing stuttering in extent and severity.

Most of these therapies, in varying measure, are also concerned with certain personal reactions of the individual to his stuttering, and with other (negative) attitudes that are presumed to be involved in the problem. Therefore, modification of such reactions and attitudes is an important part of the overall process of these therapies. We will not concern ourselves with such matters here.

Many of the variants of this approach represent differences in viewpoint regarding the etiology and nature of stuttering. However, as noted earlier (p. 4ff), these theoretical differences find little reflection in the actual therapy—the procedures are very much the same regardless of theoretical viewpoint. In some instances a theoretical rationale has been attached to certain of the therapy techniques used, but the relation of theoretic notion to therapeutic technique is more afterthought than reality. For the most part the particular techniques employed are empirical, derived over a substantial period of time through actual therapeutic effort with stutterers.

A central procedure in the reconstructive approaches is the analysis of instances of stuttering. Typically, from the beginning of therapy the patient is involved in what might be called a "symptom analysis," identification of the characteristics of his stuttering pattern. The objective is to gradually familiarize the stutterer with what takes place in the stuttering event; much attention is directed to what we have identified as accessory features.

Actually most advocates of these approaches prefer to speak of these analyses in terms of "what the patient *is doing*" at these specific times. This choice of wording conveys the interpretation that the stutter is not something that just "happens" but rather that the stutterer is in some way responsible for the events identifiable as an instance of stuttering. In fact, this interpretation is usually emphasized to the patient in the effort to persuade him that what constitutes an instance of stuttering consists of actions over which he potentially has control.

The reader should appreciate that a basic issue is being drawn in this contrast. To say that a stutter "happens" not only indicates that the event is not under the patient's control, it also clearly implies an organic origin, more specifically, that the source of the event is some neurologic anomaly. In contrast, to claim that the events of the stutter are something the person *does* suggests that, in origin as well as in function, the events are voluntary in nature and therefore essentially normal.

In many therapy approaches the patient is led to view all aspects of his stutter not only as something he does but as something he learned to do. The stutterer is misled: there is no good substantive evidence that the *core* features of stuttering are learned. It is therefore improper to lead the patient to believe that he learned to stutter.[6] The implication is unnecessary, simply because a stutterer can learn to modify and control his stuttering whether or not he thinks of it as something he learned to do. Since the cause of stuttering remains unknown, the successes achieved by the reconstructive approaches are themselves testimony to the fact that the ability to control or modify a behavior is independent of its known origin. Some sources assume that the ability to control stuttering is evidence that stuttering is learned. This is a fallacious assumption, contradicted by evidence. It should be recognized that certain known organic functions or conditions are modifiable through voluntary efforts at control. For instance, anyone can learn to inhibit or regulate his patellar reflex, which is certainly not a learned movement. We learn not to cry, or to cry in certain ways in response to certain situations or events, but we do not learn crying. The cerebral palsied child develops some control of inaccurate and abnormal movements, which were not learned patterns. Of particular relevance here is a report by Lebrun and Bayle (1973) regarding a patient who, as a result of a right cerebral lesion, tended to reduplicate strokes when writing. He stopped doing so when he discovered the examiner was interested in his mistakes; he avoided the reduplications by paying careful attention to his writing.

As noted earlier, there are several, somewhat differing variations of the reconstructive approach, but it is probably epitomized in a method described by Van Riper (1973) which, in addition to being well articulated, also is probably the method most widely followed in the United States.

As described by Van Riper (1973, p. 303) treatment by this method begins " . . . by first trying to introduce some modest changes into the stutterer's usual mode of living. The basic goal of this phase of therapy is variability." This phase consists substantially of working on "ways of behaving, thinking and feeling," particularly those that are thought to involve and affect the individual's speech. This form of psychotherapeutic effort is woven into much of the therapy program.

This first phase, with its goal of variability, also incorporates attention to changes in manner of speaking. First, the individual is assisted in the analysis of his stuttering and in identification of its features. Almost concurrently he is directed and guided in varying his stuttering, the object being to move toward a fluent (loose or easy) form of stuttering. Particular note should be made of the fact that from the beginning the procedure emphasizes cognitive process. Analysis and identification of the stuttering is based on awareness, and ability to vary the form of the stuttering requires that the patient " . . . have clearly in mind the motoric model of standard utterance" (p. 312).

The next phase of the therapy is actually the heart of the method.

Called "cancellation," it consists basically of requiring the stutterer to "re-do" the word he has just stuttered. Van Riper stresses emphatically that cancellation must not be construed as just a routine in which the stutterer simply says the word again. On the contrary, cancellation is a structured process having a definite sequence of procedures. The objective of these procedures is to help the stutterer "to learn how to unify that word" (p. 321).

The first procedure in cancellation is "the pause." Immediately after completing a stuttered word the patient is forced to endure a relatively brief silent interval[7] before making a new attempt on the word just stuttered. When he does make the new attempt, the target behavior will be "a slow-motion, prolonged sequencing" (p. 321).

Saying the word again follows a three-stage sequence. The initial stage consists of pantomime activity. The patient first pantomimes the stuttered word in an attempted imitation of the way he just said it (i.e., as stuttered); he then pantomimes a modified version of the stuttered word. In the next step he repeats the same process but now in a soft "almost inaudible whisper." The final stage calls for another repetition of the process, this time aloud (voiced).[8] In each of the steps of cancellation the rehearsals should be in a "strong, deliberate, slow-motion kind of utterance in which the sequencing of motoric components is somewhat slowed and obviously highly controlled. . . . The cancelled word does not sound the same as it would were it spoken normally. It is slower, stronger, spoken more carefully and consciously" (p. 326).

Not only is it obvious that cognitive function is integral to this method but there is clearly a concentration on slow, deliberate speaking as the means of emphasizing the appropriate patterned sequence of movements. The efficacy of this method of dealing with occurrences of stuttering is reflected in the following statement by Van Riper (1973, p. 327):

> The payoff from this training in cancellation is difficult to overestimate. We have seen many stutterers who needed very little additional therapy. Once they learned, through cancelling, other and better ways of stuttering they immediately applied this new knowledge whenever they expected or experienced disruption.

Another major phase of this therapy method, which is subsequent to cancellation, is the "pull-out." Actually, the pull-out represents an abbreviated cancellation, moved forward in time; the stutterer now begins to modify his stuttering as soon as he becomes aware of its occurrence. While the therapist continues to assist the patient in directing his efforts at modification as he moves to this phase, the transition from cancellation to pull-out very often occurs quite naturally. As indicated in the quotation above, many patients do not even need to be assisted to learn "pull-outs."

Throughout his discussion of this treatment method Van Riper mentions frequently that the patient "has to become aware of the motoric aspects of his speech." There is deliberate emphasis on proprioceptive feedback, in which the stutterer's attention is focused particularly on the movements of his peripheral speech mechanism. Van Riper believes that this proprioceptive emphasis is assisted through the use of certain adjunctive techniques, for example: various kinds of auditory masking, DAF, choral reading, the electrolarynx, pantomiming, whispering, and others. In other words, deliberate use is made of these techniques as ways of enhancing awareness of oral speech function.

Taking Van Riper's method as the best representative of the reconstructive approach, it is clear that such methods emphasize cognitive function. It is equally clear that there is definite concentration on having the patient learn about motor functions important to the activity of speaking. It is of no little interest that this skill training is implemented, in impressive part, through the technique of slowing down. Here slowing down is not used simply as control of rate; it is used for instructional purposes, that is, to emphasize to the patient the movement sequences basic to producing speech normally. This might well be an essential, though unrecognized function and value of slowing down *whenever* it is used. Additionally, it should be recalled that slowing down is expressed essentially in extended duration of the voiced elements of speech (cf. the discussions in Chapters 5, 6 and 8).

"Operant" therapy.—Therapies of the "operant" or "behavior modification" type also focus on the instance of stuttering. In fact, the focus on stuttering is emphasized: the operant approach concentrates on specific overt behaviors. Unlike the reconstructive methods, little attention is given to matters of attitude and personal reaction.

Therapies of the operant approach do not arise from a background of experience with stuttering, but rather from a rationale within the field of psychological learning theory. These therapies are of very recent origin and have gained considerable popularity by virtue of their simple format and semblance of scientific procedure.

In origin, the term "operant" denotes an hypothesized type of learned behavior.[9] Thus, references to use of the "operant" approach in stuttering therapy carry the clear implication that stuttering is learned behavior. Actually, as applied to the modification of stuttering, the term "operant" simply signifies a particular methodology. It refers to procedures borrowed from a training method utilized in work with animals in the psychological laboratory.[10]

The basic conceptual principle underlying this approach is the Law of Effect, namely, that an act tends to recur if it is rewarded, and to fail to occur if it is punished. In modern day parlance, the terms "positive reinforcement" and "negative reinforcement" are preferred over "reward" and "punishment" since the former terms are thought to avoid the subjective qualities of the latter. Two other guiding principles in this approach are "contingency" and "shaping."

Contingency means that a reinforcement should be "delivered" as soon as the behavior to be changed occurs. Inherent in the concept of contingency is the requirement that the reinforcement must follow the "target" behavior immediately.

"Shaping" is actually another word for "modification." It refers to a gradual change in behavior guided by the therapist according to a preplanned scheme.

Reinforcement and shaping are readily identified as integral features of the operant approach. However, they are not unique to it. Reconstructive therapies also employ methods and techniques that embody these concepts. Van Riper, for example, points to many effects that he considers to be reinforcements, and the gradual progressive stuttering modification in his method is certainly a form of "shaping."

Contingency does seem to represent a contribution to method; however, contingency exists as a technique quite independently of operant notions.[11] Moreover, even as used in operant method there is substantial reason to suspect that contingency does not operate in practice as it is presented in conception. First, there are problems of specifying the "target" act or behavior. For instance, is "stuttering" an adequate specification? Or should it be "syllable repetition," or "sound repetition," or "prolongation," or some combination of these three—or something else?[12] Or should one specify repetition of certain phones, or repetition of some particular syllable beginning with one of these phones? How many repetitions per instance should be allowed before delivering the contingency? Does one interrupt a prolongation or wait until it is finished? Many other relevant questions of this kind can be raised.

Technically, the operant conception should call for a quite detailed specification of the target behavior. However, certain very real limitations arise in actual practice. It is not a simple matter to regularly recognize a target behavior unless it is fairly gross in configuration. Furthermore, it is difficult to consistently recognize any particular act sufficiently quickly to deliver the supposed reinforcement *in accurate contingency.*

Considerations such as these reveal that operant procedure with stuttering is neither as highly objective nor as specific in character as it is alleged to be. In particular, the problem of accuracy in delivery of the contingent effect raises considerable question as to the way in which such contingencies actually operate. (See below.)

Operant therapies for stuttering developed rapidly from a set of experimental studies investigating the effect of operant procedures on the occurrence of stutterings and certain other disfluencies. Typically, in this work, some kind of speech activity was identified as the target behavior for some contingent effect which was presumed to have reinforcing properties. Most of these studies did indeed show that various kinds of speech acts, including stuttering, are amenable to control by the effects utilized (which ranged from enforced periods of silence, through verbal remarks such as "bad" and "not good," to substantial electric shocks).

Evidently most of these studies have been conducted with the assumption that the procedures operate in the same fashion with these human subjects as they are thought to operate with animals in the laboratory. It is assumed that the technique has some direct connection with and control of the "target behaviors"; that the procedure somehow bypasses awareness and effects change of the behaviors without the subject being aware of the process. It is further assumed that subsequent change in the behavior, such as reduction in stuttering, means that the behavior (in this case stuttering) has been "unlearned" through the agency of the contingent reinforcement.

This interpretation is highly unlikely. As noted elsewhere in this book the reinforcement notion is confounded by evidence as well as by logic. Further, it has been known for some time that many stutterers, under certain circumstances, are quite capable of controlling their stuttering for a certain length of time.

In most of this experimentation no provision was made for appraising the subject's awareness of what was going on. Actually, there is evidence that subjects are conscious of the circumstances in these experiments and of the relation of these circumstances to their stuttering. For example, in a study by Siegel and Martin (1966) an effect found to be most consistently related to reduction in stuttering was a nylon band placed around the subject's wrist and maintained in position for fairly lengthy periods. This was a very interesting finding in view of the fact that other effects in the experiment were much more dramatic and were contingent on stutterings. Most likely the effectiveness of the wrist band was due to its acting as a "reminder"; that is, it alerted the subject to monitor his performance according to what he had already deduced was expected of him.

From a slightly different direction, Cooper *et al.* (1970) found that saying the word "tree" contingent upon stutterings was as effective in reducing stutterings as saying the word "wrong." Interestingly, a comparable effect was also obtained by contingently saying the word "right." At least the words "right" and "wrong" should have produced very different effects since they should have opposite "reinforcing" properties. To find that clearly opposite words like "right" and "wrong" have equivalent effects, and that "tree" has the same effect as either "right" or "wrong," indicates that talking about "reinfocement" is at least superfluous. It seems most reasonable that in a context like this the word "tree" has the same value as "right," "wrong," "good," "bad," or any other word one might happen to use, simply because each of them has a simple cognitive value: they function as alerting and reminding signals.

In another study (Martin *et al.*, 1972) an unsolicited (and unexpected) remark from a 3½-year-old child indicated that even children of this age can become aware rather quickly of an experimental effect and its relationship to their stutterings.

In effect, then, these experiments actually provide corroboration that subject awareness is an important part of the modification process. Evidence for this effect was presented in research published by the author a number of years earlier (Wingate, 1959). In that study subjects were intentionally made aware of the procedural efforts to reduce their stuttering. Dramatic reductions in stuttering were achieved by asking subjects not to stutter and then immediately calling attention to each instance of stuttering occurrence. The results provided no evidence that the subjects had unlearned anything, but simply that they were able to control stuttering occurrence when directed to do so and given simple assistance.

Although the matter of subject awareness of procedure is typically not considered in operant type research in stuttering, the therapy efforts that have emanated from this experimental background reveal unmistakably the cognitive focus of their method. For instance, the program described by Ryan (1964) is actually an adaptation of Van Riper's method to the format of the operant approach; the program is infused with patient awareness. A program reported by Shames (1968), and an elaboration of it reported by Shames *et al.* (1969), also incorporate many features of the Van Riper method and, again, clearly specify to the patient what is to be changed and how. The program described by Goldiamond (1965), although elaborate with instruments and operant terminology, obviously involves patient awareness of objective and procedure. The system described by Andrews (1971) and Andrews and Ingham (1971) has been referred to as an instance of operant method. However, the actual substance of their system consists of a variety of therapy methods that plainly require patient awareness and active involvement. Further, the therapy methods exist quite independently of any operant scheme. The only part of their approach that resembles operant procedure is a system of reward using tokens. This is more accurately described as a system of merits and demerits; it too is obviously cognitively based, and quite detached from any contingency relationship to stutterings. It is clearly adjunctive to the actual therapeutic methods.

Certain other methods that emphasize operant principles (e.g., Mowrer, 1972) or incorporate them prominently (e.g., Curlee and Perkins, 1968) are actually forms of rate-control therapy to which certain procedural aspects of operant methodology have been added. We will have more to say about rate control presently.

The reader may have already detected that operant therapy has only a partial resemblance to the research on which it is presumably based. If operant therapy were a realistic expression of the relevant research, one should find treatment to consist simply of rigorous and systematic "negative reinforcement" of stutterings and "positive reinforcement" of periods of fluency. Obviously, much more is involved in any of the so-called operant treatment approaches.

Efforts to apply operant ideas to stuttering therapy reflect a simplistic conception that confuses procedure with process. In reality, wherever some purported operant features are said to be involved in a therapy approach they actually stand at the periphery of the modification process. *The actual modification of stuttering (or increase of fluency) is always achieved through some other means;* for example, through the use of: DAF, metronome, or slowing down (Goldiamond, 1965); Van Riper's methods (Ryan, 1964, Shames, 1968, 1969); slowing down (Curlee and Perkins, 1969; Mowrer, 1972); syllable-timed speech, DAF, etc. (Andrews and Ingham, 1971); prolonged speech, DAF, unison speech, cancellation, etc. (Ryan, 1971). In each case a process is selected which is known to enhance fluency; operant procedures are introduced into the overall scheme; the improved fluency is then attributed to the operant procedures. In actuality, the effective substance in these approaches is really some other method borrowed for the occasion; the "operant" aspects of the procedure are simply technical embellishments.

In concluding this section it is particularly relevant to comment further on two matters: (a) contingent effects, and (b) the nature of the processes exploited by the operant approach.

We have a particular interest in the so-called contingent effects, since it is through them that the operant focus on stuttering is implemented. As discussed earlier, contingencies employed with stuttering serve to call attention to stuttering and to remind the stutterer to exercise whatever control he can generate at that time. Thus, the focus on stuttering central to operant technique is also implemented through cognitive function, as it is in a reconstructive approach.

We should also have particular interest in the fact that so many of the processes exploited by the operant approach are some expression of rate control. The reader should note the frequency with which "slowing down" appears in the references cited above. He should also recall that slowing down is an essential feature of most of the other processes mentioned: DAF, use of a metronome, prolonged speech, unison speech, and syllable-timed speech. Once again we should note that slowing down is expressed essentially through extending the duration of the voiced elements of speech.

Focus on Fluency

The second form of therapy does not particularly concern itself with instances of stuttering, and only indirectly with any specific aspects of stuttering events. This therapy form consists essentially of inducing the patient to speak in a manner such that stuttering will not occur.

Representations of this approach are to be found most often in methods of foreign origin (mostly European) and in the therapy systems of the commercial schools (both in this country and abroad). We reviewed a number of such methods previously (Chapters 6, 7, and 8). Presently we will identify and briefly discuss several other methods, not previously mentioned, that also seem to represent clearly this therapy form.

The methods representing this form of approach have a more varied source than those of the form described first. Some of these methods are empirically derived; at least one originates from a very technical base; a few are founded on informed though coarse reasoning; others must certainly have evolved largely from happenstance. They differ in appearance as much as their divergent origins would lead one to suspect. Yet, in spite of their varied lineage and apparent surface differences one can find within each of them a common feature: each of these methods induces an emphasis on voicing, with concurrent modulation of prosodic expression.

Additional Procedures of the Second Form

The chewing method.—This approach to stuttering remediation, developed by Froeschels over thirty years ago, has been described in a number of sources (Froeschels, 1943, 1956; Froeschels and Jellinek, 1941; Kastein, 1947; Mohr, 1951). Since description of the method is brief, and has been very similar in content in the several sources cited, it is suitable to include here a representative description from the author of the method (Froeschels, 1956).[13]

The patient is asked to make savage-like eating movements, at first by opening the mouth and using extensive movements of his lips and tongue, then making the same sort of movement with voice emission. One must be very careful that he does not produce a stereotyped "nga-nga-nga" or "mama-mama" but really accepts the psychical situation of intending to chew food, thus emitting a great variety of speech sounds which remind one of a foreign language. In this way we seize upon a physiological function which, in the details of action, is completely unpremeditated and which presents a far-reaching similarity to speech. The identity of voiced chewing and speaking can be understood if we consider the fact that one can chew food and talk at the same time without any mutual interruption. Since we cannot execute simultaneously two even slightly different functions with one part of the body, chewing and eating movements, although they have been given different names, must be identical. The patient should contemplate this explanation but his chief job is to keep in mind that he is simply chewing his breath (voiced exhalation).

The obvious point of the method is the actual substitution of a completely unpremeditated or automatic movement (chewing), which, however, is not always accomplished at the first attempt. Once the patient has grasped the idea correctly, he is asked to do this so-called "nonsense chewing" twenty to thirty times a day for only a few seconds. After several sessions the exaggerated chewing movements should be reduced to more moderate chewing but always with voice and opened lips. Then the patient should progress into chewing his native language. The best way to do this is to have him chew a little nonsense and without voice interruption first chew number series, then days of the week, and then simple phrases. If he should persist in pausing between the nonsense (primitive language) chewing and the meaningful language, it is evident that he has not grasped the essence of the method, that is, the identity of loud chewing and speaking. In the beginning it is important to limit the patient to very short phrases and to strictly demand concentration on chewing. Otherwise he forgets to concentrate and lapses back into his old wrong function, thus confusing wrong and right ideas about the speech function. The next step would be to read simple texts, nothing in which content would be distracting, mingling the nonsense chewing in between phrases of the text. Later more can be done with conversation, with the ultimate aim of always keeping the idea of chewing in mind. The patient should be advised to continue to remind himself of the essence of speech

> by doing the nonsense chewing several times a day for a few seconds. He should be warned never to do it mechanically but always with the idea that he has food in his mouth and of course to think of chewing whenever he speaks. It is perfectly possible to keep chewing in mind regardless of the seriousness of the ideas we intend to express orally (pp. 45–47).

Reports by Froeschels and others who have used the chewing method to treat stuttering claim encouraging success. Typically the method is said to produce an immediate effect[14] and in most cases the length of time necessary to effect substantial improvement (even cure) is less than a few months. Despite such claims the chewing method never elicited much interest in the United States.

The rationale underlying the development and use of the chewing method is rather curious. The central idea is that speaking and chewing are identical processes. Ultimately this idea rests on Froeschels' conception that speech emanates from the function of chewing. Evidently the main support for this inference was derived from conjectures about the eating habits of primitive man. Additional "evidence" was said to be contained in the obvious fact that we use many of the same muscles in speaking as we do in eating. The latter observation, in particular, led to a rather unusual deduction; the following version of it is from Kastein (1947):

> We all know that we can chew and talk at the same time, despite the fact that the muscles involved in both functions are the same. Hence it follows that chewing and talking are identical. In other words, when we are able to chew we are able to talk (p. 197).

In contrast to the clear emphasis that proponents of the method placed on the identity of speaking and chewing, the reader was also advised that "a mere imitation of chewing" is not adequate. Repeatedly in the descriptions of the method one encounters the warning that the patient should not be permitted to just make stereotyped sounds like "nga-nga-nga" or "nam-nam-nam," and the like when he is being taught to chew his breath. Actually, however, these are precisely the kinds of sounds made by uninitiated persons when they first attempt to follow instructions to "breath chew." The fact that this is the typical performance produced by subjects making an untutored effort to breath chew provides a very persuasive contradiction of the supposed chewing-speaking equivalence, since one makes only the most rudimentary speechlike sounds when making chewing movements. There are, of course, even more convincing contradictions of this rationale, such as the fact that there are very different neurophysiologic patterns in chewing and speaking. However, the essential point is that, contrary to Froeschel's contention, one does not naturally emit "a great variety of speech sounds" when intending to chew. Yet, the production of "a great variety of speech sounds" is presented as the first major objective of the method, and here we come to the crux of the matter.

Routinely, in the descriptions of the chewing method, one finds emphasis on oral (i.e., articulatory) activity—the "chewing." Voicing and vocal modulation are not mentioned. They are not ignored or dismissed; they are simply taken for granted. In contrast to the emphasis placed on oral activity, the central and overriding importance of vocalization in the method is clearly revealed in the recurrent mention that the "breath" to be chewed is a "stream of sonorous breath," or "voiced exhalation," or "tonal expiration," and the like. The central importance of vocalization is also revealed in the frequent references to the "continuous stream" of speech that is induced.

In actuality, then, the first major objective of the chewing method is to induce the patient to produce sequences of articulatory postures *while modulating vocalization.* The second major objective is essentially to modify this nonsense articulatory patterning into the phonetic pattern of English; the vocal modulation aspect is continued. In effect, then, throughout the application of this method "the stream of sonorous breath" is the function really highlighted, though inadvertently.

If one observes carefully how a person speaks when using the chewing method,[15] he will be readily able to discern the predominance of voicing and the nature of its undulations. When a person undertakes meaningful verbalization with the method, the melody of the speech is similar to normal expression, but the excursion in stress change is reduced. Significantly, he also slows down considerably, and there is some slurring of articulation and more elision.

In concluding our discussion of the chewing method it is well worth noting that, in actual practice, the use of the method placed emphasis on its value as a demonstration that speaking can be easy. Although the patient was advised to repeat the fundamental activity (of "breath chewing") many times a day for very brief periods, this was not conceived as practice; the intent was to have the patient remind himself of "the essence of speech," which was assumed to be "the identity of loud chewing and speaking." But clearly the patient was practicing whether or not he conceived of the activity in this way.

The ventriloquism method.—This is another Froeschels approach, reported in 1950. Although his description of this method followed his account of the chewing method by almost 10 years, he implied that he had used both methods for approximately the same length of time.

The origins of the ventriloquism method are obscure. Froeschels did not describe a rationale for it, nor did he present an account of its development. He simply indicated that he used it with patients who did not cooperate well in the application of breath chewing. He spoke of the ventriloquism method as "more of an indirect approach than the chewing method" and stated a preference for the latter on grounds of his belief that it "offers to the patient the speech function as a whole."

Actually, the two methods have two very important features in common. One of these features should be quite evident in the descriptions given: both methods focus on oral activity—though with opposite emphases. Whereas the chewing method encourages intentional exaggeration of oral movements, in ventriloquism "inconspicuous articulation . . . is the core of the method." (See below.) The second and more fundamental common feature is revealed if one attends carefully to Froeschels' description of what the patient is led to do in the ventriloquism method. Again, one will find that, evidently inadvertently, the major focus is actually on vocalization and vocal modulation. The following is Froeschels' (1950) description:[16]

> The term, ventriloquism, signifies the use of a peculiar voice and of almost invisible movements of the articulating parts of the mouth, especially of the lips. Many writers have dealt with the voices of ventriloquists (3). It may seem that the term is not correctly applied to the method here discussed since no use is made of the artificial voice which ventriloquists produce. Inconspicuous articulation, another characteristic of ventriloquism (4), is the core of the method.
>
> The patient is first told that the modulation of the speaking voice is of great significance. The same word will transmit different meanings to the listener if pronounced with different modulations. The significance of the same words changes with the placing of stress upon one or another word. The modulation is called "speech melody."
>
> Next it is explained that articulation is not put upon the speech melody like sugar on the pie. Articulation is the speech melody modified by shaping the upper resonating cavities differently. The patient is asked to keep his lips soft while uttering a prolonged /a/. The therapist moves the patient's lips up and down, stretches and rounds them, thus changing the /a/ to different sounds. This experiment shows the patient that articulation only modifies the speech melody. At the same time he may acquire the knowledge of the kinship of all speech sounds and may partly lose his opinion that some sounds are harder to pronounce than others. If vocalization offers difficulties in vowels or in voiced consonants, the patient is told that voice and sighing are essentially the same function. He therefore should sigh if "the voice does not come out." "Sighing," one may add, "is prepared by nature just for states of distress. So if you are in 'speech distress,' why not sigh? And if you do so, speech is already in the making."
>
> The patient is then asked to read aloud with opened mouth, but to move neither the lips nor the tongue. He thus "sings" the speech melody. After a few minutes he should start moving lips and tongue slightly like a ventriloquist. Clo-

sure of the lips, touching the upper incisors with the lower lip, the upper incisors with the tip of the tongue, and the palate with the back of the tongue should be strictly avoided. The patient may be surprised at how understandable such ventriloquistic speech is. After a while the therapist starts a conversation, both he and the patient ventriloquizing. The stutterer is then told to use this method whenever possible, but certainly always at home. The parents, brothers, and sisters, should be trained in ventriloquism in order to remind him how to speak. For some days, he is required to read several times a day alternating "singing the speech melody" with ventriloquizing. After that time he is permitted to move lips and tongue a little more extensively, yet avoiding every closure and every narrow passage (fricatives). Still he should go back from time to time to ventriloquism, and even to the pure speech melody.

Normal articulation is reached step by step, slowly or rapidly, according to the clinical picture. The patient is taught by steps which are only slightly different from the preceding one, i.e., progressing from pure speech melody to ventriloquism or from just avoiding every closure to normal articulation. Therefore, difficulties are minimized.

Evidently Froeschels considered the ventriloquism method, as he did the chewing method, to be primarily a demonstration, a way of "proving to the patient that he is potentially capable of producing speech without difficulty." As in the several accounts of the chewing method, by Froeschels and others, there is little apparent recognition of the didactic aspects of the ventriloquism method. Although there is reference to teaching, even clear indication of progressive steps in training, one finds little consideration of what the patient might be learning. Actually, it would seem that the patient is not just making a use of a technique through which he can prove to himself that speech is not difficult, but that instead he is inadvertently being instructed in fundamental processes of speech production—particularly, the salience of vocal modulation.

Attentive reading of Froeschels' description of the ventriloquism method reveals that, contrary to his statement that minimizing of articulatory activity is the core of this method, the actual emphasis is on vocalization and vocal modulation.

Gadget and Scalpel.—This seems to be an appropriate time to mention two other circumstances reported to have at least a temporary salutary effect on stuttering: oral devices and surgery. We note these conditions simply to point out that their beneficial influence on stuttering, such as it was, most likely reflects the operation of the same agents presently being discussed.

ORAL DEVICES.—In the long history of the effort to cure stuttering one can find a recurring attempt to use some form of contrivance that has a direct effect on the peripheral speech mechanism. We can cite as the earliest reported example of such devices the pebbles Demosthenes is said to have held in his mouth while practicing speaking, circa 350 B.C.[17]

Most of the devices we know about were developed during the 19th and 20th centuries. Various types have appeared intermittently over the years, several in recent decades. The gadgets have varied considerably in complexity, from some simple object held loosely in the mouth to the very elaborate instrument constructed by Beattie and Peate (Figure 10:1). There is no need to attempt a complete catalogue of such devices, since almost all forms can be shown to have a common effect. However, it is appropriate to describe a representative sample of them for purposes of demonstrating the point of discussion.

Itard (early 1800s) made use of a device, made of ivory or gold, shaped something like a wishbone. It was fitted into the anterior part of the mandibular fossa, with one arm of the device passing under either side of the tongue and the heavier joint section resting under the tip of the tongue. Devices of similar construction were used by other authorities of this era. Figure 10:2 shows two items devised by Colombat that are variations on the same structural principle as Itard's contrivance.

Somewhat later, in the middle 1800s, Canon Kingsley advocated holding pieces of cork between the upper and lower molars while concurrently making an effort to hold the upper lip down a bit when speaking. In the late 1800s Robert Bates invented three corrective devices, two of which were to be worn in the mouth. The following description of the latter two items appeared in the *Journal of the Franklin Institute* in 1854. One device consisted of:

> A narrow, flattened tube of silver, 7/8ths of an inch in length, very light, thin and smooth. The diameter of the caliber of the tube, measured from the inner edge of one side to the inner edge of the other, is 3/8ths of an inch, while the depth, measured from the anterior inner edge to the posterior, is 1/16 of an inch. This is applied to the roof of the mouth, in the median line, in such a manner that the anterior end is lodged just behind the teeth, while the posterior opens into the mouth, looking upwards and backwards toward the fauces. In this position it is maintained by a delicate piece of wire or thin slip of India rubber fastened to one end of the tube, the other passing between the incisor teeth of the upper jaw.

The second device was described as:

> . . . a hollow, bi-convex disk, from one end of which protrudes a silver tube (which passes) out between the lips . . . The current of air from the glottis enters by means of a small hole at one side of the disk, and escapes through the silver tube.

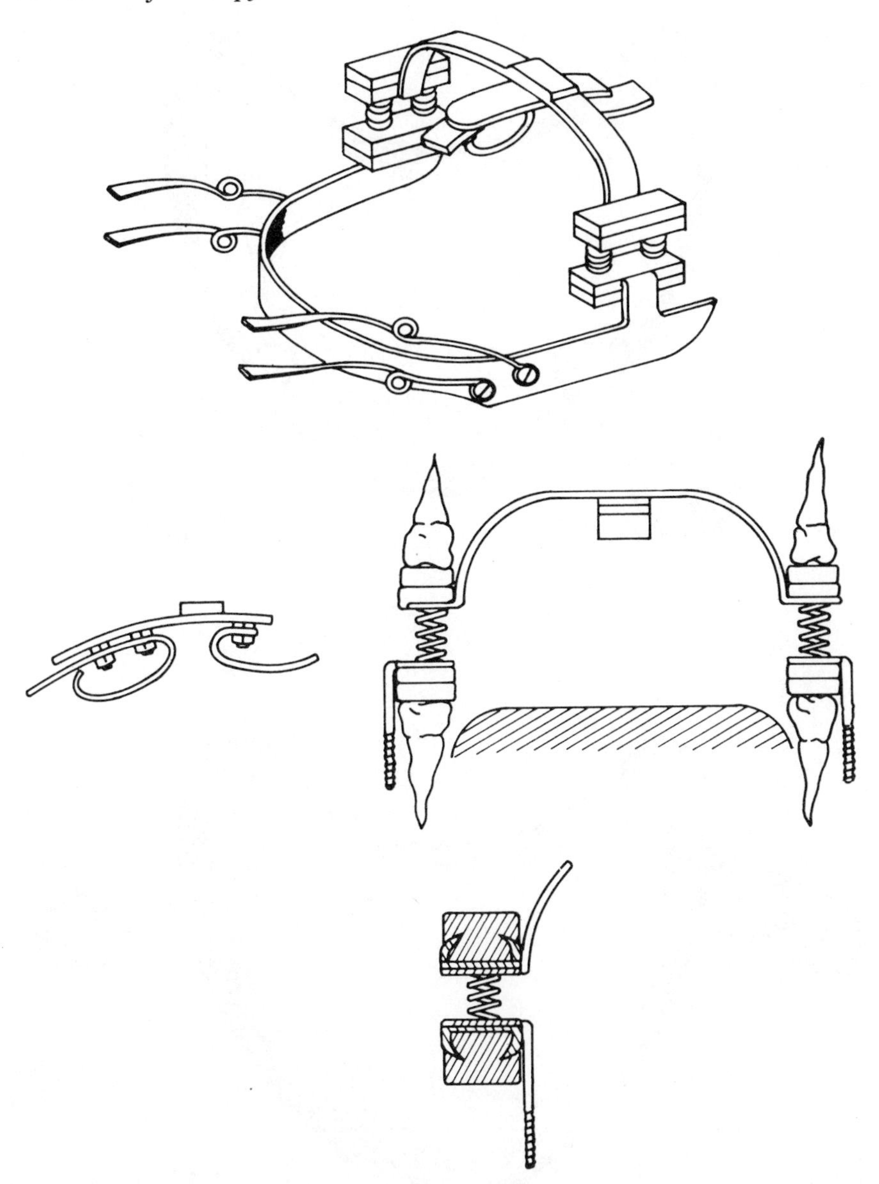

Figure 10:1 Beattie and Peate "*Device for Arresting and Curing Stuttering.*" United States Patent 1, 030, 964 issued July 2, 1912.

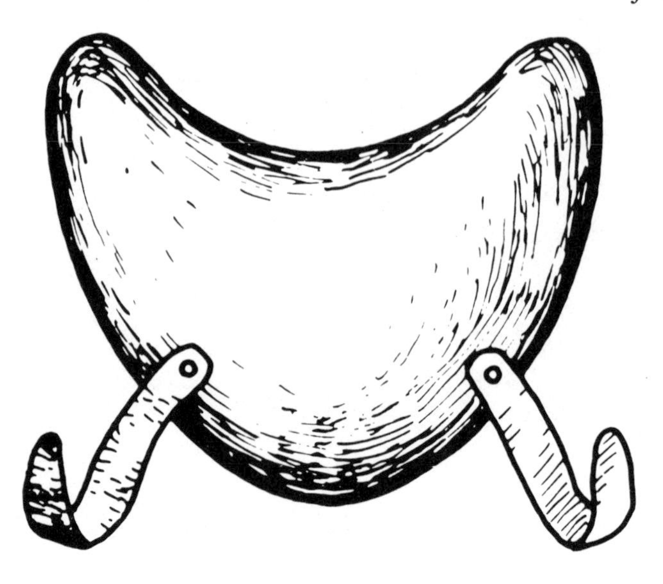

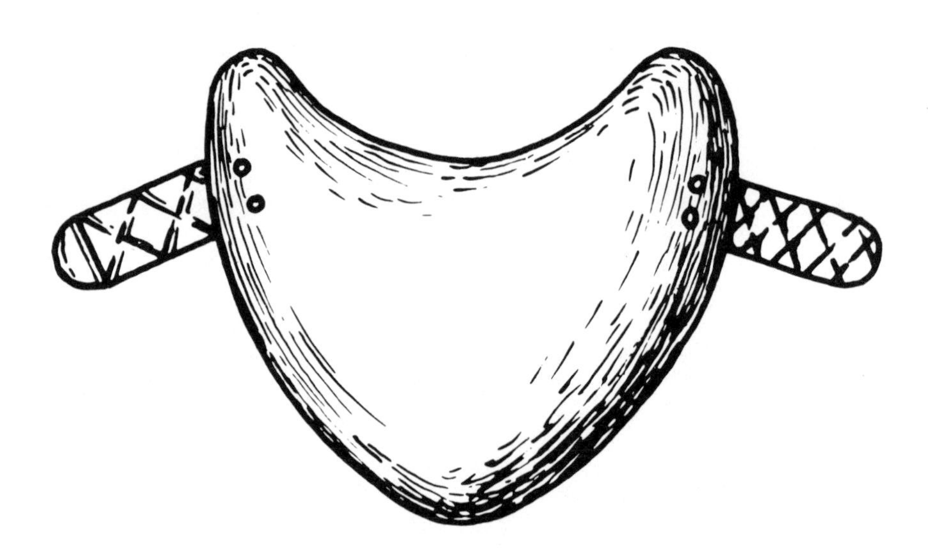

Figure 10:2 Two examples of a refoule langue. *(From Colombat, M.,* op. cit.*). The one at the top "...made of ivory, is attached to the incisors of the lower jaw by means of two little silver hooks and is placed under the tongue in order to keep the tongue held up and pushed back in the mouth." The one pictured at the bottom differs only in method of attachment; it "...is held in place by bringing together the molar teeth of the two jaws." Evidently the teeth clamped the small tabs extending from each side of the device.*

Two examples from the 20th century are the Beattie and Peate contrivance (Figure 10:1), which appeared in 1912, and the device developed by Freed (Figure 10:3), which was patented in 1957.

The latter two devices represent many that have been awarded a patent in one or another Western country. The three instruments devised by Bates also were patented, in 1851.

Of course, the issuance of a patent does not provide evidence of the efficacy of a device. Unfortunately, the recorded information about the usefulness of these instruments is very limited, and therefore we are not able to assess their effect properly. However, it seems clear that they did "work" for at least some stutters and for a period of time. Many of the individuals who developed a device were themselves stutterers (for instance: Freed, Bates, Kingsley) and it seems reasonable to assume that at least the inventor was aided by his creation. But there is also evidence that others too found some relief in their use. For example, a report on the Bates devices (Meigs, 1852) documents their successful use by persons other than the inventor, and two years later a report prepared by the Committee on Science and the Arts of the Franklin Institute (1854) announced that Bates had been awarded the Scott Legacy Prize for his "ingenious and useful invention."

Actually, we have no substantial knowledge of the course of events surrounding the usage and abandonment of oral devices. From the little available information it appears that, regardless of the immediate effect achieved with devices, their use has been typically rather short-lived. There is evidence that the effect produced while they were worn did not transfer very well to speaking without them, and this was a clear disappointment. Also, it seems most likely that people tired of having to retain the appliances in the mouth (since they are at least an inconvenience) and also that they did not look forward to wearing an appliance indefinitely.

It is safe to say that the experience with oral devices has not made much direct contribution to stuttering therapy, either in procedure or conception, largely because these techniques have received so little credence, especially in the present century. Unfortunately, no effort has been made, in any era, to investigate how these applicances might achieve the effect they evidently induce. The prevalent attitude within the profession of speech pathology has been to dismiss oral devices as being little more than a source of humor. Although their salutary effect is acknowledged, its transient character is emphasized and this is quickly explained as due to suggestion or distraction. We have already discussed (p. 187ff) the serious inadequacy of such explanations. The salutary effect of oral devices, limited as it was, cannot be dismissed so lightly.

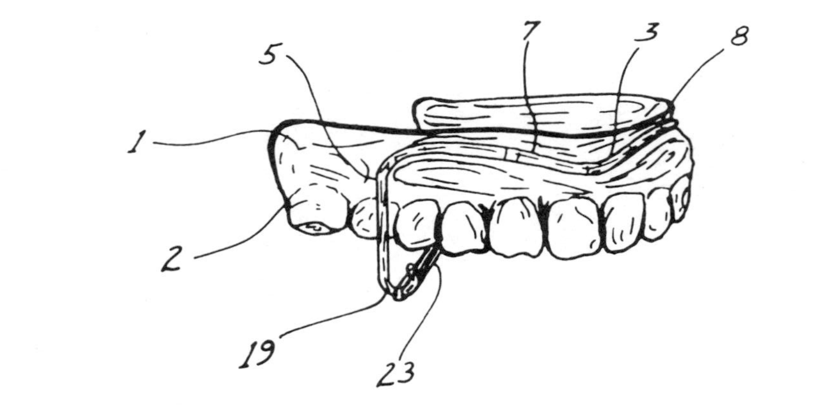

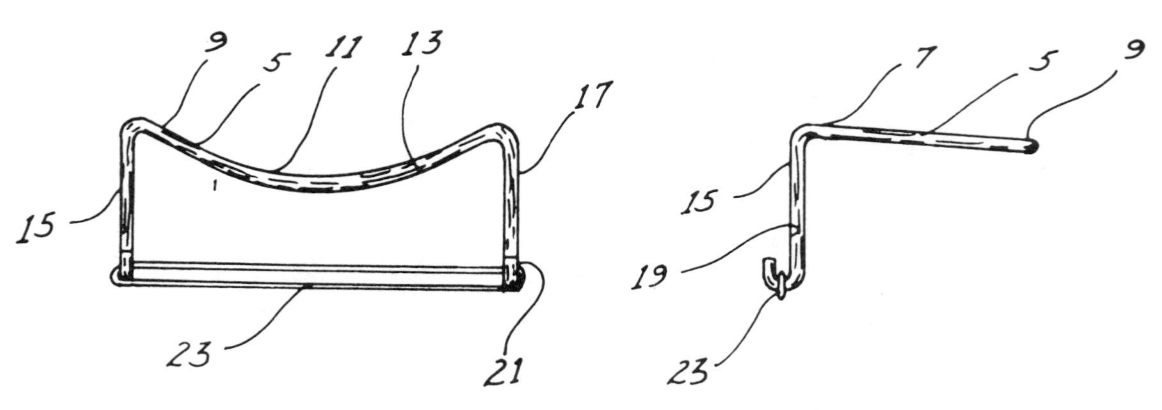

Figure 10:3 *The Freed "Anti-stammering device." United States Patent 2, 818, 065 granted December 31, 1957.*

A much more plausible explanation of the effect of the appliances is suggested in the rationales offered by some of the inventors of the instruments. To describe them briefly: the object of the Beattie and Peate apparatus was to "*minimize articulation*"; all three of the Bates appliances were devised to aid the patient in "*the maintenance of an uninterrupted current of sonorous breath*"; and Freed's device was designed "*to slow the speech movement and mechanism and require conscious effort for clear enunciation.*"[18]

Emphasis on vocalization, slowing down, minimizing articulation or articulating more carefully are features we have encountered repeatedly elsewhere in this book, particularly in Chapters 5, 8, and 9. Of special interest is the clear correspondence between these stated objectives of oral devices and the agents evidently operative in the ventriloquism method, especially the features of reduced articulation and a concurrent emphasis on vocalization.

In effect, then, it seems a reasonable inference that oral devices produce a salutary effect on stuttering by inducing what may be called "the ventriloquism effect."

SURGERY.—For several years around the middle of the 19th century surgical treatment of stuttering achieved a certain popularity. It is not certain who performed the first major surgery for stuttering, but a German surgeon named Dieffenbach is most often identified as the originator, probably because much attention was drawn to his methods. Evidently Dieffenbach was an accomplished surgeon and he was noted for his work with cleft palate. He was familiar with other kinds of speech problems and developed a particular interest in stuttering. He accepted the hypothesis, rather widely held in the 19th century, that stuttering is due to spasms of the glottis. Dieffenbach believed that these spasms also involved lingual and facial muscles.

Over some period of time Dieffenbach had encountered several patients with strabismus (crossed eyes) who also stuttered. He noticed that the extent of the strabismus in these patients waxed and waned, much like their stuttering. Evidently he interpreted this observation as corroborating his view of the cause of stuttering. It occurred to him one day that cutting into the base of the tongue might alter nervous control in the mouth and also relax the vocal folds, thereby producing a rapid cure of stuttering. He therefore developed three somewhat similar operations on the tongue; his "favorite" operation was to cut into the dorsum of the tongue and remove a sizeable section of muscle tissue.

Enthusiasm for the surgical treatment of stuttering spread rather quickly to France, England, and the United States. Surgeons in each of these countries quickly developed their own "favorite" operations, each of which had no more justification than the original one. The results achieved by surgery were said to be "immediate," and these exciting but premature claims of success were mainly responsible for the rapid spread of the method's use. However, the criteria for success were not very well thought out, and eventually it was realized that the beneficial effects of surgery were short-lived.

Some of the gory details of this sad episode are well documented by Burdin (1940). For present purposes our interest centers on two main features of this surgical treatment: (a) practically all of the surgery was done on the muscles of the tongue; (b) typically, the procedure did result in a marked reduction of stuttering; however, the improved fluency did not last very long beyond the time the patient had fully recovered from the effects of the operation.

It is not difficult to appreciate that this lingual surgery must have had the effect of markedly restricting lingual action, not so much as a direct result of the excision of the muscle tissue but indirectly because of pain and discomfort associated with tongue movement.

In view of the fact that the effect of surgery reportedly did not last much beyond the time of convalescence, it seems a reasonable deduction that, in essence, surgery-induced reduction in stuttering represented another instance of "the ventriloquism effect"—that is, the minimizing of articulatory movement and concurrent emphasis on the prosodic aspects of speech.

Accent therapy.—This treatment approach, developed in Denmark by Smith (1948, 1955) and reported to be very successful, is basically a rhythm-based therapy. However, as in other rhythm-based therapies, there is more to the system than the use of rhythm. As we have seen earlier (Chapter 7), the prominence of rhythm in a therapy approach may serve to obscure the agents or functions actually responsible for the amelioration of stuttering.

In "accent therapy" the treatment typically begins with the patient lying supine. He is assisted to attain a very relaxed condition and is then helped to become very aware of the movements of his respiration, especially the actions of exhalation. In the next stage of treatment he is instructed to "groan" on exhalation, again with his attention directed to the sensations and movements involved. Next the patient is instructed to make loose movement of the jaw and to move the articulators freely and easily while "groaning" on exhalation. This results in the production of rudimentary "nonsense syllables," in which emphasis falls naturally on the vowel-like aspects of the syllables. At this point in the therapy sequence the rhythm element is introduced into the procedure.

The rhythm is generated by the therapist beating on a type of drum that gives a deep resonating sound. The beat of this rhythm is not of a repeated, regular cadence but is varied continually. The resulting patterns have been described as resembling the pulsations of speech (Goraj, 1963) or as being "almost African in nature" (Van Riper, 1973, p. 78). Smith himself refers to these patterns as "life rhythms," a designation which suggests the fundamental significance he believes they have. Smith feels that these rhythms tap a basic action potential within the organism.

The rhythm, or "rhythms," are employed with several objectives in mind. They are intended to maintain and extend the feeling of relaxation established initially in the therapy process. Also, the patient's participation in rhythm-induced activity presumably reduces his inhibition. In fact, Smith believes the whole process has a psychotherapeutic effect. However, the principal objective of the rhythm is to serve as a focus for integrating the several motor systems involved in speech production. When rhythm is introduced into the therapy sequence, it is first related to the rudimentary speechlike performance already established. The patient "groans" his "nonsense syllables" in time to the rhythm. Thereafter, still performing in time to the rhythm, he is led to improve the quality of his articulation, gradually progressing to ordinary speaking.

Very likely the patient does feel a kind of total involvement in the whole process, which probably does support development of a positive attitude and action in speaking. However, we must not lose sight of the fact that the method centers very thoroughly on change in manner of speaking. There is a clear similarity between "moving the articulators freely and easily while groaning" and the so-called "breath chewing" in the Froeschels method described earlier. In fact, Smith acknowledges having borrowed from Froeschels. The major difference between the two methods is that accent therapy adds the dimension of rhythm, employed in a unique manner which most likely serves to further emphasize the prosodic aspects of the speech activity induced. Accent therapy appears clearly to implement the principles that have recurrently emerged in the analyses developed in this book.

Certain other European methods appear to have a good deal in common with this type of therapy approach. For instance, Stecher (1964) reported that special schools in Germany have obtained good results with programs in which the main emphasis of therapy is on relaxation and strong rhythm in speech. Van Riper (1973) mentions the use of "art song" by Fitz, also in Germany. Goraj (1963) reported that stuttering therapy in the Phoniatric Research Institute of Charles University in Prague features slow speech with normal melody pattern and emphasis on vowels. Throughout the therapy attention is directed to voicing, with the objective of producing good voice quality showing relaxation but also "life" in the voice.

The attention to voicing that seems prominent in these treatment methods may not be particularly unique to stuttering therapy. Goraj, for instance, pointed out that in Europe, where speech therapy is an offshoot of medicine, there appears to be an emphasis on voice in all treatment of speech disorders. Nonetheless, it is significant to our interests that voicing recurs so regularly in therapy methods reported to be successful.

Legato speech.—Very recently Lee *et al.* (1973) have reported the development of a therapy method which clearly appears to be based on the major principal devolved from our analyses—emphasis on vocalization and the prosodic aspects of speech.

Interestingly, this emphasis on voicing derived from a conception of speech expression developed from an engineering viewpoint (Lee, 1950). In this conception oral verbal expression is represented as a system of interrelated feedback loops (Figure 10:4) whose common junction marks phoneme, syllable, and word boundaries. Each loop has a primary source of feedback input; for example, predominantly auditory in the voice (syllable) loop, primarily kinesthetic and tactual in the phoneme loop. Within each loop neural signals, operating in reference to feedback information, actuate and regulate that part of the system under its direct influence. The voice and phoneme loops are those most intimately involved in the actual production of the audible speech signal. The voice loop provides the dominant aspect of the speech signal (i.e., speech as produced), though voice and phoneme loops must function coordinatively for speech to result.

In Lee's view of stuttering, excessive effort developed for articulation operates to prevent vocal onset. This tension, which is sometimes further increased by emotion, interferes with delicate laryngeal adjustments and their intricate coordination with the articulation systems, all of which are necessary for fluent speech. Control of vocalization is thus identified as the basic function in fluent speech and is therefore the principal focus of treatment for developing fluency.

The major technique in this approach is to teach the stutterer to speak in a manner called *legato style.* The term *legato,* adopted from the field of music, means "smooth, flowing and connected."[19] Lee *et al.* (1973) described legato style speech as:

> . . . a natural way of speaking used by many persons, such as radio announcers, and individuals who must respond with poise to extemporaneous questions. It is characterized by a brief starting of the voice before a word and maintainence of the voice throughout long connected phrases. The voice: that is, the audible or

energy carrying portions of speech, shaped by the articulatory members, waxes and wanes between words and phrases for emphasis and expression, but may not cease altogether for rather lengthy intervals for up to as much as 10 seconds.

At the beginning of training in this method the "starting of the voice before a word" is intentionally exaggerated in length. Then, as the technique is learned, the student is gradually taught to minimize the duration of the initial voicing until it is almost nonexistent. Speaking slowly and deliberately are also emphasized in this initial stage of training, providing support to the major objective of speaking in legato style.

The legato speech method makes use of recordings in a manner similar to that employed in teaching a second language. Specially prepared lessons are recorded by a voice, described as a natural legato,

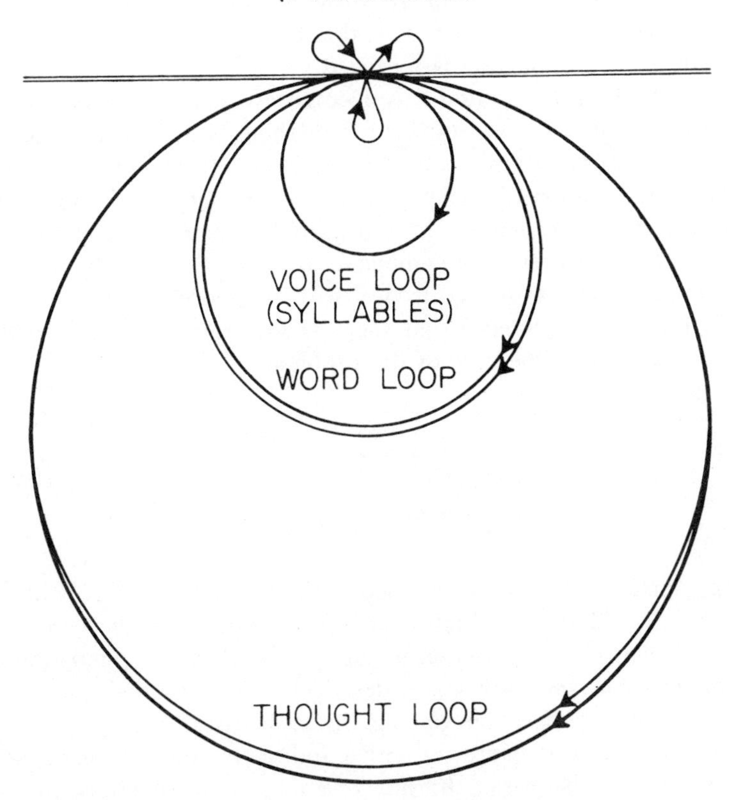

Figure 10:4 Graphic representation of speech conceived as a system of interrelated feedback loops (From Lee, 1950.)

which provides a model for the patient to emulate in carrying out the assignments and practicing the exercises presented.

After the initial training, the patient can make use of the tape-recorded lessons and exercises independently. He is to practice at home daily, responding to recordings of the model voice for half an hour, then listening to his own recordings. It is expected that, as the patient progresses through graduated assignments, comparing his performance with the recorded voice, he will acquire skill in a new mode of speaking modeled on the lines of legato form—a new mode that places emphasis on vocal modulation.

The use of "initial vocalization" or "a starting sound" has been the focus for criticism of this method, the complaint being that this is simply a modern version of an old "trick," such as the use of an initial /i/ sound advocated over a century ago by Neil Arnott (cf. Klingbeil, 1939). However, rather than dismiss the use of initial vocalization as a trick, it would seem more appropriate to seriously consider how it functions to support fluency. The analyses developed in this book indicates that fluency is enhanced because phonation is focalized.

In concluding this section it is necessary to point out a very significant feature about the effect of therapy methods that focus on fluency. These methods have a direct and decisive effect on the entire stuttering: not only is the stutterer aided to speak fluently but, in addition, whatever accessory features might have occurred as part of the individual's overall stuttering pattern are eliminated as well. Thus, with the use of these methods there is no need to deal with accessory features. This fact alone is impressive evidence that there is something common to these methods that gets to the core of the problem.

INTEGRATION

This chapter has been concerned with an analysis of forms of stuttering therapy. Many seemingly different therapy methods were found to have, at their core, a common feature: an emphasis on phonation and vocal modulation. In a few cases description of a method and its use reveals a direct emphasis on voicing. In most cases, however, the emphasis on phonation is expressed either indirectly, through such means as slowing down, the use of rhythm, or attention to vowels; or inadvertently, through techniques such as "breath chewing," or the use of appliances.

The principle derived in the present chapter is the same one that has recurred consistently in earlier analyses of other therapy methods (Chapters 5, 6, 7) as well as in the analysis of conditions that have a salutary influence on stuttering (Chapter 8).

The fact that we can repeatedly find substantial indication that amelioration of stuttering is linked to induced emphasis on vocalization is compelling evidence for the validity of vocal modulation as a fundamental therapeutic principle. This conclusion receives additional complementary support from the analysis, developed in Chapter 9, that stuttering is most appropriately conceived as a disturbance in control of vocalization. Again it should be noted that various lines of evidence converge on the same focus.

We will return to this topic again in Chapter 12, where we will consider implementation of the vocal modulation principle within an overall management approach.

Notes

1. We have already dealt with the contradictions and unrealities inherent in this view (pp. 64–66).
2. Neither does "play therapy," no matter how intricately it is rationalized. Play therapy may have some value in certain isolated cases of stuttering in children but it is by no means routinely justifiable. Also, there is good reason to suspect that those successes claimed to result from play therapy might well represent children who would have recovered without any kind of treatment.
3. The specific objective—no stuttering—is usually identified. However, it need not be. For instance, use of one of the fluency-inducing procedures, such as rhythm, need not reveal the objective. This might be an important consideration in certain plans for management.
4. That is, therapies that deal directly with stuttering, as contrasted to "purely" psychotherapeutic efforts.
5. Variants of this approach are represented in the methods of Van Riper, Bryngelson, West, Eisenson, Johnson, Bloodstein, Starbuck, Sheehan, and others. The description given by the authors of some of these approaches is heavily overlaid with abstracted explanations of one kind or another, but the common element of the actual speech therapy is very much the same throughout.
6. Cf. in particular, Wingate (1966a, 1966b). Also, this counsel may have an unfortunate bearing on the patient's eventual adjustment to his problem and his ability to deal with it.

7. Regardless of the interpretations that might be offered regarding the significance of this pause, it seems evident that the individual has at least the opportunity, if not the requirement, to immediately retrospect and reflect on what he has just done.

8. One is reminded here of the "dry run" technique passed on by word of mouth on a Portland, Oregon, street corner. Cf. pp. 118–119.

9. Distinguished from "respondent" behavior. Simply put, a "respondent" is elicited by an identified stimulus; an "operant" is said to be "emitted," i.e., there is no readily identifiable eliciting stimulus and, moreover, there is no need to be concerned about its possible existence.

10. Actually, the essential method has been used for years by animal trainers in circuses and other trained-animal shows.

11. In fact, contingency was the immediate procedural objective of an alerting device the present author developed some years ago (1967) as a therapy aid. The objective of the device was to help stutterers isolate and analyze instances of stuttering in "natural" circumstances, such as during ordinary conversation. See further description in Chapter 12, page 345.

12. Considerations such as these underscore the importance of an appropriate definition of stuttering.

13. Reprinted by permission from E. F. Hahn, (ed.), *Stuttering: Sigificant Theories and Therapies.* Stanford: Stanford University Press, 1956.

14. In my own experience, a very credible claim.

15. Once again we encounter the error made in the interpretations offered for so many other conditions found to have a salutary effect on stuttering: the failure to carefully observe and describe the nature of the patient's manner of speaking under the condition. Cf. Chapter 8.

16. Reprinted by permission from the *Journal of Speech and Hearing Disorders*, **15**, 1950.

17. We have no idea how frequently this simple remedy has subsequently been attempted, nor with what success. I have known of two stutterers who reported the successful use of such objects held in the mouth. One of them knew the Demosthenes story, the other did not but had tried the technique at the suggestion of a friend. The latter case, a mechanic, had used three ball bearings because of their weight, saying that he was less likely to swallow them than similar objects of lighter weight, such as marbles. He had used the ball bearings successfully for close to three years and would have been willing to continue to use them except that they were eroding the lingual surface of his mandibular incisors and canines.

The likelihood of swallowing an oral device is a concern mentioned by several inventors of oral appliances and this was considered in their design of the device.

18. Italics mine.

19. Refer to earlier discussion, p. 195.

References

Andrews, G. Token reinforcement systems. *Australian and New Zealand J. Psychiatry*, **5**, 135–136, 1971.

———and R. J. Ingham. Stuttering: Considerations in the evaluation of treatment. *British J. Dis. Commun.*, **6**, 129–138, 1971.

Burdin, G. The surgical treatment of stammering, 1840–1842. *J. Speech Dis.*, **5**, 43–64, 1940.

Colombat de l'Isere, *Traite de tous les vices de la parole et en particulier du Begaiement*, Bechet et Labe, Paris, 1840.

Committee on Science and the Arts, Report on Robert Bates' Instruments for the Cure of Stammering. *Journal of the Franklin Institute of the State of Pennsylavania*, 5–8, 1854.

Cooper, E. B., B. B. Cady, and C. J. Robbins. The effect of the verbal stimulus words *wrong*, *right*, and *tree* on the disfluency rates of stutterers and nonstutterers. *J. Speech Hearing Res.*, **13**, 239–244, 1970.

Curlee, R. F. and W. H. Perkins. Conversational rate control therapy for stuttering. *J. Speech Hearing Dis.*, **34**, 245–250, 1969.

Froeschels, E. A technique for stutterers—"Ventriloquism." *J. Speech Hearing Dis.*, **15**, 336–337, 1950.

———In Hahn, E. F. (Ed.), *Stuttering: Significant Theories and Therapies* (2nd Ed.), Stanford Univ. Press, Stanford, 1956, pp. 41–47.

———Pathology and therapy of stuttering. *Nerv. Child*, **2**, 148–161, 1943.

———and Auguste Jellinek. *Practice of Voice and Speech Therapy*, Expression, Boston, 1941.

Goldiamond, I. Stuttering and fluency as manipulable operant response classes. In Kranser, L. and L. P. Ullmann (Eds.), *Research in Behavior Modofication*, Holt, Rinehart and Winston, New York, 1965.

Goraj, J. T. A report on three European speech facilities, ASHA, **5**, 860–864, 1963.

Kastein, Shulamith. The chewing method of treating stuttering. *J. Speech Dis.*, **12**, 195–198, 1947.

Klingbeil, G. M. The historical background of the modern speech clinic. *J. Speech Dis.*, **4**, 115–132, 1939.

Lebrun, Yvan and Madeline Bayle. Surgery in the treatment of stuttering. In Lebrun and Hoops (Eds.), *Neurolinguistic Approaches to Stuttering*, Mouton, The Hague, 1973.

Lee, B. S. Effects of delayed speech feedback. *J. Acoust. Soc. Amer.*, **22**, 824–826, 1950.

———W. E. McGough, and Maryann Peins. A new method for stutter therapy. *Folia Phoniat.*, **25**, 186–195, 1973.

Martin, R. R., Patricia Kuhl, and S. Haroldson. An experimental treatment with two preschool stuttering children. *J. Speech Hearing Dis.*, **15**, 743–752, 1972.

Meigs, J. A. Clinical report on Robert Bates's cure for stammering. *Clinic of Jefferson Medical College*. Surgeon General's Office Library, Feb. 21, 1852.

Mohr, Erika. Chewing therapy in stuttering. In Weiss, D. A. and H. H. Beebe, *The Chewing Approach in Speech and Voice Therapy*, S. Karger, Basel–New York, pp. 28–30, 1951.

Mowrer, D. E. *Technical Research Report S-1: Reduction of Stuttering Behavior.* Arizona State University Bookstore, Tempe, 1972.

Ryan, B. P. Operant procedures applied to stuttering therapy for children. *J. Speech Hearing Dis.*, **36**, 264–280, 1971.

———The construction and evaluation of a program for modifying stuttering. Ph.D. dissertation, University of Pittsburgh, 1964.

Shames, G. Operant conditioning and stuttering. In *Conditioning in Stuttering Therapy*, Publication 7 of the Speech Foundation of America, Memphis, 1968.

———D. H. Egolf, and R. C. Rhodes. Experimental programs in stuttering therapy. *J. Speech Hearing Dis.*, **34**, 30–47, 1969.

Siegel, G. M. Punishment, stuttering and disfluency. *J. Speech Hearing Res.*, **13**, 677–714, 1970.

Smith, S. The pedagogic treatment of stuttering. In *Nordisk Larebog for Talepedagoger*, Rosenkilde og Baggers Forlag, Copenhagen, 1955.

———The treatment of stuttering: therapeutic exercises. *Report of the Conference on Speech Therapy*, Tavistock, London, 1948.

Stecher, Sylvia. Speech therapy techniques in Germany. ASHA, **6**, 157–159, 1964.

Van Riper, C. *The Treatment of Stuttering*, Prentice-Hall, Englewood Cliffs, 1973.

Wingate, M. E. Alerting device for stuttering therapy. ASHA, **9**, 375, 1967 (abstr.).

———Calling attention to stuttering. *J. Speech Hearing Res.*, **2**, 326–335, 1959.

———Stuttering adaptation and learning: I. The relevance of adaptation studies to stuttering as "learned behavior." *J. Speech Hearing Dis.*, **31**, 148–156, 1966.

———Stuttering adaptation and learning: II. The adequacy of learning principles in the interpretation of stuttering. *J. Speech Hearing Dis.*, **31**, 211–218, 1966.

IV

MANAGEMENT

11

ASSESSMENT OF STUTTERING

An adequate assessment of stuttering has several interrelated objectives. The fundamental and primary task is the correct identification of the speech problem; the considerations necessary to this task were covered in Chapter 4. A second objective is to obtain a larger picture of the individual who comes, or is brought, for an evaluation. A closely related third objective is to obtain information relevant to purposes of counseling—of the stutterer, and parents, and others who may deal extensively with the stutterer (such as teachers). It should be made clear that "counseling" is intended here in the broad sense: it includes the activities of giving information and advice as well as making the effort to deal with feelings and attitudes.

At the end of this chapter is an *Evaluation Form* designed as a guide for recording comprehensive data about any individual who stutters. It can be used in direct interview with older stutterers and in direct examination with supporting parental interview in the case of children. The format provides a means for organizing information from past and present relevant to the objectives cited above. Most of the inquiry concerns the first three objectives, directing attention to potentially significant aspects of the case which might have a bearing on management.

Part I of the *Evaluation Form* seeks background information, a relatively standard part of the identifying data for any case record. Information on such matters as family structure may sometimes be of orienting value in respect to counseling; most often, of course, in cases involving a child. The material contained in the remaining sections has been arranged in a manner found to be conducive to a smooth flow of topics in the interview. Some of these data may be omitted as circumstances indicate; for instance, the material on birth conditions and on early speech and language development in the case of an adult stutterer, who is not likely to have such information available.

Part II of the *Evaluation Form* represents the essential core of the appraisal, in that it explores the major outlines of the stuttering problem and certain relatively immediate related circumstances. Part III deals with various aspects of the history of the problem, areas that always have some bearing on therapy and counseling. Part IV is directed to important qualifying information that is particularly relevant to management.

CONDUCTING THE APPRAISAL

The examiner's initial objectve is to elicit a substantial amount of spontaneous speech in order to provide an adequate sample of the stuttering for purposes of observational description of its nature and severity. It is a good idea to obtain this sample from conversation in which the patient is likely to be relatively at ease. This can be done by orienting the initial content of the interview to some appropriate topic other than the speech problem; for example, following up the identifying information with questions regarding occupation, interests, avocational activities; or, in the case of a child, family, school, and play activities. Later, the examiner should confirm whether the sample of stuttering observed is representative of the individual's typical performance in respect to both frequency and extent of the stuttering. In the case of adult and teenage stutterers this can be done by direct inquiry; with children the query should be directed to the accompanying parent. In the case of older children (ordinarily, approximately age 8 or older) one might ask both child and parent. Answers given by the stutterer himself, whether adult or child, need not be taken completely at face value in respect to accuracy, but the replies are of significance in the total scope of the appraisal.

Description of Present Stuttering

The examiner's description.—The *Evaluation Form* contains space for recording a description of the patient's stuttering, which should include notation of the type of speech symptom (repetition or prolongation and which is the more prominent), the frequency of occurrence, the amount of effort, and the nature and extent of accessory features. A rating of severity should also be included. The examiner will find it helpful to utilize the scheme presented in the *Severity Rating Guide*, which follows the *Evaluation Form* at the end of this chapter.

The first column of the *Guide* calls for an overall judgment of severity. The remaining columns are self-explanatory and contain reference to the several dimensions that usually comprise a single judgment of severity. Column 1 is intended for purposes of recording one's subjective judgment and this rating can be made independently of the other three.

For any one individual, ratings in the Frequency, Effort, and Accessory Features columns often vary. It is as important to identify and record this pattern as it is to make an overall judgment of severity. It is instructive to identify, over a period of time, the patterns of ratings in the last three columns that coincide with the subjective judgments of severity level. One will find that different patterns coincide with the same overall severity level judgment, but also that certain aspects of the patterns are less important than others.

One will find that frequency alone is seldom the principal criterion of overall severity. In fact, judgments of severity depend much more on the amount of difficulty the individual is perceived to have with instances of stutter. Columns 3 and 4 in the *Guide* deal with the dimension of difficulty. The contents of these two columns are closely related, inasmuch as accessory features are evidently often elaborated signs of effort. Yet evidence of effort is not routinely expressed in accessory features; indication of effort may well be limited to actions involving only the musculature of the speech apparatus. Although the more dramatic type of accessory feature, such as a head jerk, quickly prompts a judgment of "severe," the fundamental criterion of severity is the amount of apparent effort involved, and often considerable effort is apparent without the occurrence of an accessory.

The frequency ratings are expressed in ratio form, which is easier to manage than the percentage mode used in some rating scales.[1] The assessment of frequency is intended as a *rating*, not an actual count. It is literally impossible to keep a record of the number of words spoken as well as the number of words stuttered, with the intent of making a percentage estimate, while at the same time attempting to attend and respond appropriately to the content of what the person is saying. As indicated earlier, the speech evaluation should be made of spontaneous conversation; the ratio form provides a simpler and more efficient reference frame for in vivo assessment. Even the ratio form is not likely to be very accurate for the "Very Mild" to "Mild" levels. However, this is not a particularly serious problem. Also, the examiner can always arrange for a concrete count (and check his rating skill as well) by recording the interview.

It sometimes happens, particularly in the case of young children, that no stuttering is evidenced during the examination. This occurrence has sometimes led an examiner to conclude erroneously that the child does not in fact stutter. Actually, such events usually reflect the variability in stuttering occurrence that is reported for many stutterers. In such instances the parent will invariably remark that the child did not stutter on this occasion.[2] Careful inquiry should be made of the parent as to what they have observed in their child's speech that they call stuttering. Most often they speak of it in the terms of common parlance, referring to repeating, hesitating, blocking, getting stopped, getting stuck, "can't get the words out," and the like. If they use only the first two terms, care should be taken to identify explicitly the character of the "repetitions" and the "hesitations."

In some cases the parent is not able to give a satisfactory description of the speech features that concern them. This problem can be handled readily by asking the parent to imitate what the child does when he is stuttering. Usually this is sufficient to resolve the issue. In those rare cases where even this approach is not productive the examiner should provide examples of different kinds of disfluencies, imitating several instances of unitary repetitions and prolongations and also some normal nonfluencies. He can then ask the parent to identify which of these disfluency types is characteristic of the child's fluency irregularity. Occasionally this may serve as the point of departure for edifying parents in the matter of distinguishing normal and abnormal disfluency. Should the examiner be convinced that the parent is actually concerned about normal nonfluencies, he can then counsel the parent directly regarding appropriate measures for dealing with them. However, one should always be judicious about both the judgment and counsel given in situations like this, and the parents should be afforded the opportunity to return for further appraisal if they continue to remain concerned.

Most often it will be found that when parents use the term "stuttering" they mean the kind of disfluencies which the speech therapist also recognizes by this name. This observation, found repeatedly in the clinical setting, is strongly corroborated by the results of much formal research, as reviewed in Chapter 4.

The patient's description.—The *Evaluation Form* also provides space for recording the patient's own description of his stuttering, and an attempt should be made to obtain such description from anyone who is old enough to know why he comes to the clinic. An examiner should make it clear that he is attempting to elicit as comprehensive a statement as possible regarding the patient's awareness of what is happening and what he is doing when he stutters.

With stutterers who are self-referred the reason for their presence in the examination is obvious and the examiner can readily broach an open discussion of stuttering. The reason for the appointment may be equally obvious in many cases of children who are brought to the clinic by a parent. However, in such instances it is advisable to obtain from the patient his own statement as to why he is there. This is best done after an initial period of casual conversation, which usually permits an easy entry into discussion of the problem. Usually, valuable qualitative information is obtained in this procedure. For example, many youngsters are quite straightforward about talking about their stuttering and this tells something very important about the child, his general attitude, and his reaction to his stuttering. Other children may seem to be evasive, or feign ignorance, or register irritation about the examination, or acknowledge the problem but be simply indifferent to the whole matter.

One need not have any serious reservations about use of the word "stuttering" in these discussions. Despite the still widely held belief that use of this "label" has some sort of magical effect in producing, or at least exacerbating, stuttering, the relevant research (cf. Chapter 4) contradicts this notion. Realistically, it seems evident that use of the term is rather immaterial. With young children who do not use, or perhaps actually do not know, the term, one can speak in a simple descriptive manner. The essential point here is that if an individual knows he is being seen in regard to a speech problem, there is little reason to be evasive or guarded about it. In fact, doing so may convey an unwarranted air of mystery or carry the implication that there is something unspeakable about the problem. Further, one of the objectives of the appraisal is to attempt to determine the extent to which the patient is aware of the problem.

It is surprising how frequently the stutterer can give only a vague or general descriptive statement about his stuttering. This is true of older stutterers as well as children. Often he will simply say that he "gets stuck," or that he cannot say the word, or that the word "won't come out." Sometimes he will mention that he repeats, or "blocks," or forces the word out, but unless he has had therapy in the relatively recent past, he will rarely give any specific description of his actions or sensations while stuttering. At times, more careful, probing questions will reveal that the stutterer has more awareness of his stuttering than might appear from his initial statement, but it is not often that a stutterer's description will match what the careful examiner is able to observe.

As might be expected, children in the early grades are less able than older children and adults to describe or imitate their stuttering. At the same time they reveal some knowledge of their stuttering by being able to identify instances of it denotatively. That is, a child who is not able to describe his speech anomaly on request will "point to" it by saying "Like that" in reference to a stutter he has just experienced. This capability can also be found in even younger children. Generally speaking, however, it is not productive to probe for such information with youngsters of kindergarten age or younger.

Variability and relativity.—In many individuals stuttering occurs with some amount of variability, which may be related to personal matters, external influences, or unknown circumstances. It is advisable first to attempt to elicit a spontaneous statement from the patient, or his parents, regarding the matter of variability. To the extent that this initial statement does not yield information relative to the subheadings in this part of the outline, specific questioning can then be directed to these areas.

Inquiry should be made regarding whether the stuttering shows fairly regular fluctuations over certain intervals of time. Stutterers vary a good deal in this respect: some cannot report any periods of this kind at all; others report "good" and "bad" periods which may last for weeks or months; and others show variations covering spans of a few days. A periodicity may sometimes be found to be related to environmental or situational factors of which the individual or the family may not be aware. However, in many instances the periodicity has no definable relationship to external events, or to the individual's psychological state, even in cases where the stutterer, or his parents, have made it a point to watch for some. Although we do not as yet have any adequate means for assessing it, there exists a reasonable suspicion that some kinds of periodicity may have a physiological basis related to individual organismic rhythms.

There are a number of circumstances for which many stutterers report similar variations in stuttering. For instance, it is common to find reports of less stuttering when relaxed, speaking with spouse or close friends[3], and so forth; and increased stuttering when speaking to an authority figure, or in a group of persons largely unknown to them, and so on. Such reactions most likely reflect a simple stress reaction. On the other hand, the influence of certain circumstances may be unique to the individual. Some such effects seem to be of a "conditioned" character; others may be more dynamic in nature, having a personal emotional significance to the individual.

It is important that the examiner be circumspect in his inquiry in this area, being careful to avoid suggesting ideas or otherwise contributing bias. It is best to begin by asking for an overall description and, for whatever probing is necessary, to phrase queries in a general way and avoid leading questions.

The stutterer should be asked for his own explanation of the variation he reports, and his statement should be taken into account in the overall analysis of the reported variability. Sometimes his explanation will be consistent with that deduced by the examiner, but at times it will be at variance. The credibility of the explanation should be weighed judiciously. It is the professional obligation of the examiner to avoid bias and to be scrupulously objective in assessing the significance and import of the variability reported. Generally speaking, it is most sensible to favor the simplest explanation.

Inquiry should be made regarding circumstances in which the stuttering is worse and when it is better, in the event that this information has not been revealed in the spontaneous statement. These points are essentially refinements of the matter of situational relativity. One should also inquire about whether stuttering is ever completely absent and under what circumstances. Although many stutterers do report clearly fluent periods, it is rather illuminating, especially in reference to assertions made in the literature, to find how many stutterers do not claim that they are at some times completely fluent.

Inquiry regarding the incidence of stuttering in such special circumstances as speaking alone, on the telephone, reading aloud, etc., was originally included as a kind of casual research questionnaire item. However, it has been found to have value from a counseling standpoint on several dimensions, particularly with older stutterers. For instance, as we have seen earlier (p. 25) the claim of no stuttering when speaking alone is very likely to be unrealistic. The extent to which any particular stutterer contends this for himself should be compared to his awareness of the stuttering he evidences in the presence of the examiner. This provides an assessment of his reliability in self-observation of stuttering. It will be found that many stutterers are not as alert to instances of their stuttering, even in conversation, as they are routinely believed to be.

There are other ways in which information in this category has counseling value. For example, many stutterers seem to be mollified, or feel a spirit of community with other stutterers, to learn that many others report less stuttering when alone, or that they do not stutter when singing, etc. Somewhat differently, for many stutterers a feeling of uniqueness is reduced by the discovery that normal speakers also report that they are less comfortable speaking on the telephone than speaking face-to-face. Also, in respect to speaking on the telephone, or speaking to groups, or some other category in this section, the examiner may learn something of specific value regarding the particular individual's personal reactions to, and interpretations of, the effects of such circumstances on himself and his stutter.

A last item to consider in this general area is the matter of stuttering relative to particular sounds or words. Again, stutterers show a considerable variability on this dimension. Some stutterers will indicate that they "can stutter on anything"; others may identify particular sounds, and sometimes special words, that are troublesome for them. Whenever special sounds or words are mentioned, the examiner should make note of these with the intention of verifying the report in his observation of the patient's speech. That is, the examiner should be alert to record whether the individual's stutterings do involve, disproportionately, the sounds or words claimed.[4] In most instances it will be found that the individual is only partly correct; i.e., stutterings do not involve the sounds he mentioned as frequently as claimed. In cases where the stutterer's contention is not borne out by observation, the discrepancy can serve as a point of direct counseling that usually leads to at least some change in the stutterer's perception of his problem. If it is found that he does tend to have trouble "with" certain sounds it may be appropriate to undertake an analysis of his points of difficulty, which may then lead to intensive work on the motor patterns involved in these particular sound sequences.

Techniques of control.—An examiner should inquire whether there are any means whereby the stutterer can reduce the extent, or minimize the severity, of his stuttering. While this inquiry is generally most appropriate in respect to older children and adults, one can nevertheless gain similar information from parents in cases of younger children. The examiner should be interested in learning about anything that has been found to be helpful in mitigating the stuttering, whether this be related directly or indirectly to some previous therapy, the result of lay suggestions, or some adventitious discovery. The value of any such technique should be carefully appraised by the clinician. In view of the essentially pragmatic base for stuttering therapy, it is reasonable to adopt the position that any technique having a demonstrated benefit on stuttering, and no untoward effect on the person, deserves consideration in the overall management picture. Many of such techniques will be found to reflect the principles illuminated in this book. As might be expected, "slowing down" is one technique reported frequently.

Relevant History

History of the stuttering.—One is interested in the age of stuttering onset for research purposes and the contribution this eventually will make to improved understanding of the problem. However, information regarding age of onset also has considerable practical value. One is particularly interested in the nature of stuttering at the time of onset, in possibly relevant circumstances which obtained at the time, and in the subsequent course of the disorder and potential influences on it.

There has been a good deal of quibbling and confusion generated about this matter of onset of stuttering. Essentially, the problem created here was propagated by the "evaluational" viewpoint of stuttering, which contended that at the time of "original diagnosis" of stuttering (by a parent) the nonfluency observed was actually normal in character. The justification for this claim was based on the finding that in many cases parents cannot readily designate a specific date of stuttering onset. However, if this finding is viewed realistically, it simply means that, in general, parents are not particularly attentive to the early instances of stuttering symptoms and do not become attentive to them until they are quite persistent or recurrent.

Actually, this is clearly indicated in Johnson's (1959) own work on stuttering onset. (Cf. discussion of this matter in Chapter 5.) Many of the parents participating in that study identified stuttering in their child several months before they considered it a problem. This is a rather common finding in actual practice. Frequently parents will indicate that although the stuttering was quite obvious to them for some time, they expected that it would eventually subside. In fact, in a number of such cases a parent will report having been led to make this assumption because an older sibling of the child in question had stuttered for a period of time but had subsequently "outgrown it."

In some cases parents will report a fairly definite time of onset, often associated with certain external events or circumstances. While the examiner must be attentive to such testimony, he should also be very circumspect in his appraisal of it. It has been my experience that accounts of this kind are generally quite suspect. Many parents, in their search for an explanation, are unwittingly inclined to search for something dramatic. Unfortunately, the appeal of the dramatic also influences the speech pathologist, who is not only likely to encourage such interpretation by the parent, but also subsequently passes it on to his colleagues.

Particularly since material of this kind may substantially influence treatment plan and counseling, one should be very guarded about accepting such information at face value. Careful inquiry will many times reveal that there is actually considerable temporal dislocation between the apparent onset of stuttering and the event supposedly responsible for it as given in the initial parental report. In some cases certain events might possibly have been related to an exacerbation of the stuttering, yet careful questioning indicates that identifiable stuttering was present previously.

In clarifying time of onset a very valuable procedure for the temporal ordering of events is to help the informant organize his recollection by relating events to historical "highpoints" such as holidays, birthdays, vacations, school entrance, change of residence, and so forth. Such procedure often reveals, to the informant as well as the clinician, that the sequence of events reported for stuttering onset is at least not very clear—and therefore not likely to be valid.

The examiner should be particularly interested in changes in nature and frequency of the stuttering that have occurred since its time of reported onset. As we have seen in Chapter 5 the course of stuttering, contrary to prevalent belief, is not invariably one of progression. Over the long term there is more frequently a general picture of stability, if not mitigation, of the symptoms.

In the case of children one will most often find report of either periodic fluctuation in the stuttering, no substantial change over fairly extended periods, or evidence of gradual improvement. Exacerbation in frequency or character of the stuttering is reported much less frequently. When periodicity in occurrence of stuttering or variability in extent or severity are reported, one should take care to identify possible related circumstances. Not infrequently, one will obtain report of increase in stuttering associated with events containing a subtle yet pervasive atmosphere of general pressure or excitement. The most common of these is an increase of stuttering at the beginning of the school year compared to a relative absence during the summer vacation period. Also, special holiday periods will tend to have an associated increase in stuttering.

In respect to the finding of periodicity, a most favorable prognostic pattern I have found is one in which the stuttering is reported to be episodic, relatively uninfluenced by associated circumstances, and with evidence of increasing length of the periods between recurrence of the stuttering. However, we do not as yet have any reliable prognostic indices.[5]

The overall situation is not too much different among older stutterers. A few may report exacerbation or a change in the nature of the symptoms over a period of time, and others will tell of periodic variations in occurrence of their stuttering. However, most older stutterers can report no substantial change in their stuttering over long periods of time, and some will report a gradual improvement. Again, whenever there is report of change, an effort should be made to identify possible related external circumstances or changes in the stutterer's personal life or adjustments. The examiner should also attempt to elicit the stutterer's own explanation for such changes, even though he need not accept this account literally.

Language development.—This information is most likely to be of significance in respect to children. Evidence of delay in language development would suggest a need for assessment of language function. Such appraisal may reveal a need for language training in the overall management program.

Similarly, the presence of other speech problems is most likely to have significance for management in respect to children. However, one does occasionally find some persisting articulatory error in an adult who stutters. Cluttering features are another type of speech defect found occasionally with stuttering. Any current speech problem other than stuttering also deserves attention in the overall management of the patient.

Medical history.—The medical history is important for its possible relevance to the problem. It is not known that stuttering is caused by particular circumstances of a medical nature; however, there are certain kinds of events which are clearly suspect. Perinatal difficulties, accidents involving head injury, and severe illnesses involving high fever may well have at least a contributory effect on the appearance of stuttering. Berry (1938) and Milisen and Johnson (1936) have reported an elevated occurrence of such conditions in the medical history of stutterers. Also, one finds in many other sources reports of stuttering occurrence subsequent to head injury and illnesses involving the central nervous system.

As yet there is no known medical treatment appropriate for stuttering. However, in cases having a suspect medical history treatment of other possible sequellae, such as seizures, may be found to have an effect on the stuttering.

Unfortunately, the major value of a medical history is for counseling purposes, and even there its value is not too definitive. Yet, simply stated, the presence of a suspect medical history has possible explanatory value, which is often important to parents.

School problems.—In this category interest is again focused primarily on the child stutterer, particularly the young child. One is interested in the matter of school adjustment from the standpoint of functioning in the classroom and also peer relationships, particularly as these activities might involve the child's stuttering.

The experiences and adjustments of the stuttering child represent another area in which professional as well as lay folklore is very often contrary to fact. Stuttering does not necessarily create significant problems for a child.

Generally speaking, young children are not critical of others. They are often inquisitive and may ask frank questions or make direct comments about anything they observe. But they are not likely to make much issue of personal differences or oddities they perceive. Particularly with youngsters through at least the second grade level, one finds that they can be quite aware of something unusual in a peer without showing much reaction to it. Although children of this age range are known to be well aware of stuttering, they are most likely to be either indifferent to it or matter-of-fact about it.

Problems related to the stuttering may be more likely to arise at a somewhat later age. However, even in this period it is by no means certain that difficulties will develop. Much depends on circumstances, such as where the child lives and who his friends are, his personality characteristics, the personalities of at least certain of the other children with whom he is in frequent contact, and a number of other variables. Some child stutterers happen to be leaders among their peers and are popular and well-liked. Most of them, like most nonstuttering youngsters, are accepted pretty much as is, with their stuttering evoking little more reaction than extensive freckles or an oddly shaped nose. The stuttering child who is seemingly the object of ridicule because of his stuttering may well have personal characteristics that would invite this treatment regardless of his speech.

Although a stuttering youngster may sometimes be subjected to teasing, quite often this is not malicious or particularly insensitive in nature, and many stuttering youngsters accept it as such. While some children who are teased do react negatively, many are not particularly affected by teasing, or are bothered by it only at certain times, or from certain individuals. Similarly, while one sometimes encounters a stuttering child who is reluctant to recite in class because of his stuttering, one will also find those who have no such reticence.

One should be interested in the child's school adjustment in ways that go beyond the possible involvement of the stuttering. The topic of school problems also encompasses matters of academic function. One should be cognizant that academic learning depends heavily on language capability, specifically reading and spelling. Regardless of the equivocal research findings regarding reading and spelling problems among stutterers, some children who stutter also give evidence of language limitations. It would seem prudent that efforts be made to afford special help to the stuttering child who evidences problems in language function, for what this might contribute to the overall program of stuttering management.

Personality description.—The examiner should first attempt to get a general description of the personality of the person in question, whether he is inquiring about the individual himself or about a child in interview with a parent. One is interested primarily in an overall statement about what the individual is like—his typical moods, ways of behaving, manner of relating to others, etc. In the case of direct interview with the stutterer it is important to know how he views himself as an individual. We are also interested in knowing how he sees his stuttering in relationship to his view of himself.

Again, one will find a great deal of variation. Many individuals are rather forthright and seemingly honest in self-appraisal; others are reticent or not capable of very much self-analysis. In cases where the individual has difficulty giving a reasonably adequate personal description the examiner can inquire about those things which the stutterer either considers personally, or has been told by others, are his characteristic traits or ways of feeling or acting.

Once more, contrary to the image perpetuated in both professional and lay literature, stutterers are not typically shy, retiring, or inhibited. Neither are they typically fearful, anxious, or burdened with guilt, shame, or any other unique emotion. As revealed in the evidence presented in Chapters 2 and 3, stutterers show considerable variation in personality. The examiner must be prepared to consider each stutterer as an individual.

It is valuable to obtain from parents a similar kind of personality description of child stutterers. On occasion it may be worthwhile to take separate statements from each parent. In addition to the features mentioned regarding older stutterers, in the case of children we are particularly interested in identification of certain characteristics that have been reported to occur more commonly among stuttering youngsters, namely, a tendency to be sensitive, nervous, etc. One should be particularly alert to such characteristics in regard to recommendations for management both at school and at home. In some cases where such patterns attain particular prominence, as for example in association with a number of other symptoms as listed, a referral for psychologic evaluation might well be indicated. Of course, serious consideration of such referral should be made in view of much case material.

Laterality (Sidedness).—In present-day practice no one seems to give much consideration to the matter of laterality; the general persuasion seems to be that it is an irrelevant matter. Concern with laterality faded for a number of reasons but primarily because its presence and potential effect could not be demonstrated regularly in cases of stuttering. Still, there exists some rather persuasive evidence that laterality may be directly influential in some cases of stuttering.

Currently the role of laterality in stuttering is primarily of theoretical interest. However, it seems that we do not yet have justifiable grounds for disregarding it entirely at a practical level. If a practitioner is to be responsibly thorough he should not ignore factors that might reasonably have a contributory significance to a problem. The simplest measure to be taken along these lines is to permit and encourage a youngster to function in accordance with his natural sidedness preference.

Family history.—The material in this section has its most direct practical application for purposes of counseling.

One is particularly interested in the matter of familial incidence of stuttering. There is a good deal of evidence which indicates a genetic factor in stuttering, although the pattern and mechanism of transmission are not very well understood. While attempts have been made to account for the finding that stuttering "runs in families" on the basis of social or nongenetic features, these attempts provide a feeble and wholly inadequate explanation. They do not account for the fact that stuttering skips generations, that only certain members of the family are afflicted, and that there is a very uneven sex ratio in stuttering occurrence.

It is not at all uncommon to find a report of current stuttering in some other member of the immediate or extended family. One will not infrequently find that some other member of the immediate or extended family, including the child's parents or siblings, stutters now or stuttered for some length of time in childhood. Even in cases where there is no reported incidence of stuttering in the family background one cannot therefore assume that there is no hereditary influence. It should be kept in mind that, for several reasons, one always obtains minimum evidence regarding the familial incidence of a disorder like stuttering. Family size is clearly a limiting circumstance to uncovering reports of stuttering in the family line, since there is less probability that it will be manifest in a small family. Also, the informant (the patient himself or his parents) often has limited information beyond the immediate family. Further, childhood stuttering is sometimes forgotten after a lapse of several years.

Sinistrality (left-handedness) and twinning are two other characteristics that have been identified as occurring more frequently in the family history of stutterers. As indicated earlier, there is a basis for formulating a connection between sinistrality and stuttering, although this relationship is presently not clear. The connection between stuttering and twinning is less well documented, but again the evidence of some relationship is persuasive and it seems possible that this element may be interrelated with that of sinistrality. Although the actual nature of the relationship between stuttering, sinistrality, and twinning is presently only conceptual, their concurrence does lead to the suspicion of some common genetic base.

The information gathered regarding family history is of great value in counseling. Some parents will report having heard, or deduced, that stuttering is "hereditary." Others will indicate that this implication comes as a surprise. Nonetheless, many of them are relieved to learn that there is a substantive basis for suspecting a constitutional cause of stuttering. This allows some parents to unburden themselves of feelings of self-doubt, guilt, and self-recrimination. As noted in the *Introduction* of this book, a large majority of present-day parents have accepted an account of stuttering as due to something "psychological." Many will reveal having made a search for circumstances that "brought it on," or will have wondered what they have done, or are doing, that caused the child to stutter.

As noted previously, stuttering does appear superficially to be "due to" emotional effects or psychological influences. Additionally, both the professional and lay literature have long been saturated with explanations of stuttering as a psychological problem. Having the opportunity to seriously consider the stuttering as a constitutionally conditioned problem allows parents the freedom of looking at the disturbance more objectively. They are not as likely to feel confused and frustrated about it, and many have the opportunity to feel some relief from a burden of self-doubt or self-blame they have accrued. Most parents are thus in a better position to work constructively with the clinician.

Among teenage and adult stutterers one may expect to find less readiness to accept the possibility that stuttering is a physiological problem. There are several reasons for this reluctance. In substantial measure it is due to the prevalent explanations of stuttering as a psychological problem, which many stutterers find credible because of certain impressive aspects of their own personal experience. Additionally, the prospect of a physiological basis for stuttering often suggests a pessimistic outlook; i.e., that the disorder is not remediable. It is thus more attractive to believe that the cause of stuttering lies hidden in one's psychic past, either in the form of an emotional problem or as the effect of some particular circumstances that somehow interfered with learning to talk correctly. Such beliefs are often accompanied by the anticipation that the stuttering can be completely eliminated if only the right solution is found.

Discussion of the nature of stuttering is often precipitated when gathering the family history material. It is preferable to defer this discussion, if possible, until near the end of the evaluation, when inquiry is made regarding the patient's or parent's view about the cause of stuttering (see below).

Experience and Reaction

Attitude toward stuttering.—Special attention should be given to the matter of attitude toward stuttering, not only of the individual himself but also of those close to him. The attitude of the stutterer himself is most important; the attitude of others is a secondary consideration, to be dealt with in relationship to the stutterer's own attitude.

Attitudes may be a detriment or a support to therapy and it is important to know beforehand what adjustments might need be made. In certain cases it may be necessary to deal with attitudes prior to initiating actual work with speech.

It is necessary that one recognize that attitudes toward stuttering are very much an individual matter, and vary a good deal from one person to another. The examiner should take care to obtain a stutterer's own statement of attitude toward his stuttering and avoid perceiving in the statement some translation of a supposedly common pattern. A realistic assessment is necessary to efficient and realistic management.

The major attitude among adult stutterers is often reflected in the reason they come for help. Some of them will emphasize their reaction to the problem, complaining of the limitations stuttering imposes on feelings of freedom within their personal and social relations. They will mention embarrassment, social sensitivity, a reluctance to speak at some times when they otherwise might, or something similar. Others will indicate that they view the impediment as having an annoyance character but not necessarily one that creates in them a good deal of stress or "painful reaction."

One should listen well to the statement of attitude registered by children, and be willing to take the statement at face value until such time as a child might indicate something different. Of course, it is prudent to take into consideration the personal characteristics of the child who makes the statement; one must be reasonably sure that the statement is sincere. Still, the major point is that one must avoid imputing a common set of feelings and reactions to every child who stutters.

It has been my experience that most youngsters register a relative indifference to their stuttering. Such notable reaction as they may have is ordinarily relative to particular circumstances and, in some few cases, to certain individuals. In the case of children one should be prepared to differentiate between the attitude reflected by the child and that revealed by the parents. Not infrequently one will find that a parent's report of a child's attitude toward his stuttering is more a projection of the parent's feeling than it is an accurate description of the child's actual reaction.

Usually it is appropriate, within this context of attitude, to inquire about the patient's (and if indicated, the parent's) assessment of the severity of the problem. The examiner should encourage a narrative description regarding the perceived extent of the problem, but also obtain, for comparative purposes, a rating judgment utilizing the descriptive designations included in the Severity Rating Guide.

It is also important to inquire about the attitude of other persons—as perceived by the stutterer. As discussed earlier, the situation with children is not typically one in which the child stutterer is subject to abuse, nor feels that he is. However, if circumstances of this sort do obtain, it will be necessary to consider management assistance through parents and teachers, as well as helping the child to deal with the situation himself.

Some older stutterers project a negative reaction from other people. These are the stutterers who often serve as textbook examples and who do indeed need help in respect to restructuring their distorted perceptions. On the other hand, many stutterers do not share these unrealistic persuasions and therefore do not need counseling in respect to them.

It should be kept clearly in mind that, in the final analysis, the importance of attitude is not paramount. Attitudes are only one aspect of the overall problem. They must be taken into account, they are often important in determining patient involvement in treatment and therefore therapeutic progress, but one must be careful not to overvalue their contribution in the overall problem.

Treatment or management.—It is valuable to know what assistance the stutterer has had previously, how long ago, for what length of time, and with what results. Of principal interest here are those techniques reported to have had a beneficial effect, regardless of their nature or origin. At the same time we should also take note of techniques reported to have been ineffectual or detrimental. An inventory of past successes and failures is of value in both direct treatment and for purposes of counseling and guidance.

Explanation of cause.—We are interested in the patient's and parents' ideas about the reason he stutters primarily for purposes of counseling. Many times none of them will have given much thought to the matter. This in itself suggests a good deal about the attitude, reaction, and adjustment to the problem. On the other hand, ideas about the cause of the stuttering may be pretty well developed. This is most likely to be encountered among certain adolescent or adult stutterers. It is encountered less frequently among parents and, expectedly, it is very rare among children.

As indicated earlier, ideas about the cause of the problem have an effect on the adjustments made to it. Sometimes these views determine assumptions and anticipations regarding therapeutic method; they may also considerably influence expectations of therapeutic effort. Cases showing little interest or concern with cause present a very different management prospect than those which reveal a preoccupation with it. The clinician is much better able to deal effectively with a patient or parent when their views about cause are known.

Counseling in regard to the nature of stuttering, i.e., giving information about the disorder and dealing with ideas, beliefs, and attitudes toward it should be a routine part of the management process. It is usually at least initiated at the time of evaluation, if the format suggested here is used. Depending upon individual circumstances, such counseling may even be substantially completed at that time. In other cases this aspect of management may persist for some time into the period of actual therapy. Some patients will cling to their preferred conceptions, particularly if encouraged or permitted to do so through an harmonious bias of the clinician. In some cases this may work out to the satisfaction of all concerned. However, it should be recognized that in the final analysis the whole matter should be approached honestly and realistically. The honesty lies in the acknowledgment that we do not really know what causes stuttering; the realism lies in accepting the significance of the available evidence, unselected by preference and uncomplicated by conjecture.

Evaluation of Stuttering

I. *Background Information*

Name ______________________ Age ________ Sex ________ Educ. ________ Rel. ______________

Address ______________________________ Tel. ______________________

____

Father ______________________ Age ________ Educ. ________ Occup. ______________

Mother ______________________ Age ________ Educ. ________ Occup. ______________

	brothers	sisters
Siblings (age)		
Other persons in the home		

II. *Present stuttering: description. Speech symptoms (predominant type), accessory features (nature and extent), severity (cf. Severity Rating Guide)*

A. *Examiner's description*

B. *Patient's description*

C. *Variability-reltivity*
  1. narrative description
  2. specific topicy
     a. periodicity
     b. situations or individuals
     c. extremes (when worst, when best; ever absent)
     d. special circumstances
        when alone ______ with pets ______, young children ______ telephone ______ to groups ______, reading aloud______, singing ______, when angry ______ excited ______, relaxed ______, tired ______, good mood ______

D. *Techniques of control*

III. *Relevant History*
  A. *History of stuttering:*

B. *Language development*

	-12	12-17	18-23	24-29	30-35	36-41	42-48
1. use of: words							
word combinations							
relating experiences							

  2. other speech problems (as a child ________; presently ________)

C. *Medical History*
  1. natal conditions
  2. accidents
  3. illnesses

D. *School problems*
   1. academic
   2. adjustment

E. *Personality description*
   1. general
   2. characteristic traits
   3. special features: "nervous" ________ "sensitive" ________ thumbsucking ________ nailbiting ________ nightmares ________ enuresis ________ eating problems ________ fears ________ other ________

F. *Laterality*

G. *Family History*

	patient	*immediate family*	*father's side*	*mother's side*
stuttering				
sinistrality				
twinning				
other speech defect				

IV. *Experience*

A. *Attitude toward stuttering:*
   1. patient's
   2. parents
   3. others (siblings, teachers, peers, employers)

B. *Treatment or management:*

C. *Explanation of cause:*
   1. patient's
   2. parent's

Severity Rating Guide

Overall Rating	*Descriptive Assessment*		
	Frequency (per words spoken)	*Effort*	*Accessory Features*
Very Mild	1/100 (1%)	no perceptible tension	none
Mild	1/50 (2%)	perceptible tension but "block" easily overcome	minimal (staring; eye blinks or eye movement or slight movement of the facial musculature)
Moderate	1/15 (7%)	clear indication of tension or effort; lasts about 2 seconds	noticeable movement of facial musculature
Severe	1/7 (15%)	definite tension or effort; lasts about 2-4 seconds; frequent repeat attempts	obvious muscular activity, facial or other
Very Severe	1/4 (25%)	considerable effort; lasts 5 seconds or more; consistant repeat attempts	vigorous muscular activity, facial or other

Notes

1. Cf., for example, Johnson, Darley, and Spriestersbach (1963), Riley (1972), and Van Riper (1971).

2. This clinical observation, whereby parents reveal that they make a distinction between stuttering and normal speech (with its normal nonfluencies), offers additional commentary on the identifiability of stuttering.

3. However, some stutterers report the opposite, and will acknowledge that they stutter more under these conditions because they make less effort to monitor themselves.

4. This information may occasionally have particular significance, as in the following case in which difficulty associated with a specific sound reflected emotional dynamics.

A late-teen-age stutterer did not realize that his difficulty with "r-words" occurred most frequently with words like "rich," "Republican," and "relative." This young man and his mother were dependent for a considerable amount of their comfortable support on a wealthy uncle who subtly exacted compliance from both of them through the leverage of his financial support. The young man felt very hostile toward the uncle because of the constrictive pressures the uncle imposed, but at the same time felt intimidated. He reacted by being subtly resistive in "understandable" ways, one of which was by espousing very liberal political views. However, the resistance he could express in such ways was hardly sufficient to resolve the frustrations he felt.

This is the type of case that one finds too often in the literature presented as an example of the psychological basis of stuttering. In this particular case (and, I suspect, in most cases) there was only a superficial connection between the patient's stuttering and his conflicts. The latter were manifested in ways other than through his stuttering. Further, the conflicts did not "cause" him to stutter, even with the words cited; these stuttering instances are better viewed as a coalescent product of two vulnerabilities. Also, a better understanding of himself and his personal problems did not "cure" his stuttering, although by being less tense in certain situations he then stuttered less in them.

5. The only definitive indication of this kind is the spectrographic pattern reflecting transition failure, reported in a follow-up study by Stromsta (1965). Cooper (1973) has recently compiled a provisional list of criteria gathered from suggestions made in various literature sources; their validity is unknown.

References

Berry, Mildred F. A study of the medical history of stuttering children. *Speech Monogr.*, **5**, 97–14, 1938.

Cooper, E. B. The development of a stuttering chronicity prediction checklist: A preliminary report. *J. Speech Hearing Dis.*, **38**, 215–223, 1973.

Johnson, W. *et al. The Onset of Stuttering*, Univ. of Minnesota Press, Minneapolis, 1959.

Johnson, W., F. L. Darley, and D. D. Spriestersbach. *Diagnostic Methods in Speech Pathology*. Harper and Row, New York, 1963, p. 281.

Milisen, R. and W. Johnson. A comparative study of stutterers, former stutterers and normal speakers whose handedness has been changed. *Arch. Speech*, **1**, 61–86, 1936.

Riley, G. D. A stuttering severity instrument for children and adults. *J. Speech Hearing Dis.*, **37**, 314–322, 1972.

Stromsta, C. A spectrographic study of dysfluencies labelled as stuttering by parents. *De Therapia Vocis et Loquelae*, **1**, B16–Aug., 1965

Van Riper, C. *The Nature of Stuttering*, Prentice-Hall, Englewood Cliffs, 1971, pp. 223–227.

12

THERAPY AND COUNSELING

The management of stuttering should be approached with realism. We must be honest not only with ourselves but with our patients.

The most important reality to face and remain aware of is that we do not know what causes stuttering in the sense of its ultimate source.[1] The various theories of stuttering are attempts to explain ultimate cause, and the explanations presented, though in some respects persuasive, are highly conjectural. As discussed in earlier chapters, these attempts to explain stuttering origin, i.e., the "nature" of stuttering, do not have very substantive support in the research literature.[2]

Theories of stuttering are actually not of much help to therapy; in fact, a good case can be made that theories of stuttering are more confounding than facilitative in their contribution to management practice (Wingate, 1975). Therefore, clinicians must be guarded in the extent to which they are influenced by any particular explanation of stuttering, and they should be suspect of management methods determined by such explanations.

As a rule the various explanations of the "nature" of stuttering cast stutterers into some kind of common mold, in which one presumably can expect to find a standard set of attitudes, experiences, action tendencies, feelings, reactions, hopes, wishes, and the like. Of course, many stutterers may show certain similarities in variables of this kind, but there is no justification for believing that any such features will necessarily be found routinely or regularly in individuals who stutter. Furthermore, some of the variables frequently said to be important in the genesis and maintenance of stuttering—such as fear, sensitivity, and so forth—have been elaborated far beyond their appropriate relevance (cf. Chapters 2 and 3). "The stutterer," and most of what is typically included in this image, is an unfortunate overgeneralization. The only thing we can be certain is common to stutterers is that they have a unique type of speech disturbance.

There are three essential points intended in the preceding paragraphs. First, stuttering is principally a *speech* problem. Second, for no individual stutterer is there a known basic *cause* of his stuttering. Third, for any particular stutterer one cannot predict what the *effects* of his stuttering might be.

The facts of unknown cause and indeterminate effect are of equal importance in dealing honestly and realistically with patients and their families.

COUNSELING

It is appropriate to deal first with the topic of counseling, even though it is not the aspect of management considered to be first in order of importance.

The overall management of stuttering involves dealing with the stuttering itself, the individual who stutters, and the people close to him, particularly parents and teachers. Which of these dimensions is emphasized depends upon circumstances, including the age of the patient. In most cases the major management focus is on the patient's speech.

Dealing with the individual and his attitudes is subsidiary to the primary focus of working on his stuttering and his speech. At the same time, we are interested in the individual stutterer as a person, and over the long term we must remain alert to his individual psychology, with all that this implies. Maintaining a sensitivity to, and consideration of, the individual is not only a continuing matter in stuttering therapy, it is also one that should be developed early in the management approach, simply because the kind of person with whom one is dealing will have some influence on how the treatment proceeds. One will need to recognize the individual differences that exist among stutterers and make whatever adjustments in management plan seem indicated by such differences. This means that one cannot expect to deal with the personal aspects of stuttering from an orientation which assumes that stuttering has a similar significance for all stutterers. It also means that one cannot assume that personal aspects of stuttering are always important variables in the overall picture; one must be careful not to perceive more than is really there.

Much has been written about counseling in stuttering therapy and a very substantial portion of this literature deals with counseling as almost equivalent to psychotherapy. Certainly the kind of relationship that one can expect will develop in stuttering therapy should be attentive to very personal feelings and attitudes of the patient. However, even more importantly, counseling involves the professional functions of supplying information, providing appropriate explanation, and giving advice. I believe that such functions should constitute the predominant activity in the speech clinician's counseling of the stutterer. Speech pathologists typically are not adequately trained to manage a psychotherapeutic relationship, in spite of the fact that some aspects of their activities can lead to positive psychological change for the patient. In many helping relationships—including those of the ministry, law, medicine, practical nursing, and so on—events transpire which are psychologically beneficial to the patient, even though the primary aid he receives has another focus. Psychological benefit derives through the course of speech therapy as well; however, aid of a psychological nature ordinarily should not be the major focus of the therapy.

I do not wish to minimize the importance of dealing with psychological aspects of stuttering, but I think this matter should be approached in its proper perspective. Certain stutterers will need considerable attention to the psychological aspects of their problem; in fact, in some few cases referral to a clinical psychologist or a psychiatrist may be quite appropriate. Also, there are many stutterers who need help with attitudes and feelings that have developed as a result of their experiences, which may affect their lives directly or indirectly. A good management program should incorporate work with such matters as an integral part of the therapy.

I have chosen not to consider at any length the topic of dealing with attitudes and reactions, since this topic is covered adequately in many sources. Instead, I wish to emphasize that the clinician must not make routine assumptions about the psychology of stutterers but should deal with each patient individually. Therapeutic activity based on routine assumptions often is likely to be superfluous, wasteful, or in error. For example, lack of adequate motivation is frequently interpreted as a sign of resistance—but resistance to what? In certain literature sources the resistance is explained in terms of covert or devious personal feelings of the patient; i.e., he is resisting therapy because of some hidden motivation to not relinquish his stuttering. Actually, the "resistance" may very well be much more prosaic in nature. Stuttering therapy can be expected to be long-term and to require of the patient a great deal of application and initiative—so much, in fact, that the demands of treatment will often outweigh the discomfort value of the stuttering. In effect, it is simply that the effort required of the patient is too much like work; the "resistance" is quite straightforward.

The willingness of a patient to participate actively in therapy is a persisting concern in management. Often the actual level of motivation is not particularly evident in the beginning; it may be revealed only after the patient has come to realize the extent of the commitment required of him.

Many aspects of individual differences go beyond matters of personality features or aspects of attitude and are of special relevance to stuttering management. A particularly important domain centers on the individual's knowledge of his stuttering, including not only his personal experiences of it but also what he believes about it, his own thoughts and awarenesses.

The stutterer's knowledge of his stuttering as he has experienced it and the set of beliefs he has about it serve as points of departure for helping him understand it more fully and realistically. At one level, it is likely that he is unaware of many aspects of his stuttering as it occurs. Familiarity with these features will be helpful to him in learning to manage his stuttering. At another level, the stutterer and his parents are also likely to be poorly informed or misinformed about stuttering in a broad sense. Some of their knowledge will be consistent with reliable information about the disorder, but probably a good deal of it will be distorted or partial information.

We have already covered, in Chapter 11, many of the important areas that need to be incorporated into the counseling. There are, in addition, certain other matters that contribute importantly to a realistic base for helping the patient and his parents (and others) to understand his stuttering.

To begin with, it is appropriate to emphasize that we must acknowledge stuttering to be basically a speech problem. It is, in essence, a defect in the fluent production of audible language. Instances of stuttering represent an inability to proceed at certain points in the speech sequence. The speech flow is interrupted, from some unknown source. The principal "markers" of this interruption are events which indicate that certain parts of the speech production system are temporarily in a steady-state condition (prolongation) or a state of oscillation (elemental repetition).

It is most realistic to understand this defect, in its observable occurrence, as something that *happens*. It is not meaningfully understood as essentially something one *does*—unless we are willing to speak in the same manner about such other actions as stumbling, yawning, hiccoughing, trembling, and the like. To the extent that the individual stutterer is aware of his stuttering instances he experiences them as events that happen during the course of his speaking.

The only justifiable motivation to impute to a stutterer relative to his stuttering is an intention to continue speaking in spite of an event that interrupts the continuity of his speech. This description is also what a stutterer (at least an unsophisticated stutterer) is most likely to report himself.

The interaction of these two events—the stopping versus the motivation to continue—may often lead to certain other manifestations. The first order of such subsequent events is effort—effort to continue an intended act (or acts) of the speech sequence. An increase in effort to speak, perhaps developing into what might be called struggle, is a natural adjustment to being stopped in the act of speaking. Consider for instance what happens in similar circumstances: a drawer that sticks, a door that resists opening, a pen that does not write, etc. In all of these examples the person faced with the difficulty is immediately induced to exert more effort in the attempt to resolve it. Most often the effort begins gently but increases in vigor if the difficulty is not overcome. Evidently the same thing occurs in stuttering. It is important to remember that acts identifiable as effort, or struggle, represent immediate motor adjustments which occur in response to an event that has already happened.[3]

Another dimension of importance in dealing with stuttering has to do with the matter of the expected outcome of treatment. There exists a curious inconsistency in the attitude of most clinicians regarding the anticipated results of treatment. Within the profession there is a widespread and well-established suspicion of any claim for a cure for stuttering. In fact, professionals are clearly skeptical of claims for treatment methods that imply any result even tantamount to cure.[4] In spite of this attitude, most clinicians undertake therapy with a stutterer with an implicit assumption, or at least the aspiration, that the anticipated goal of the treatment is cure of the stuttering. To be realistic, one should anticipate that the actual eventual goal is more likely to be something short of cure. Some stutterers, most likely young ones, will attain a level of essential cure or something very close to it, but as yet we have no means of discerning who these individuals might be. In general, it would seem appropriate that the goal for stuttering therapy is simply maximum improvement, even though that is not a very well-defined goal.

One area of professional knowledge in speech pathology bears indirectly, though importantly, on this matter of realism—what we now know about the structure and nature of language. In view of what the speech clinician should know about the nature of language it is time to abandon approaches to stuttering therapy which encourage the stutterer to think in terms of returning to the "automaticity of speech." Everyone in the field should know by now that verbal expression in its usual sense—meaning spontaneously formulated propositional language—is not automatic. "Automaticity" hardly can be said to characterize formulated speech at any level of analysis, even certain types of everyday greetings or remarks. The only potentially "automatic" speech is limited to the brief, highly routinized utterances of the order of epithets and exclamations. Moreover, several lines of evidence from work in linguistics and speech science clearly indicate that even the sequencing of speech units below the level of the word does not run off automatically. It is thus unrealistic to lead a patient to believe that there lies within him a capability for fluency that can be "unlocked." It is also improper to lead the patient to believe that speech clinicians have the capability, in any therapy program, of reinstating or developing a facility which in essence is not attainable even for the normal speaker.

A similar error is contained in the assumption that in stutterers normal speech or normal speech potential lies somewhere below the surface and will emerge as the stutterings are removed. The question has not yet been resolved whether the speech of stutterers is basically normal in quality during intervals between episodes of stuttering, but even if it is, this does not mean that the stuttering is simply a circumstance overlaid on a basically normal capability. The findings obtained from recovered stutterers bear cogently on this matter: the reader will recall that many of the persons identified as recovered stutterers still reported a residual tendency to stutter or to experience intermittent recurrences of stuttering.

The studies of stuttering recovery have yielded certain other findings that are also particularly relevant for counseling purposes. Almost always recovery was said to have taken place gradually, including those cases in which individuals reported having worked diligently at improving their speech. Too often stutterers who come for help—particularly young adults—hope for rapid improvement or cure. Many of these individuals are looking for a "key" to their problem, some special method or some psychological revelation that will enable them quite suddenly to be relieved of their stuttering. Stutterers accepted for therapy should realize that, in all likelihood, a great deal of time, as well as considerable application, will be required in order to achieve a substantial, enduring improvement in their fluency. They should also recognize that the rate and extent of progress is an individual matter related to many aspects of themselves as individuals.

The reader may recall earlier mention (Chapter 10) of two forms of approach in stuttering therapy: endeavoring to remove (reduce) the stuttering or improving speech fluency. Although the eventual objective is the same, the means of attaining it are different. The former approach directs attention to modifying the instances of stuttering; the latter approach works toward improvement of the person's speech. The two orientations can be used conjointly, but preferably with the former subsidiary to the latter.

A therapy approach that deals with instances of stuttering tends to be too circumscribed and cumbersome. For instance, approaches of this form typically spend considerable time working on the features of the stuttering event, identifying, cataloging, analyzing, and explaining them. This activity includes a lot of attention to the accessory features, and often efforts are made to reduce these features before undertaking to attenuate the speech features. Therapy of this kind can be quite effective; however, reservations about it are that: (1) it tends to be needlessly detailed, and (2) more importantly it is addressed to the modification of stutterings rather than primarily to the improvement of speech.

The therapy approach developed in this book focuses principally on generating the experience of fluency and helping the patient to understand the basis for how fluency is achieved. The patient is helped to experience fluency through the use of various procedures which directly induce and support fluent speaking. Since fluency results immediately from the use of these procedures, it is not necessary to deal separately with most aspects of stuttering events. In particular, there is no need to direct attention to whatever accessory features may occur as part of a patient's stuttering, since these features are simply eliminated by the effect of the fluency-inducing procedures. Actually even therapeutic attention to the speech features of the stuttering event is reserved primarily for purposes of illustration and contrast; that is, to help the stutterer contrast what *is* happening when a stuttering event occurs with what *should be* happening. His experience of what should be happening is objectified in the effect generated by the fluency-inducing procedures, and the character of this effect should be clearly identified by the clinician. Ordinarily this experience of fluency should be augmented by helping the patient to understand how it is effected.

The basic principles of this therapy approach have been discussed in detail in Chapters 9 and 10. The object of the present chapter is to discuss the procedures for implementing these principles. The reader will find that he has already encountered most of these procedures in several other places within this book, where our interest focused on deriving an explanation of their effect. This chapter presents a format for the use of these procedures and others, couched in a rationale that centers on the principles which they evidently embody.

OVERVIEW OF THE THERAPY FORMAT

The ultimate yet fundamental objective is to educate the stutterer regarding motor aspects of speech expression. In particular he should come to appreciate the central importance of vocal modulation as the vehicle of fluency.

Vocal modulation implies prosody or melody of speech, which is the (vocalized) "tune" that underlies the words and phrases of connected speech. This tune, sometimes referred to as intonation pattern, consists primarily of variations in syllabic stress.

Therapeutic attention centers around speech melody for several reasons. First, there is compelling evidence that prosodic features are critical determinants of the locus of stuttering events; specifically, that stuttering occurrence is some function of stress prominence. Second, prosodic change is evidently the principle common to so many ameliorative influences on stuttering. We need not elaborate further on these matters here. The reader is referred to Chapters 9 and 10 for a review of the relevant analyses and principles; later sections of the present chapter will develop the application of these principles to actual therapeutic practice.

At some point, which will vary with circumstances, the patient should come to understand the important role of speech melody in supporting fluency. The extent of the patient's understanding may well vary as a function of several variables, the most obvious of these being his age. However, it will be found that the essential ideas can be communicated effectively to youngsters of at least school age, particularly when the explanations are accompanied by demonstrations and actual involvement of the patient in the execution of the principles.

We will develop the discussion of this therapy format in a general way, considering that what will be said can be applied easily to most individuals above the age of approximately 7 or 8. By this age children can be expected to be reasonably accessible to some level of explanation regarding the execution of skilled acts, can identify sources of sensations of many bodily activities, and can also be expected to be somewhat sophisticated in regard to the structure of words—or at least the fact that words have structure. The clinician may be surprised to find that even kindergarten age youngsters can appreciate and follow an explanation of the central features of this therapy approach.

The patient should be given as full an explanation as possible of (a) what evidently occurs in stuttering and (b) how this method of therapy works to correct it. The ultimate objective in this respect is that the patient should be helped to understand the essential content of Chapter 9: that is, that stuttering is localized at certain points of linguistic stress, and that linguistic stress reflects the melody of speech, which is predominantly a function of vocalization.

A preliminary feature in stuttering management[5] is to identify how well the individual knows his stuttering. As mentioned in earlier chapters, it is surprising how poorly most stutterers are acquainted with their own difficulty. Getting the person to attend to and be able to analyze what happens when he stutters, what he senses and feels, where his stuttering happens, and so forth, are desirable first steps in developing his understanding of the stuttering event, and subsequently, the means of its correction. Awareness of this kind can be used to set the contrast to what he is not doing—and what he should be doing—in order to speak fluently. As we have indicated earlier, it is not necessary to analyze this event exhaustively; it is sufficient to have the stutterer identify the broad outlines of how he feels "stopped." We are most interested in helping him to recognize that the essential problem is that he is not moving on in the sound pattern sequence.

At the outset the patient should be instructed, in simple terms, about the phonatory mechanism, essentially the action of the lungs and vocal folds. The patient should understand the action of the lungs in providing a stream of air which sets the vocal folds in motion and thus produces sound. He should be helped to physically experience his own phonatory activity, paying special attention to the sensations that are thereby produced. Instruction at this stage should emphasize the basic aspect of phonation as well as the understanding that articulation is an aspect of speech production which is a modification of the primary (vocal) vehicle of oral expression. The credibility of this explanation can be communicated by pointing out that, to begin with, human communication is a truly vocal process. (Infants initially make only phonated noises and then only gradually do they come to modify the stream of sound by articulatory gestures.)

From here the initial instructions should move to the use of demonstrating the basic character of phonation and its importance in sustaining fluency. Here the therapist can lead the patient though a progression of fluency-inducing procedures (identified later, p. 334ff) which are used at this stage as a means of illustration. However, use of these procedures should not be limited to demonstration; any of them can play a significant role in the treatment process. Indeed, they provide an available fund of techniques, which embody the common principles, and from which one can draw selectively over the course of therapy as occasion permits or suggests. The fact of overlap among these procedures is actually a positive feature for therapy; in fact, the overlap should be emphasized to the patient as illustration that the various procedures represent the same basic principles which he must come to understand as a fundamental aspect of his therapy.

The next stage in the instruction process begins the emphasis on the basic principles of this therapy. Objectives here are to develop the patient's awareness that the central feature in speech is its melody, which is an undulating pattern of tone and intensity. The central point to be communicated here is that voicing is the foundation of audible speech and that it is through voicing that the pattern of speech, the melody, is expressed. Subsequent instructions center on the equivalence of linguistic stress to speech melody, the relationship of stuttering to linguistic stress, and the role played by speech melody in supporting fluency.

It is at this point that the detailed analysis of the stuttering event, presented in Chapter 9, should be brought into the instructional sequence, and the individual's familiarity with his own stuttering is then related to the analysis. An important focus of this assessment is the locus of stuttering occurrence. If the individual does not already recognize it, one can easily point out to him that most stuttering occurs in the initial parts of words and never on final parts of words. From here it is a short step to relating the locus of stuttering occurrence to points of linguistic stress, or, in the terms that have already been used in explanation of the nature of speech, the points where the melody "peaks." It is easy and particularly worthwhile, to review a recording of the patient's spontaneous speech with him, pointing out that his stutterings indeed do occur at such points. Many stutterers will be able to connect this finding with their personal observations that in many instances, once they have "got going" in saying a word or phrase, they have no trouble saying the rest of it. Often this approach may also have relevance to longer groups of words as well.

The crucial point to be emphasized here is that stuttering almost always occurs at certain points of linguistic stress, and that linguistic stress is predominantly a function of vocalization. From this follows the central principle of the therapy approach: namely, the need to develop control of vocalization in expressing appropriate speech melody, with particular awareness to dealing with stress prominences. Further demonstration, utilizing certain of the procedures used previously, should be undertaken here.

At this point the patient will have moved into the process of therapy, which will endeavor to help him consolidate his "feel" for the technical aspects of the principles embodied in these procedures, and to expand their use into an increasing span of his speech performance.

TREATMENT METHOD

The format of the direct treatment involves two phases that differ in focus but clearly overlap in substance. The first phase is primarily instructional; the second phase consists of implementation of procedures.

The First Phase: Instruction

The initial objective is to inform the patient of (1) the central importance of vocalization in maintaining fluency and (2) how linguistic stress is related, on one hand, to stuttering, and on the other hand, to vocal modulation. The ultimate objective of this initial phase is to develop an understanding of what seems to turn fluent speech into stuttering and how this can be contravened quite naturally by implementing certain fundamentals of the speech process.

The significance of vocalization.—The first step is to teach the patient something about how the motor speech system functions in respect to phonation. He should understand the essential process in which air is expelled from the lungs, passes between the vocal folds and sets the folds in vibration when they are sufficiently close together. This vibration produces a sound which is the beginning of voice and which takes on its full character from being "shaped" by the cavities and structures of the nose and mouth.

In making this explanation, particular attention should be directed to the action of the vocal folds. One should take care to explain that the folds are subject to both reflexive and voluntary control. The patient should understand the position and action of the vocal folds under various conditions: that they are open during quiet breathing; closed firmly in order to support muscular exertion; alternately opening and closing vigorously during coughing; and brought together when producing sound. Graphic displays are always helpful in communicating this information. Physiologic models and other media should be used if one has access to them. However, the essential points can be explained with rather simple maneuvers. For instance, the first two fingers of either hand can serve as a crude but adequate means of portraying the opening and closing of the glottis. A very simple but clear analogue of the relation between expiration and vocal fold function can be conveyed through the use of a balloon. By this means one can show unobstructed air flow, generation of sound by approximation of the "folds," and complete stoppage of air flow.

The patient should be required to reproduce all of these functions and should be directed to attend carefully to the sensations he experiences in doing so. A reflexive closure of the glottis is effectively demonstrated by having the patient attempt to lift something heavy. Voluntary control of the vocal folds is demonstrated clearly by having the patient produce easy vocal onset many times at his natural pitch level. Throughout these "exercises" emphasis is placed on the patient's awareness of the sensations he experiences, primarily the feedback from the area of the larynx. It is particularly important that he become very aware of the vibration that is associated with vocalization. This awareness can be enhanced by having the subject lightly place thumb and forefinger on either side of the throat at the level of the larynx. This maneuver should be used often in ongoing therapy.

During this phase continual emphasis should be made of the fundamental importance of vocalization in speech. The patient should recognize that phonation provides the basic "carrier" of the verbal message; that vocal pattern is the original means of expressive communication in the young human (as well as other animal species); and that information is carried by voice tone and pattern in addition to the message conveyed by words per se.

Demonstration of vocal support of fluency.—In this second step the patient is led through a sequence of fluency-inducing procedures to demonstrate to him their effect in generating fluency and to impress him with the fact that phonation is the feature common to all of these procedures.

THE EFFECT OF SINGING.—Most stutterers seem to be aware of the fact that they do not stutter when they sing. Those who do not already know this should be made aware of it. It is particularly worthwhile to create actual demonstration as well as telling the patient about the effect of singing. The clinician should be willing to help the patient overcome any embarrassment or reluctance about singing by initially singing himself, alone or with the patient.

It has been found worthwhile to emphasize to the stutterer that, in the effect produced by singing, generation of sound is the important vehicle supporting fluency rather than some other factor such as, for instance, the memorization of the words of the song. This can be demonstrated quite effectively by supplying the patient with other words to sing to the tune he knows. This requires a little ingenuity on the part of the clinician, but one or two new lines for a song should be sufficient for this purpose.

USE OF THE ARTIFICIAL LARYNX.—An artificial larynx of the vibrator type developed by Western Electric Corporation provides a good source for demonstrating that vocalization is important in stuttering. The stutterer will be able to speak without stuttering when using the artificial larynx as the source of generated sound for his speech. This particular demonstration has been found to be very impressive if done well. The clinician should become familiar with the use of the artificial larynx and be able to create reasonably intelligible speech with it himself before attempting its use in demonstration. A little practice in use of the instrument is necessary in order to be able to produce intelligible speech. Demonstration is not likely to be as impressive to a stutterer if the speech he hears produced in this way is not very understandable. In addition to the overall effect of this particular demonstration, there is also something to be learned, by the stutterer, from the sensation of vibration that is generated in the pharynx. It is an experience that can be likened to the vibration produced by the vocal folds themselves in generating their natural sound source.

VOICE CHEWING.—This demonstration employs the Froeschels method described earlier (Chapter 10). However, one can show the patient what he is expected to do without making actual reference to the type of description presented by Froeschels (for instance, chewing like a savage). The patient should be led through the range of sound formation that can be made in this manner. The clinician should carefully model all levels of performance of this technique. He should begin with the simple "moaning" type of oral noises, then proceed to the level of producing nonsense syllables, and finally to performances at the level of approximating actual words in sequence. Throughout, the patient's attention should be directed to the ease, looseness, and slowness of movement, and especially to the prominence of vocalizing in the total procedure.

SPEAKING TO A DEFINITE RHYTHM.—The patient should be exposed to several of the rhythm-based methods. For instance, one should make use of the desk metronome or a "Pacemaker," and syllable-timed speech supported and unsupported by some other activity. Actually it is valuable to use all these methods, especially with more severe cases. In such instances one should begin with a desk metronome and then progress to some other externally supported source of pacing, and finally to internally regulated syllable-timed speech.

Generally it seems best to begin with some mechanically supported performance. Also, the use of syllable-timed speech is enhanced by initially having the patient accompany the performance with some other motor act, such as tapping a surface with the hand or finger, or "keeping time" with his foot. At the same time, before completing this demonstration the patient should have had a reasonably lengthy experience of speaking to rhythm without external support. Moreover, he should have experience speaking to several different rhythms other than the basic one-syllable-per-beat. It is not necessary to become too elaborate in this demonstration that different rhythms are effective; the essential objective is simply to make the patient aware of the fact that fluency can be achieved even with varying patterns of rhythmic beat. It is particularly important to use this aspect of the rhythm demonstration to emphasize that the induced fluency is not strictly dependent on the beat per se, but evidently centers on the vocal control the patient is induced to express in following the regularized pattern.

VENTRILOQUISM MODE OF SPEAKING.—Again, the technique used here is essentially the one described by Froeschels (Chapter 10). The technique should be described and modeled for the patient and he should be coached in it until he is able to perform it satisfactorily. The essential objective here is to emphasize to the patient that the manner of speaking induced by the ventriloquism technique centers on phonation, occasioned by the deemphasis of the articulatory aspect of speaking.

SPEAKING IN A FOREIGN DIALECT.—Most older individuals should be able to make an attempt at speaking in the manner of certain non-native speakers of English. Most persons can be expected to be at least familiar with the speech distortions thought to be typical of an Irishman, Italian, Frenchman, or German. Actually, it does not make much difference whether the patient does a believable rendition of the dialect; the important thing is that he make a clear effort to do so, since in this effort he will be induced to implement vocal control, which is of course the actual objective of the procedure. The clinician should provide initial demonstration in order both to clarify what is meant and to obviate any feelings of embarrassment in the required attempt. He should also continue to support the patient's effort, intermittently employing choral speaking of a dialect if this seems necessary to help the patient overcome reluctance. At the same time this exercise need not be carried on long, since its use is principally for demonstration. Unlike the other procedures, it is not utilized in ongoing therapy, except perhaps as occasional didactic reference.

OTHER FLUENCY-INDUCING PROCEDURES.—The other fluency-inducing procedures discussed earlier—auditory masking, delayed auditory feedback, and shadowing—may also be used for purposes of demonstrating the important effect of phonation (and reduction of rate as well) in supporting fluency. However, these procedures are not generally as impressive for demonstration as the others, largely because the patient is not well able to perceive their effect immediately. Under auditory masking, DAF, and shadowing the patient's awareness of his speaking adjustments are at least partially obscured by the condition responsible for the effect. For this same reason these procedures have less value than the others for extended use in therapy. Moreover, both auditory masking and delayed auditory feedback require instrumentation, which not only may not be available in many places, but in the final analysis is superfluous if the desired effect can be achieved without it.

Melody, stress, and stuttering.—In all of the foregoing demonstrations the patient should be continually reminded of the central role played by phonation. In the next instructional phase the objective is to emphasize speech melody; to help the stutterer understand the relationship between phonation, melody, linguistic stress, and stuttering, and how control of stuttering is based on the understanding of this relationship.

SPEECH MELODY.—It is possible that, in going through the demonstrations of the preceeding stage, the matter of speech melody already may have been introduced, perhaps in the course of discussing the effect of certain demonstrations with the patient. The matter of speech melody should now be emphasized, with the patient told that all speech has a pattern or melody. This can be demonstrated in many simple ways, drawing examples from short sentences or phrases in the ongoing conversation between patient and clinician.

A particularly good means of illustrating the melody of speech is through use of a technique I call "sounding." Sounding is to ordinary speech as humming is to song; it consists of producing the melody without the words. The clinician should demonstrate sounding, using samples from several different sources. A good point to begin is with the use of simple rhyme. Nursery rhymes are good; so are very lyric kinds of poems such as "The Village Blacksmith." This should be followed by examples from less metered poetry and then some prose, including bits of ordinary conversation.

Sounding is presented at this point for purposes of illustrating the melody in speech. Later it is useful as a therapy technique as well. It is particularly valuable with certain stutterers: those who seem to have trouble expressing the appropriate melody in at least certain of the assignments they are given.

MELODY AND LINGUISTIC STRESS.—The clinician should next clearly identify speech melody as the expression of linguistic stress. This provides the transition into the topic of locus of stuttering occurrence and related matters. Care should be taken to point out that stress is related to syllables, that the points of stress are developed in respect to vowels, which are the focal aspect of syllables, and that vowels are the major speech expression of phonation. Again, graphic aids are very helpful. The clinician should draw, on blackboard or paper, a wave form representing the changes in stress of a phrase or a simple sentence (see Figure 12:1), spoken at the time, and pointing out to the patient the correspondences between the audible and the graphic pattern. One should make it a point to distinguish particularly the contrast between syllables receiving first-level stress—what will be called stress "prominences" or stress "peaks"—and syllables that are not stressed. The principal reason for making this distinction at this time is to relate it to locus of stuttering occurrence.

STUTTERING AND LINGUISTIC STRESS.—The most effective means of demonstrating that stuttering is associated with stress prominence is to play back a sample of the patient's speech and identify with him the loci of stuttering events. It should be impressed upon him that stuttering occurrence is clearly related to stress increase. This finding can be contrastively supported by pointing out that stuttering does not occur where stress decreases, i.e., in unstressed syllables. One can then review the material covered in the foregoing sections as a base for developing the patient's understanding that stuttering evidently occurs in the effort to move into a stress peak. With what he should know now about the speech process he should be able to understand that this activity heavily involves vocal function.

This is a good time to point out to the patient that stuttering does not occur *on* a sound, as it might appear, but that the crux of the difficulty is in *moving on* in the sound sequence. When he is "stopped" or "blocked" in his forward progress, as reflected in either elemental repetitions or prolongations, he is not making the necessary transitions into the next sound. Almost invariably, this next sound will be a stressed vowel. Now while "shaping" of the vowel will involve certain oral movements, the predominant adjustments required in producing a stressed vowel are phonatory, and not simply the act of phonation but, additionally, an increase in volume, duration, and pitch. Actually, the increase in volume and duration are the important variables to identify to the stutterer. Patients are well able to appreciate that stress regularly involves an increase in these dimensions, but they are not especially alert to the attendent changes in pitch. The patient should then recognize that this difficulty in moving on, this transition failure, evidently centers in the attempt to execute those phonatory acts necessary to produce a stress prominence. This description identifies the essential problem that must be dealt with.

A final step here is to point out that the solution to the problem relates very intimately to the identification of its nature. The clinician should explain that control of stuttering can be effected through proper execution of speech melody, particularly as this activity centers on moving smoothly into stress prominences. Here one should again make use of certain of the procedures used in the earlier demonstrations, but this time emphasizing in particular how the procedures induce expression of a pattern or melody. I have found that the use of various rhythms and of the ventriloquism technique are particularly good for this purpose.

This is a good point to introduce the notion of ballistic movements and their application in speech activity. Ballistic movements not only have the quality of smooth and continuous motion, but they also carry with them the quality of ease of action and a relatively relaxed kind of motion. Both of these qualities are important for the stutterer to learn to experience.

The general idea of ballistic movements should be explained carefully, with appropriate illustrations from various activities, particularly sports. In many cases it seems worthwhile to have the stutterer experience the feel of ballistic movement in gross muscle action, such as in pretended movements of a golf or tennis swing, or contrived exercises that convey the essential experience. He should then be coached to experience a feeling for a ballistic quality in speech movement. Once again, rhythm in particular provides a very good vehicle for this feature of speaking. It should be stressed to the patient that this fluid, "follow through" quality of movement should be incorporated when focusing on the melody of speech, especially in the acts of moving into stress peaks.

The Second Phase: Implementation

The activities of the instructional phase have provided the fundamentals, the groundwork, on which the treatment process is based. Actually, of course, the therapy has begun with the activities of the first phase; the second phase is simply that indeterminate period during which various procedures are brought to bear on helping the patient achieve increasingly more fluent speech.

Among the procedures used in demonstration during the instructional phase, the following are usable as part of the continuing therapy: (a) voice chewing, (b) sounding, (c) rhythms, (d) ventriloquism.

Two other procedures become relevant once speech melody has been identified as the ultimate focus. One is the reading of poetry. The objective here should be obvious: much poetry is constructed to capitalize on the melody patterns of the language, particularly very metered or lyric poetry. Use of poetry thus helps to emphasize to the patient the whole notion of the melody that lies within phrases and sentences. One should begin with very simple poems having a definite kind of beat and gradually move to blank verse. A good example of progression would start with a poem such as Longfellow's "The Village Blacksmith" or Henley's "Invictus," through poems such as Masefields's "The West Wind" and Frost's "Stopping by Woods on a Snowy Evening," and then on to poems such as Goldsmith's "The Deserted Village." In reading poems the objective is to speak them with expression and "feeling," to generate an emphasis of the feeling for the melody that is in the *message*. This type of procedure presents a transition phase into performing similarly with casual, conversational speech.

A second additional procedure follows quite naturally from the foregoing and, in a very real sense, is the epitome of all of the procedures in this method. It is a simple one, consisting of the technique of speaking with intentional exaggeration of the melody contained in what is being said. To do this the patient must sense the melody of what he is speaking; it so happens that in doing so his attention falls most naturally on the activity involved in moving into stress prominences. A third technique incorporated in the extended therapy process is also a simple one: slowing the speech rate. Many stutterers do speak or attempt to speak at a faster rate than they can handle. For all patients slowing the speech rate is substantial aid in developing a feel for the primary effect that is induced by the other procedures. Actually one will often find that a slower rate results indirectly from application of the other procedures, especially the procedure of emphasizing speech melody.

Throughout all this activity the patient's attention is to be maintained on the "carrier tone," which he is encouraged to sense particularly from the laryngeal area feedback. To this end, it is often necessary to encourage the patient to develop slightly more volume and to perform what has often been described in speech training as "projecting." He is also coached in developing a smooth vocal tone that is neither initiated nor terminated abruptly. Special attention is continually directed to the management of moving into stress prominences. Here the coaching emphasizes easing into the movement, and to "swell" into the vowel sound whose peak is the "target" in the stressed syllable.

Throughout the continuation of therapy the core objective remains the same. The various procedures identified can be used as necessary to support the objective of emphasizing speech melody. In fact, one of the major advantages of this method is that any of the procedures can be brought into play and used as seems necessary at the time. For instance, in certain cases it may be intermittently necessary to revert temporarily to one of the more basic procedures, such as voice chewing, in order to dramatically emphasize phonation and looseness of oral movements. However, it has been my experience that the mainstay procedures are the following: intentional exaggeration of the speech melody, implemented in the ordinary discourse of a therapy period; intentional maintenance of a slower rate, which articulates neatly with the exaggeration procedure; and occasional reversion to ventriloquism as a support procedure to emphasize the prominence of the phonatory aspect of speech and compare it to articulation, which is being done with minimal movement and effort.

Quite regularly the patient should be encouraged to enhance his feeling of vocal control by developing "an assertive posture." By this I mean essentially a positive attitude and manner, a "leaning forward" psychologically, with an intent to "speak out." Where necessary the patient should be strongly encouraged to maintain an assertive attitude of a more general nature in his speech relationships with others. Many stutterers have developed a feeling that they need to reply quickly to questions put to them, or they may be otherwise vulnerable to a sensed pressure to express quickly what they have in mind. Any susceptibility to yield to such pressure must be counteracted; the stutterer must learn to resist this feeling of pressure and to employ his new skills with care and deliberateness. The speech capability generated by the techniques of this therapy approach provides a base for the necessary confidence to reply with improved fluency; the stutterer needs to give himself a chance to perform satisfactorily.

The major objective of this method is to develop skill in sequential speech movements that encompass phrases and sentences. However, there are times when it is necessary or important to deal immediately with a specific instance of stuttering. This problem can also be handled through application of the essential principle identified here. In dealing with a specific instance of stuttering the stutterer is enjoined to focus on moving into the vowel sound of the stressed syllable, with the idea that the objective is the stress peak and that he should direct his attention to integrating those movements necessary to achieve that goal. I have found stutterers well able to appreciate that, for example, in a word like "ninety" or "ninetieth" they are able to deal appropriately with the stressed syllable by focusing specifically on its execution, and once this has been achieved the rest of the word flows easily. One should emphasize to the patient that this technique is simply a focalized application of the same principles that are being implemented in development of the speech melody.

This method of therapy usually results in a rapid change in level of fluency and ease of dealing with instances of stuttering, and there is no need to work at modifying the stuttering in a piecemeal fashion. As might be expected, rapid improvement is noted especially in oral reading; however, some individuals show immediate gains even in their efforts with spontaneous speech. Most stutterers are genuinely impressed with the dramatic change that is wrought and may become very excited about it. Although one must support this enthusiasm, it is necessary to point out to the patient that, most likely, a good deal of work lies ahead.

Generally speaking, it is not an easy matter for most individuals to maintain the achieved level of fluency continuously in casual speech, primarily, it seems, because the new method of speaking is not quickly incorporated as a mode of speaking. Thus, there is a sort of "on-off" nature to the improvement, evidently a reflection of the fact that the improvement depends upon conscious control. The stutterer should be clearly encouraged to look upon this therapy as skill development: I like to draw the analogy that it is like learning to perform any other complicated skilled activity, such as playing the piano, or even learning certain sports, such as golf. This means that improvement requires substantial practice that is fairly continuous and on-going.

Once he has reached a certain level of understanding and coaching, there is much the patient can do on his own. In fact, he has little limit on his spontaneous application to the desired activities. He should be required to do a lot of "homework," which should include a certain amount of reading aloud of poetry and prose material, alternating between the two with the intent of consolidating his feel for the inherent melody. He should also be encouraged to soliloquize, taking advantage of times of the day when he is alone and able to talk out loud to himself. In fact, the latter circumstance provides very good practice opportunity for overexaggeration of the speech melody in spontaneously formulated speech, the objective being, of course, to continually develop the feel for the experience in a circumstance closer to ordinary speaking. He should also seek out actual speaking experiences, with the same objectives in mind.

For some stutterers, particularly children, it is necessary for the clinician to make up assignments for gaining such experiences. However, older stutterers should be capable of developing sufficient initiative to devise their own opportunities, although the therapist can of course make helpful suggestions. The current availability and relatively low cost, of cassette tape recorders make these machines a valuable adjunct to the therapy process. It is desirable that the patient have access to a recorder for his own use. Use of a recorder enables him to take with him modeled examples of speech from the clinician which he can then attempt to reproduce, as well as creating his own tapes on different material, which can be brought back for joint appraisal with the clinician. The patient can also make use of the recorder to "eavesdrop" on himself in various speaking situations and utilize these samples as an ongoing form of double monitoring.

Where possible the therapy regimen should attempt to enlist the cooperation of other persons. The patient should be encouraged to solicit monitoring feedback from members of his family, friends, and coworkers. In the case of children such external sources should probably be limited to members of the family; however, one can envision circumstances in which a very close friend (or friends) could be similarly helpful.

The idea of enlisting the aid of others carries the implication of continuous and absolute monitoring of the individual's speech. Complete monitoring might be an ideal objective and perhaps it would be particularly productive if incorporated in a concentrated, intensified, residential program lasting several weeks or more. As yet we have not had occasion to undertake this sort of program. Short of that, it seems most suitable to consider the involvement of other persons more from the standpoint of the number of persons supporting the therapy, without, however, expecting that all (or even almost all) instances of stuttering will be monitored. In other words, under ordinary therapy circumstances it seems that one should be judicious in respect to the rigor of the demands placed on the patient. To some extent expected performance is presently a matter of the attitude of the therapist and the tolerence level of the patient. Further study may change what now seems appropriate to do. It may be that better results will be obtained through rather absolute monitoring, even incorporating a contingency system or token economy of some sort. However, it does seem that this sort of scheme is best suited to intensive therapy, and there are few situations that provide this opportunity.

Especially in the early period of therapy the effort to change is particularly demanding. Since the realistic goal of therapy is a substantial but continuing *improvement* over the long term, and not necessarily a "cure," one should not anticipate "turning off" the stuttering in a short time. Particularly in view of this goal the therapy should not be made an ordeal, even though the patient should remain clearly aware that personal commitment is necessary and continuous application is desirable. It is a reasonable expectation that, with sincere application, the new way of speaking will eventually become a kind of "second nature" performance that the stutterer will be able to employ with increasing capability and satisfaction.

Presumably the more continuously the patient exercises this form of speech the sooner he will incorporate it more extensively into his regular activities. Also presumably, the more he maintains it during the therapy session, the more he is likely to persist in it in intervening periods. Nonetheless, the clinician has to make a judgment about the extent to which he should be a "taskmaster" during the therapy sessions.

In the early stages of therapy, especially, some stutterers slip out of "control" more easily than others. Lapse in control is likely due to several factors. Among them, certainly, is the matter of the patient's awareness of his stuttering. Another is the aspect of the balance between the annoyance value of stuttering and the effort required to maintain fluency. A number of factors may need to be taken into account. The extent to which a clinician should require continuing performance will vary with the individual stutterer, the stage of treatment he is in, the relationship that has developed, "good days" and "bad days," and sometimes very special considerations of the moment; for example, it would not be conducive to a good therapeutic relationship to insist on rigorous self-monitoring of stutters that occur while the patient is confiding some very personal feelings.

There are several ways to get the stutterer to implement the method, if he lapses. The simplest means is to tell him that he is not performing as he should. Usually this is a feasible method with a stutterer who performs well for extended periods but then has a short interval of lapse. On the other hand, if it is necessary to intervene often, a good way of helping the stutterer maintain the method is through the use of a reminder system. A reminder could consist of a simple signal such as raising one's hand. However, a hand signal usually is not quick enough for effective intervention; also, it has the distracting effect of interfering with the conversational relationship. The clinician should keep in mind that an objective of this therapy method is to have the subject apply it in as "natural" a setting as possible. For this reason, no auditory or visual signal is particularly suitable. It is better to devise some means of tactile contact. Actually, a string tied to the subject's finger and held by the clinician provides a simple device of this sort. However, in order to transmit the signal quickly the string must be held in such a manner that there is very little slack in it. Since body movements are a natural and common occurrence during conversations, problems arise in respect to maintaining the string in appropriate tension. The most effecient system is a modification of a "reminder" device reported some time ago by the author (Wingate, 1967). The original device delivered a mild electrical surge which could be adjusted by means of a potentiometer to the sensitivity level of the subject. The variable control permitted delivery of a simple tingling sensation just slightly above awareness for any particular individual. The device worked well with most patients, but since some people were unable to dismiss the association of "shock," the device has been modified so that the battery-supplied charge operates a simple vibrator held by the patient.[6] The advantages of this device are that it is quick, flexible, and usable in any situation. A particular value of the device, as mentioned in the initial report, is that markedly improved fluency evidently results from simply having this sort of physical tie between patient and clinician. This result has tremendous value for at least demonstrating to the stutterer that he is capable of the control necessary to produce at least very improved, if not continuously fluent, speech. I have found that use of the reminder is not frequently necessary, although it is appropriately used from time to time as a kind of "booster shot." If the stutterer is one who can markedly improve his speech when hooked up with the device, his attention should be directed emphatically to what he is doing at that time which results in the fluent speech he achieves. The device thus becomes a very potent means of intensifying feedback awareness.

Dealing with children of primary grade level.—As mentioned earlier, working with school-age children should ordinarily not present any particular problem, since they seem well able to grasp the essential ideas of this method, if it is presented in terms within their level of comprehension. Knowing the principles of the method allows for innovation and creativity in the development of procedures. One public school therapist of my aquaintance has reported considerable success with youngsters as young as kindergarten level through use of what she calls a "talkogram." Using a roll of adding machine tape which provides a surface of sufficient length, the child is asked to record with a pencil a trace of the undulating movement he experiences as he is speaking. This procedure provides graphic and physical support to the performance as well as incorporating a ballistic aspect of gross movement.

An important dimension to consider in dealing with the school-age child is the counseling of the teacher. Teachers vary in their knowledge and beliefs about stuttering; some teachers may have acquired fairly definite ideas about stuttering during the course of their own professional education, and these ideas may well reflect the current biases found among speech pathologists. The clinician should make the effort to apprise the teacher, in summary at least, of the rationale and background for the treatment method being employed. It is to be expected that activity in the classroom will have the objective of supporting or augmenting the work of the speech clinician.

Generally, teachers have two major questions about dealing with the stuttering youngster: one has to do with the matter of speaking in class, and the other is in regard to the reaction of other children. Consideration of both matters should proceed from the common base of being able to deal with the stuttering in a straightforward and matter-of-fact manner. The management should be adjusted to the individual child and the particular circumstances at the time. In my experience stuttering youngsters are not regularly as unwilling to speak in class or in groups as we have been led to believe. Of course, a child should not be required to speak if he is reluctant to do so; adjustments in this attitude will be an objective of the direct speech therapy and should be approached through coordinated efforts of clinician and teacher. At the same time, many youngsters who stutter are not unwilling to recite, and they should be permitted, even encouraged, to do so. Particularly if achievements are being gained in speech therapy, speaking in class can become an opportunity, a positive learning experience, for both the child and his classmates, regardless of whether the youngster was originally reluctant to speak.

In respect to the reaction of other children one must first question whether this is a problem as regularly as it has been said to be. Testimonies of having been teased or ridiculed are naturally touching, and they fit in with a (too) often voiced remark that "children can be cruel" in their reactions to others. But this is an overstatement. Children are typically curious, honest, and candid. Some of their candor, particularly about handicaps, is frequently interpreted as cruelty by adults because of attitudes adults have developed about such matters. However, children are also generally quite capable of being sympathetic and supportive along with their frankness and openness, and these benign inclinations can be nurtured and developed.

Undoubtedly there are instances in which peer reactions present an unsettling experience for the stuttering youngster. Certainly when this does happen measures must be taken to minimize the situation and then turn it around. But one cannot anticipate that the reaction of other children will be routinely negative. Again, the situation must be dealt with individually, in terms of the dimensions that are present or that develop. In general it is best to deal with the matter of stuttering as openly as circumstances require, neither making a particular issue of it nor trying to obscure or evade it. If properly handled in an open and casual manner, the child's experiences in the classroom, with teacher and peers, can be a supportive adjunct to the therapy efforts of the speech clinician.

Dealing with the preschool-age child.—The situation is somewhat different in dealing with the preschool child, since in such cases there is more reason to work with the parents. Much of what is relevant to counseling with parents has been covered in Chapter 11, but there are certain matters that deserve restatement or addition.

It is rare to find a parent who is not unduly concerned about the presence of stuttering in a young child, and one should be careful not to attempt to dismiss it lightly nor to "normalize" the disfluency. Parents should be advised that, technically and scientifically, we are not certain what it is necessary to do for stuttering at this age level. At the same time, there is a commonsense basis for following certain seemingly appropriate procedures.

In general, it seems to make good sense to avoid bringing pressure on the child, particularly if there is some indication that pressure leads to increased stuttering. There are also certain indirect management procedures that seem indicated on these grounds. For instance, it seems advisable to discourage speaking or to manipulate circumstances such that opportunity to speak is reduced during episodes when the stuttering is pronounced. Generally speaking it seems appropriate to minimize the amount of excitement the child is subject to, again especially if it is known that stuttering increases under levels of excitement. Of course, it should be obvious that the child should not be forced to speak or to "perform" with speech.

If the stuttering is mild, it seems that the best course of action is to follow very indirect procedures, at least for a trial period of perhaps several months while the status of the stuttering is kept under observation. This observation can be accomplished by the parents, with the understanding that they have access to the clinician for indirect consultation or subsequent direct evaluation of the child if they so wish.

In some cases a more direct kind of intervention may seem indicated. If so, it should be understood that the direct management is to be undertaken on a trial basis. The parents should be advised that the methods to be attempted are based on a rationale rather than on a history of extended use and proven effect, although they can be reassured regarding the efficacy of the methods with older stutterers. In some cases it may be desired to conduct the direct management through the parents alone; in other cases the therapist may participate in the therapy, providing demonstration and modeling of methods for the parents, in addition to the couseling.

Whenever direct intervention of some degree is undertaken, the parents should of course understand what is being attempted. To this end they should be apprised of the rationale for the method used, which means taking them through the essentials of the instructional phases discussed earlier in this chapter. They should understand that the general objective of the direct management will be to communicate to the youngster the importance of voicing and something about the existence of melody in speech.

One of the simplest techniques is to present to the child a speech model that is slow in rate, somewhat measured, easygoing, and resonant in quality. The parents should make efforts to take advantage of times when they are involved in conversations with the child to speak in this manner and indirectly encourage him to do likewise.

A way of bringing the matter of phonation and phonatory control to the child's awareness is provided in play that imitates different kinds of animal voices. This sort of thing can be done while looking at picture books or through the use of dolls or puppets. Children themselves provide another avenue of approaching implementation of the methods espoused here. From time to time youngsters spontaneously produce a sort of "fun" speech that is usually accompanied with gross motor movements having a definitely ballistic character. Not only can parents seize upon such occurrences but they can also make a point of introducing this form of play more frequently, taking advantage of the opportunity to introduce awareness of the melody pattern and voicing control that is involved in the activity.

The foregoing suggestions have to do with generating or supporting ongoing speech through the emphasis of melody or patterning of a spontaneous sort. There are times when specific intervention during instances of stuttering may be appropriate. These techniques should be undertaken by the clinician first and modeled for the parents through observation. One level of intervention requires that the clinician be able to anticipate the actual word on which the youngster is having difficulty. This technique calls for intervening in the form of choral speech; the object is to lead the child into saying the word by clearly "swelling" into the stressed syllable, mildly exaggerating the development of the vowel in that syllable. The objective here, of course, is to teach the child, by example, to grasp a feeling for the pattern for dealing with the stress prominence. A second level of dealing with instances of stuttering is similar to the foregoing but is retroactive. In cases where the clinician cannot anticipate the word with which the child is having difficulty a similar approach can be introduced following the youngster's eventual production of the word. For instance, if a child has difficulty moving from the /h/ phoneme in saying "house," the clinician can enter in immediately after the word has finally been said, saying it in a manner that emphasizes the diphthong. One can also make a point of verbally identifying the existence of the diphthong in its prominent place in the syllable, and again reproduce how one moves into producing this particular sound. Sometimes the youngster may seem relatively impervious to this "instruction"; however, he may also intermittently show a definite curiousity about it and at these times seem able to follow what is being suggested.

The foregoing suggestions regarding direct work with preschool youngsters must be understood to be preliminary attempts to develop some sort of direct management to which one can have recourse in cases where indirect management approaches do not seem to support improvement or where the stuttering may seem to be getting worse. The techniques have not as yet been employed with a sufficient number of very young stutterers to document their efficacy. However, they are expressions of the same principles that underlie the methods to be used with older stutterers and, at the present time, their use with a few young children has been encouraging. At the same time, it may well be that at this level, as well as at somewhat older ages, the most beneficial effect is occasioned by circumstances well beyond our control—namely, the influences of maturation. It will be a long time before we can know with any certainty whether or not such procedures will have real value in dealing with stuttering at this age level. For the interim, they do provide an avenue of approach that is at least consistent with a rationale having a defensible basis and which one might therefore anticipate should have some positive effect. Nonetheless, anyone making use of such procedures, clinicians and parents alike, should recognize their source and their provisional status and make use of them judiciously.

EPILOGUE

This book has been concerned with the development of an approach to stuttering therapy founded on broadly supported principles. A major contribution of the book lies in the integration that underlies the identification of these core principles for stuttering therapy.

The therapy program advocated in this final chapter includes procedures that embody these principles, follows a sequence that is logically consistent and has been found to be effective. At the same time, as suggested earlier in this chapter, I do not believe that stuttering therapy need be limited to the procedures, or sequence, presented in the preceding pages. In fact, the overall policy in respect to therapy should permit flexibility in the use of appropriate available procedures. Certain methods not incorporated in the present chapter, though mentioned earlier in the book as exemplifying major aspects of the basic principles, should not be overlooked. For instance, the legato-speech method developed by Lee *et al.* (1973) could well constitute a major dimension of a therapy program under certain circumstances.

Since feedback, particularly immediate feedback, is a very valuable aspect of the training, instrumentation utilized specifically to enhance feedback can be a significant therapeutic adjunct. Occasionally I have made use of auditory amplification to heighten the patient's awareness of his ongoing speech. This can be done very simply with an ordinary tape recorder, using an earphone in place of the recorder's speaker as the monitor. The patient's ongoing speech is returned at increased volume through one earphone; using only one earphone is sufficient and permits use of the technique while speaking conversationally with the therapist.

Closed circuit television is similarly useful for training purposes. Its suitability and advantages should be obvious.

More sophisticated forms of instrumental aid are available. Massengill (1970) has reported the use of the polygraph to supply stutterers with feedback about their speech performance. Gautheron *et al* (1973) report the successful use of a glottograph and oscilloscope to monitor laryngeal action. Most recently Agnello (1975) has developed instrumentation specifically designed to assist the stutterer to develop skill in control of voice onset[7] and Guitar (1975) has reported the use of surface electrode myography as a feedback source.

Mention of instrumentation always recalls the instrument that has reappeared so frequently in the history of stuttering therapy—the metronome. There are many cases in which it may be advisable to make extended use of the metronome as a supportive aid. In fact, one should face the possibility that for certain cases the optimal solution may lie in the long-term use of an aid such as the Pacemaster. Mr. Libby, developer of the Pacemaster, has reported that many stutterers say they are very satisfied with their use of the device, and accept it in much the same way as people accept the use of eyeglasses or a hearing aid.[8]

Generally it seems preferable to conduct therapy with a minimal use of instrumentation. The ideal objective of therapy is to enable the stutterer to have command of his speaking performance in as "natural" a way as possible. Achievement of this goal depends on the development of internal sources of information and motor control. The patient must develop the "feel" of the total activity of fluent expression. Also, from a practical standpoint, instrumentation, particularly the more sophisticated type, may not be readily available to a clinician. Most of the procedures covered in this book do not require instruments, a valuable advantage to clinician as well as patient.

There are occasions when the use of "progressive relaxation" procedures (see Jacobson, 1957) can be very worthwhile as adjunctive aid. The primary objective is to apply these procedures to the musculature of the speech apparatus, especially of the face and neck; however, it is usually expedient to begin with one of the extremities,[9] since patients seem better able to grasp what is expected of them when "trained" with a large muscle system. Patients should be advised that these procedures represent a form of skill training in muscular control, identifying acquisition of this skill as consistent with other aspects of the therapy. Use of these procedures can be incorporated readily into the overall therapy approach; they are particularly compatible with such procedures as "breath chewing," ventriloquism, and the exercises designed to develop a sense of ease in vocal control.

As a final important consideration we must call attention to the advantages of therapy in groups. Group therapy for stutterers provides the usual benefits to the individual that are inherent in the group experience, such as the opportunity for identification with, and support from, others. In stutterer groups there are special benefits to be derived from a spirit of common effort with a particular problem. In the course of group work patients can share experiences that are highly relevant to each other, perceive contrasts as well as similarities among themselves, and compare beliefs and attitudes. Such activities are routinely found to have some degree of personal benefit to most participants.

But there are other advantages to group work which relate particularly to the therapy approach presented here. The didactic features of this approach can be implemented with groups as well as with individuals; in fact, certain advantages accrue through a group experience of the instruction and demonstrations. Questions posed by group members contribute to clarification and help accentuate the points and principles being presented. Usually the demonstrations are additionally impressive when one witnesses them performed by others as well as by oneself. Also, group involvement often enhances the individual's performance of a demonstration. Additionally, group members can serve as effective monitors of each other during the course of therapy.

Group participation also provides the best vehicle for role playing, in which certain problems can be worked out in a controlled rehearsal of reality. Role playing is particularly worthwhile for working on commonly occurring problems, such as the "time pressure" experience (in which a person feels impelled to respond quickly), or the "tentative attitude" condition (the insufficiently assertive psychological posture that is mirrored in an ineffective control of voice).

In sum, there are a number of procedures that can be incorporated supportively into the therapy approach developed here. Throughout, however, the central orientation remains focused on implementation of the basic principles of vocal control and modulation in the expression of the melody of speech.

Notes

1. In contrast to the *immediate* source, which we have already identified as some phonatory dysfunction.

2. This includes the theories currently in favor, namely, those that explain stuttering as an emotional problem, or as learned behavior.

3. It should also be kept in mind that certain acts occurring at the time of a stutter, such as a brief staring, eye blink, or certain movements of the facial musculature, may be aspects of the "happening" (the blocking) rather than the immediate efforts at adjustment as described here.

4. Tacit professional recognition of the essential intractability of stuttering is reflected in the fact that stuttering is the only speech defect accepted within the professional ranks. That is, persons who stutter are permitted, even encouraged, to pursue a career in speech pathology. In fact a sizable number of them are quite successful in the field; many have evidently experienced considerable improvement in their stuttering but most of them are not actually "recovered" in a literal sense. In contrast, persons having articulation, voice, or language problems are typically advised not to consider a career as a speech pathologist until their own problems are corrected.

5. This will depend to some extent on the stutterer's age. It is difficult to set a lower age limit but one should feel free to make the attempt with children of school age, and perhaps younger, if the child gives indication of understanding what is being sought.

6. Commercial models will be available soon.

7. A commercial model of the instrument, called the Speech Onset Comparator, is available from Xetron Corporation, 11079 Reading Road, Cincinnati, Ohio.

8. Personal communication. These clients are located predominantly in foreign countries (particularly Germany), where the use of a device is more widely accepted by practitioners, who recommend it.

9. In some cases it may seem advisable to take the patient through the whole Jacobson "course."

References

Agnello, J. G. Larynegeal and articulatory dynamics of dysfluency interpreted within a vocal tract model. In Webster, L. M. and L. C. Furst (eds.), *Vocal Tract Dynamics and Dysfluency*, Speech Institute: New York, 1975.

Gautheron, B., A. Liorzou, C. Even and B. Vallancien The role of the larynx in stuttering. In Lebrun, Y. and R. Hoops (Eds.), *Neurolinguistic Approaches to Stuttering*, Mouton: The Hague, 1973.

Guitar, B. Reduction of stuttering frequency using analog electroymographic feedback. *J. Speech Hearing Res.*, **18**, 672–685, 1975.

Jacobson, E. *You Must Relax*, 4th ed., McGraw-Hill, New York, 1957.

Lee, B. S., W. E. McGough, and Maryann Peins. A new method for stutter therapy. *Folia Phoniat.*, **25**, 186–195, 1973.

Massengill, R. Use of the polygraph in speech therapy with stutterers. *J. Speech Hearing Dis.*, **35**, 96, 1970.

Wingate, M. E. Alerting device for stuttering therapy. *Asha*, **9**, 375, 1967 (abstr.).

———The relationship of theory to therapy in stuttering. *J. Commun. Dis.*, (in press).

AUTHOR INDEX

SUBJECT INDEX

PRODUCTION NOTE

This book has been set in Janson
by Cemar Graphic Designs Ltd. of Rockville Centre, N.Y.
Printing and binding were done by Quinn & Boden Company, Inc., Rahway, New Jersey
Book designed by Raymond Solomon